T0214778

Lecture Notes in Computer Science 11795

More information about this series at http://www.springer.com/series/7412

Qian Wang · Fausto Milletari ·
Hien V. Nguyen et al. (Eds.)

Domain Adaptation and Representation Transfer and Medical Image Learning with Less Labels and Imperfect Data

First MICCAI Workshop, DART 2019
and First International Workshop, MIL3ID 2019
Shenzhen, Held in Conjunction with MICCAI 2019
Shenzhen, China, October 13 and 17, 2019
Proceedings

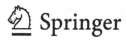 Springer

Editors
Qian Wang
Shanghai Jiaotong University
Shanghai, China

Fausto Milletari
NVIDIA GmbH
Munich, Germany

Hien V. Nguyen
University of Houston
Houston, TX, USA

Additional Workshop Editors see next page

ISSN 0302-9743   ISSN 1611-3349   (electronic)
Lecture Notes in Computer Science
ISBN 978-3-030-33390-4   ISBN 978-3-030-33391-1   (eBook)
https://doi.org/10.1007/978-3-030-33391-1

LNCS Sublibrary: SL6 – Image Processing, Computer Vision, Pattern Recognition, and Graphics

This Springer imprint is published by the registered company Springer Nature Switzerland AG
The registered company address is: Gewerbestrasse 11, 6330 Cham, Switzerland

Additional Workshop Editors

Challenge Chairs

Qian Wang
Shanghai Jiaotong University
Shanghai, China

Bram van Ginneken
Radboud University
Nijmegen, Gelderland, The Netherlands

Tutorial Chair

Luping Zhou
University of Sydney
Sydney, NSW, Australia

First MICCAI Workshop on Domain Adaptation and Representation Transfer, DART 2019

Fausto Milletari
NVIDIA GmbH
Munich, Germany

Shadi Albarqouni
Technical University Munich
Munich, Germany

M. Jorge Cardoso ⓘ
King's College London
London, UK

Nicola Rieke
NVIDIA GmbH
Munich, Germany

Ziyue Xu
NVIDIA
Santa Clara, CA, USA

Konstantinos Kamnitsas
Imperial College London
London, UK

First International Workshop on Medical Image Learning with Less Labels and Imperfect Data, MIL3ID 2019

Hien V. Nguyen
University of Houston
Houston, TX, USA

Vishal Patel
Johns Hopkins University
Baltimore, MD, USA

Badri Roysam
University of Houston
Houston, TX, USA

Steve Jiang
UT Southwestern Medical Center
Dallas, TX, USA

Kevin Zhou
Chinese Academy of Sciences
Beijing, China

Khoa Luu
University of Arkansas
Fayetteville, AR, USA

Ngan Le
University of Arkansas
Fayetteville, AR, USA

Preface

Computer vision and medical imaging have been revolutionized by the introduction of advanced machine learning and deep learning methodologies. Recent approaches have shown unprecedented performance gains in tasks such as segmentation, classification, detection, and registration. Although these results (obtained mainly on public datasets) represent important milestones for the MICCAI community, most methods lack generalization capabilities when presented with previously unseen situations (corner cases) or different input data domains. This limits clinical applicability of these innovative approaches and therefore diminishes their impact. Transfer learning, representation learning, and domain adaptation techniques have been used to tackle problems such as: model training using small datasets while obtaining generalizable representations; performing domain adaptation via few-shot learning; obtaining interpretable representations that are understood by humans; and leveraging knowledge learned from a particular domain to solve problems in another.

The first MICCAI workshop on Domain Adaptation and Representation Transfer (DART 2019) aimed at creating a discussion forum to compare, evaluate, and discuss methodological advancements and ideas that can improve the applicability of machine learning (ML)/deep learning (DL) approaches to clinical settings by making them robust and consistent across different domains.

During the first edition of DART, 18 papers were submitted for consideration and, after peer review, 12 full papers were accepted for presentation. Each paper was rigorously reviewed by three reviewers in a double-blind review process. The papers were automatically assigned to reviewers taking into account and avoiding potential conflicts of interest and recent work collaborations between peers. Reviewers have been selected among the most prominent experts in the field from all over the world. Once the reviews were obtained the area chairs formulated final decisions over acceptance or rejection of each manuscript. These decisions were always taken according to the reviews and were unappealable.

Additionally, the workshop organization granted the Best Paper Award to the best submission presented at DART 2019. The Best Paper Award was assigned as a result of a secret voting procedure where each member of the committee indicated two papers worthy of consideration for the award. The paper collecting the majority of votes was then chosen by the committee.

We believe that the paper selection process implemented during DART 2019 as well as the quality of the submissions have resulted in scientifically validated and interesting contributions to the MICCAI community and in particular to researchers working on domain adaptation and representation transfer.

We would therefore like to thank the authors for their contributions, the reviewers for their dedication and professionality in delivering expert opinions about the submissions, and NVIDIA Corporation, which has sponsored DART, for the support, resources, and help in organizing the workshop. NVIDIA Corporation has also sponsored the prize for the best paper at DART 2019, which consisted of a NVIDIA Titan V GPU card.

November 2018

Fausto Milletari
Nicola Rieke
Shadi Albarqouni
Ziyue Xu
Konstantinos Kamnitsas
M. Jorge Cardoso

Organization

Organization Committee

Fausto Milletari · NVIDIA GmbH, Germany
Shadi Albarqouni · Technical University Munich, Germany
Maximilian Baust · NVIDIA GmbH, Germany
M. Jorge Cardoso · King's College London, UK
Konstantinos Kamnitsas · Imperial College London, UK
Abood Quraini · NVIDIA Corporation, USA
Nicola Rieke · NVIDIA GmbH, Germany
Daguang Xu · NVIDIA Corporation, USA
Ziyue Xu · NVIDIA Corporation, USA

Program Committee

Azizi, Shekoofee · University British Columbia, Canada
Bagci, Ulas · University of Central Florida, USA
Bai, Wenjia · Imperial College London, UK
Bragman, Felix · University College London, UK
Dorent, Reuben · King's College London, UK
Dou, Qi · Imperial College London, UK
Ferrante, Enzo · Universidad Nacional del Litoral, Argentina
Gao, Mingchen · University at Buffalo, USA
Huang, Ruobing · University of Oxford, UK
Ledig, Christian · Imagen Technologies, USA
Lewis, Kathleen · Massachusetts Institute of Technology, USA
Liang, Jianming · Arizona State University, USA
Paschali, Magdalini · Technical University of Munich, Germany
Prevost, Raphael · ImFusion, Germany
Ross, Tobias · German Cancer Research Center, Germany
Sarhan, Mhd Hasan · Technical University of Munich, Germany
Shin, Hoo-Chang · NVIDIA Corporation, USA
Simson, Walter · Technical University of Munich, Germany
Tsaftaris, Sotirios · The University of Edinburgh, UK
Varsavsky, Thomas · University College London, UK
Xia, Yong · Northwestern Polytechnical University, China
Xu, Yan · Beihang University, China
Zettinig, Oliver · ImFusion, Germany

Area Chairs

Fausto Milletari   NVIDIA GmbH, Germany
Shadi Albarqouni   Technical University Munich, Germany
M. Jorge Cardoso   King's College London, UK

MIL3ID 2019 Preface

MIL3ID 2019 is the First International Workshop on Medical Image Learning with Less Labels and Imperfect Data. The MIL3ID 2019 proceedings contain 16 high-quality papers of 8 pages each, which were selected through a rigorous peer-review process.

We hope this workshop will create a forum for discussing best practices in medical image learning with label scarcity and data imperfection. This forum is urgently needed because the issues of label noises and data scarcity are highly practical but largely under investigated in the medical image analysis community. Traditional approaches for dealing with these challenges include transfer learning, active learning, denoising, and sparse representation. The majority of these algorithms were developed prior to the recent advances of deep learning and might not benefit from the power of deep networks. The revision and improvement of these techniques in the new light of deep learning are long overdue.

This workshop potentially helps answer many important questions. For example, several recent studies found that deep networks are robust to massive random label noises but more sensitive to structured label noises. What implication do these findings have on dealing with noisy medical data? Recent work on Bayesian neural networks demonstrates the feasibility of estimating uncertainty due to the lack of training data. In other words, it enables our classifiers to be aware of what they do not know. Such a framework is important for medical applications where safety is critical. How can researchers of MICCAI community leverage this approach to improve their systems robustness in the case of data scarcity? Our prior work shows that a variant of capsule networks generalizes better than convolutional neural networks with an order of magnitude fewer training data. This gives rise to an interesting question: are there better classes of networks that intrinsically require less labeled data for learning? Humans always have an edge over deep networks when it comes to learning with small amounts of data. However, recent work on one-shot deep learning has surpassed humans in an image recognition task using only a few training samples for each task. Do these results still hold for medical image analysis tasks?

The proceedings of the workshop are published as a joint LNCS volume alongside other satellite events organized in conjunction with MICCAI. In addition to the LNCS volume, to promote transparency, the papers' reviews and preprints are publicly available on the workshop website. In addition, the papers, abstracts, slides, and posters presented during the workshop will be made publicly available on the MIL3ID website.

August 2019

Hien V. Nguyen
Vishal Patel
Ngan Le
Badri Roysam
Steve Jiang
Kevin Zhou
Khoa Luu

Organization

General Chair

Hien Van Nguyen — University of Houston

Program Committee Chairs

Vishal Patel	Johns Hopkins University
Badri Roysam	University of Houston
Steve Jiang	UT Southwestern Medical Center
Kevin Zhou	Institute of Computing Technology, Chinese Academy of Sciences
Khoa Luu	University of Arkansas
Ngan Le	University of Arkansas

Program Committee

Aditi Singh	University of Houston
Anjali Balagopal	UT Southwestern Medical Center
Chi Nhan Duong	PdActive, Inc.
Chuong Huynh	VinAI Research
Daguang Xu	NVIDIA Corporation
Haofu Liao	University of Rochester
Jiayi Shen	Texas AM University
Jinghui Guo	UT Southwestern Medical Center
Kha Gia Quach	Concordia University
Pengyu Yuan	University of Houston
Qiming Yang	UT Southwestern Medical Center
Rajeev Yasarla	Johns Hopkins University, Whiting School of Engineering
Siqi Liu	Siemens Healthineers
Ti Bai	UT Southwestern Medical Center
Xiao Liang	UT Southwestern Medical Center
Xiaoqian Jia	UT Southwestern Medical Center
Yigong Wang	UT Southwestern Medical Center
Yuankai Huo	Vanderbilt University

Contents

MIL3ID 2019

DART 2019

Noise as Domain Shift: Denoising Medical Images by Unpaired Image Translation

Ilja Manakov[1,2]([⊠]), Markus Rohm[1,2], Christoph Kern[2], Benedikt Schworm[2], Karsten Kortuem[2], and Volker Tresp[1,3]

[1] Chair for Database Systems and Data Mining, LMU Munich, Munich, Germany
ilja.manakov@med.uni-muenchen.de
[2] Department of Ophthalmology, LMU Munich, Munich, Germany
[3] Siemens AG, Corporate Technology, Munich, Germany

Abstract. We cast the problem of image denoising as a domain translation problem between high and low noise domains. By modifying the cycleGAN model, we are able to learn a mapping between these domains on unpaired retinal optical coherence tomography images. In quantitative measurements and a qualitative evaluation by ophthalmologists, we show how this approach outperforms other established methods. The results indicate that the network differentiates subtle changes in the level of noise in the image. Further investigation of the model's feature maps reveals that it has learned to distinguish retinal layers and other distinct regions of the images.

Keywords: Optical coherence tomography · Generative Adversarial Networks · Image denoising

1 Introduction

Medical imaging is one of the great pillars of modern diagnostics. Clinicians rely on it to obtain information from inside the patient's body in a non-invasive way. However, noise in the images erodes their quality and makes their interpretation difficult. Moreover, it can cause algorithms, designed to automatically extract measurements from those images, to be inaccurate or fail outright. In this paper, we focus on the domain of retinal optical coherence tomography (OCT) [11], a standard diagnostic tool in ophthalmology. Retinal OCT produces a series of 2D slices (b-scans) that display the depth profile of the retina, thus enabling clinicians to detect many sight-threatening diseases early in their progression. The dominating type of noise in OCT is called speckle. The speckle noise pattern depends on the imaged tissue and is highly sensitive to its position and orientation. Since signal and speckle noise originate from the same physical process,

---

Electronic supplementary material The online version of this chapter (https://doi.org/10.1007/978-3-030-33391-1_1) contains supplementary material, which is available to authorized users.

Q. Wang et al. (Eds.): DART 2019/MIL3ID 2019, LNCS 11795, pp. 3–10, 2019.
https://doi.org/10.1007/978-3-030-33391-1_1

distinguishing signal from noise is particularly challenging. Interested readers are referred to [8] for more details.

Current popular methods for denoising OCT scans, such as BM3D [2] or wavelet denoising [1], neither incorporate knowledge about the OCT process nor about structures of the human eye. We argue that such knowledge should help in this task, given the complex and sample-dependent nature of speckle noise. On the other hand, methods emerging from the field of deep learning [4,14] have demonstrated precisely this ability, i.e. to learn the semantic characteristics of their input domains. We, therefore, aim to leverage deep learning to create a method that can denoise retinal scans by utilizing knowledge it has gained about this domain.

While writing this paper, we discovered recent work from Halupka et al. [5] and Huang et al. [7], in which they investigated a different GAN-based approach to retinal OCT denoising. Their approaches require paired training images, which can lead to problems with inaccurately registered images. Additionally, in their works, the denoised domain is constructed by registering and averaging samples from the noisy domain. Constructing denoised samples in this manner is not always feasible or possible and registration of images from different domains will likely not work well.

Our approach casts denoising as a domain translation problem. We demonstrate that, with some modifications, the cycleGAN model, introduced by Zhu et al. [14], can learn a mapping between a low and high noise domain from unpaired training data.

We introduce our method, the HDcycleGAN model, in Sect. 2 and evaluate its performance quantitatively and qualitatively in Sects. 3.2 and 3.3. In Sect. 3.4, we take a closer look at what our model has learned by inspecting its feature maps.

2   Methodology

Initially, we started by directly applying the cycleGAN model to the problem of learning a mapping between images of a high noise (HN) domain $h \in H \subset \mathbb{R}^{h \times w}$ and a low noise (LN) one $l \in L \subset \mathbb{R}^{h \times w}$. However, we soon discovered that this model does not perform well on our problem as is. Therefore, we made some modifications to the existing cycleGAN framework and developed our final model, the Hybrid Discriminator cycleGAN (HDcycleGAN). Figure 1 shows a pass through our model, starting from an HN image. In the following, we briefly summarize the required knowledge about the cycleGAN and highlight the changes we made and why we made them.

The cycleGAN combines two Generative Adversarial Networks (GANs) [4] into one two-way Autoencoder. Here, the generator of each GAN learns the mapping from one image domain to the other. In combination, they act like encoder and decoder of an Autoencoder. This framework allows two directions of traversal; going from domain one to domain two and back to domain one or vice versa. The paper also introduced the cycle consistency loss, which corresponds to the reconstruction loss in the standard Autoencoder setting. The goal of this loss function is to achieve consistency when transforming an image from one domain to the other and back. The generators in the cycleGAN down-sample the input image using strided convolutions, pass it through a series of residual blocks [6] and finally use fractional-strided convolutions for up-sampling. The discriminators down-sample their inputs through strided convolutions to produce a scalar output.

Using a cycleGAN-based approach allows us to train the network on unpaired images. In this way, registration of images becomes obsolete and we can avoid uncertainties that arise due to interpolation in affine transformation or in cases of mismatch between the images. An additional benefit of this framework is the cycle-consistency loss; although we are primarily interested in the mapping from HN images to LN, this added loss function provides a training signal to the network that is more stable than that of the discriminator alone.

We made three adjustments to the original cycleGAN model:

Skip Connections. In our first experiments, the vanilla cycleGAN generated blurry images. The sharpness of the image and clarity of visual features with small spatial extent play a crucial role when it comes to image quality. To address this problem, we added skip connections to the generators, which concatenate the output of each down-sampling layer to the input of the corresponding up-sampling layer.

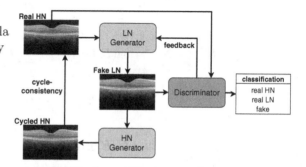

Fig. 1. Schematic overview of the HDcycleGAN model. The path starting from HN is shown here. Starting from LN works analogously

Resize-Convolutions. Additionally, we noticed checkerboard-like artifacts in the generated images. Following an investigation by Odena et al. [10], we replaced each fractional-strided convolution with a combination of bilinear up-sampling and a padded convolution to remedy this issue.

Shared Discriminator. Even after the first two modifications and testing different hyper-parameters, the model failed to consistently improve image quality when mapping from HN to LN. We then noticed that both discriminators learn the characteristics of real OCT b-scans independently. The two image domains are almost identical in terms of image content. Consequently, the discriminators could not pick up on the subtle differences between the domains (see Fig. 1 in the supplementary material). As a remedy, we utilized a single discriminator that is shared between both generators. The discriminator can thus focus on the differences between the two domains instead of the full range of characteristics of each.

This change resulted in the most significant improvement in visual quality of the generated images.

This shared discriminator acts as a three-way classifier, outputting the class probabilities for real HN, real LN and fake. As the discriminator now has to discriminate between more samples, we increased its complexity by adding a residual block with two convolutions in between each down-sampling layer.

The loss function of our model can thus be written as follows: Let $G_H : L \rightarrow H$ and $G_L : H \rightarrow L$ denote the generators that learn a mapping from LN to HN and from HN to LN respectively and $D : \mathbb{R}^{h \times w} \rightarrow \mathbb{R}^3$ the discriminator. Let $t_h, t_l, t_f \in \mathbb{R}^3$ be the one-hot encoded vectors that represent the classes real HN, real LN and fake. Then the loss of the network is:

$$\mathcal{L} = \lambda_{GAN} \left(\mathcal{L}_G \left(l, h \right) + \mathcal{L}_D \left(l, h \right) \right) + \lambda_{cycle} \mathcal{L}_{cycle} \left(l, h \right), \text{ with} \tag{1}$$

$$\mathcal{L}_G(l, h) = -\sum_{j=1}^{3} t_{hj} \log(D(G_H(l))_j) - \sum_{j=1}^{3} t_{lj} \log(D(G_L(h))_j) \tag{2}$$

$$\mathcal{L}_D(l, h) = -\sum_{j=1}^{3} t_{fj} \log(D(G_H(l)_j) - \sum_{j=1}^{3} t_{fj} \log(D(G_L(h)_j) \\ -\sum_{j=1}^{3} t_{hj} \log(D(h)_j) - \sum_{j=1}^{3} t_{lj} \log(D(l)_j) \tag{3}$$

$$\mathcal{L}_{cycle}(l, h) = \|l - G_L(G_H(l))\|_1 + \|h - G_H(G_L(h))\|_1 \tag{4}$$

Here λ_{GAN} and λ_{cycle} are hyper-parameters for weighting discriminator and cycle-consistency loss respectively. For our model, we set $\lambda_{GAN} = 1$ and $\lambda_{cycle} = 10$ following [14]. Our implementation of the described methodology is publicly available at github.com/IljaManakov/HDcycleGAN. We also provide implementation details in the supplementary material.

3   Experiments and Results

After training the HDcycleGAN for 245 epochs with an Adam optimizer and a learning rate of 5×10^{-4}, we performed both quantitative and qualitative analyses on the test set, which we explain in Sects. 3.2 and 3.3. In the quantitative analysis, we compared our approach to popular denoising methods using several measurements of similarity between real LN images and denoised ones. For the qualitative analysis, the similarity between real LN images and images produced by BM3D [2], wavelet denoising [1] and our method was assessed by three ophthalmologists independently. Finally, in Sect. 3.4, we inspect the learned feature maps of the LN generator. We start by describing our dataset.

3.1   Dataset

We acquired the data for this task in-house, using a SPECTRALIS OCT+HRA from Heidelberg Engineering, as part of the general diagnostic workflow for macular diseases. We did not select patients based on any further traits. As such, the scans in the dataset show various kinds of diseases in all stages and are representative of the typical imaging data generated at our hospital. To gather the images belonging to the high noise domain, we followed the hospital protocol, using 30° ART Volume acquisition with 12 frames averaged for each b-scan. The low noise domain consists of acquisitions that follow the same protocol except that we set the number of averaged frames to 60. We obtained both HN and LN images from the same patients on the same visit. As the proprietary software of the device manufacturer handles the frame averaging, we did not have access to the individual frames. In total, we gathered 23030 b-scans in 470 volumes from 235 patients for each noise domain. We used 90% of the volumes for training and the remaining 10% for testing. Before passing the images through our model, we scaled the 496×512 images to a pixel intensity range between 0.0 and 1.0.

3.2   Quantitative Evaluation

To asses our model's performance, we evaluated the similarity between the generated images and the ground truth LN images in the test set. Since we acquired HN and LN scans pairwise, we registered the images employing a registration algorithm based on discrete Fourier-transform [12]. After registration, we calculated the peak signal-to-noise ratio (PSNR) and structural similarity index (SSIM) between the two images. Additionally, we used the Marching Cubes algorithm [9] to find the contour of the retina. Inverting the selection yields a background mask, while reapplying Marching Cubes on the retinal layers with a different level finds contours in highly reflective parts of the retina. We designated these regions as signal. This process is illustrated in Fig. 3 of the supplementary material. Using the signal and background regions, we then calculated the mean-to-standard-deviation ratio (MSR) and contrast-to-noise ratio (CNR). To better gauge the performance of our approach, we included median filtering, wavelet denoising [1], bilateral filtering [13], non-local means [3] and BM3D [2] in the comparison. The results are displayed in Table 1. We can see that our model outperforms the other methods in all measurements except SSIM, where BM3D is slightly ahead. Overall we find that the performance of BM3D and our model is very close in inter-image measurements (SSIM and PSNR). In intra-image measurements (CNR and MSR) the margin between our approach and the others widens. It is also worth noting that our algorithm requires 30% less time to run on CPU than BM3D and beats all other algorithms by almost an order of magnitude on a low-end GPU (see Fig. 2 in the supplementary material). Although PSNR, SSIM, MSR and CNR are standard metrics of image quality, there is a caveat to these results; since HN and LN samples stem from independent acquisitions the noise in them is uncorrelated. This might explain why the overall improvement in these metrics is relatively low for all algorithms.

Table 1. Results of the quantitative analysis. Values are shown as mean ± standard deviation.

Method	CNR	MSR	PSNR	SSIM
Raw	3.66 ± 2.21	3.96 ± 1.73	21.99 ± 1.33	0.662 ± 0.055
Median	3.82 ± 2.36	4.25 ± 1.92	22.32 ± 1.45	0.682 ± 0.051
Wavelet [1]	3.81 ± 2.37	4.23 ± 1.86	22.34 ± 1.41	0.690 ± 0.053
Bilateral [13]	3.78 ± 2.33	4.28 ± 1.93	22.29 ± 1.40	0.690 ± 0.053
nl-means [3]	3.78 ± 2.33	4.43 ± 2.12	22.32 ± 1.40	0.702 ± 0.051
BM3D [2]	3.87 ± 2.44	4.39 ± 1.97	22.50 ± 1.45	**0.708 ± 0.052**
Ours	**4.00 ± 2.51**	**4.73 ± 2.23**	**22.58 ± 1.41**	0.706 ± 0.050

3.3 Qualitative Evaluation

Because of this caveat, we asked three expert ophthalmologists to visually assess the quality of our results. We provided them with 150 real LN images from the test set and images generated from the corresponding real HN images using BM3D, wavelet denoising and our method. For each such sample, the clinicians rated the methods by their similarity to the real LN images. We ordered the images in each sample randomly and did not provide any indication as to which model generated which image. The results of this evaluation, displayed in Fig. 2, confirm the findings of the quantitative evaluation. The experts unanimously agree that our approach outperforms the benchmarks.

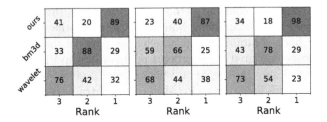

Fig. 2. Results of the qualitative evaluation by three experts.

3.4 Feature Map Inspection

We attempted to understand how the model is approaching the task of image enhancement by looking at the feature maps that it has learned. We did this by passing a sample through the LN generator and extracting the neuron activations at every layer. Due to the convolutional nature of the generator, these layer outputs are shaped like images with many channels. Hence we can view each channel in the activations of a layer as a gray-scale image which we refer to as a feature map.

By up-scaling the feature maps to the size of the input, we then checked for spatial correlations. For visualization purposes, we show some feature maps from different layers, which highlight distinct regions of the retina, in Fig. 3. Many more can be found in the supplementary material accompanying this paper.

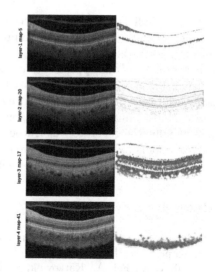

We observed that the feature maps at the output of the deeper residual blocks become increasingly abstract and spatially uncorrelated with the input. The feature maps at the outputs of the first four layers (initial convolution and downsampling 1 to 3) and shallower residual blocks exhibit a strong spatial correlation with the input. Moreover, the different channels seem to correspond to anatomically distinct regions in the b-scan, although segmentation was never part of the training objective.

Fig. 3. Example of the feature maps. On the left, the input image is overlaid with the map. On the right, the feature map is shown by itself.

We think that this finding is relevant when viewed from two perspectives. Firstly, it shows that the model has gained some domain specific knowledge about the structure of macular OCT scans, which general methods such as BM3D and wavelet denoising are lacking. Secondly, this property can prove useful from the viewpoint of transfer learning, i.e. when applying this model to other tasks. The feature maps themselves can also be used for other tasks.

An example of the second point can be found in Fig. 11 in the supplementary material. We discovered a feature map that appears to track the positions of the Inner Limiting Membrane (ILM) and the Retinal Pigment Epithelium (RPE) (the inner- and outermost layers of the retina) (see Fig. 10 in the supplementary material). We then multiplied the feature map with its corresponding b-scan, applied the image mean as a threshold and skeletonized the remainder. The resulting lines can be used to estimate retinal thickness. This method seems to work well even in the presence of pathologies, such as myopia (row 4, col. 4) or vitreous detachment (row 1, col. 4 and row 5, col. 3), which are typical causes for segmentation errors in commercial segmentation algorithms.

4 Discussion

In this paper, we applied the HDcycleGAN model to the problem of image enhancement. In medical imaging, reduced image noise typically comes at the cost of increased acquisition time, radiation dose or other detrimental effects. Our model can learn a mapping between domains that correspond to different settings of those costly acquisition parameters.

Additionally, our approach learns the structural characteristics of the medical imaging domain, which further improves its usefulness as it can be leveraged for other tasks in that domain. As part of future work, we wish to study the transferability of our approach to other imaging modalities, such as Ultrasound.

As is the case with all GAN-based methods, the training of this model is not straightforward and the performance does not appear to increase monotonically throughout training. Nevertheless, our approach allows us to pre-train the parts individually; the generators as Autoencoders and the discriminator as a classifier between domains. In the future, we also plan to test if pre-training can improve training stability and model performance.

References

1. Chang, S.G., Vetterli, M.: Adaptive wavelet thresholding for image denoising and compression. IEEE Trans. Image Process. **9**(9), 1532–1546 (2000)
2. Dabov, K., Foi, A., Katkovnik, V., Egiazarian, K.: Image denoising with block-matching and 3D filtering, vol. 6064 (2006)
3. Darbon, J., Cunha, A., Chan, T.F., Osher, S., Jensen, G.J.: Fast nonlocal filtering applied to electron cryomicroscopy. In: 2008 5th IEEE International Symposium on Biomedical Imaging: From Nano to Macro, pp. 1331–1334 (2008)
4. Goodfellow, I., et al.: Generative adversarial nets. Adv. Neural Inf. Process. Syst. **27**, 2672–2680 (2014)
5. Halupka, K.J., et al.: Retinal optical coherence tomography image enhancement via deep learning. Biomed. Opt. Express **9**(12), 6205–6221 (2018)
6. He, K., Zhang, X., Ren, S., Sun, J.: Deep residual learning for image recognition. In: The IEEE Conference on Computer Vision and Pattern Recognition (CVPR), June 2016
7. Huang, Y., et al.: Simultaneous denoising and super-resolution of optical coherence tomography images based on generative adversarial network. Opt. Express **27**(9), 12289–12307 (2019)
8. Joseph, M., Schmitt, S.H., Xiang, K.M.Y.: Speckle in optical coherence tomography. J. Biomed. Opt. **4**(1), 95–105 (1999)
9. Lorensen, W.E., Cline, H.E.: Marching cubes: a high resolution 3D surface construction algorithm. In: Proceedings of the 14th Annual Conference on Computer Graphics and Interactive Techniques, pp. 163–169 (1987)
10. Odena, A., Dumoulin, V., Olah, C.: Deconvolution and checkerboard artifacts. Distill **1**(10), e3 (2016). http://distill.pub/2016/deconv-checkerboard
11. Podoleanu, A.G.: Optical coherence tomography. J. Microsc. **247**(3), 209–219 (2012)
12. Reddy, B.S., Chatterji, B.N.: An FFT-based technique for translation, rotation, and scale-invariant image registration. IEEE Trans. Image Process. **5**(8), 1266–1271 (1996)
13. Tomasi, C., Manduchi, R.: Bilateral filtering for gray and color images. In: Sixth International Conference on Computer Vision, pp. 839–846 (1998)
14. Zhu, J.Y., Park, T., Isola, P., Efros, A.A.: Unpaired image-to-image translation using cycle-consistent adversarial networks. In: The IEEE International Conference on Computer Vision (ICCV) (2017)

Temporal Consistency Objectives Regularize the Learning of Disentangled Representations

Gabriele Valvano[1,2]($\boxtimes$), Agisilaos Chartsias[2], Andrea Leo[1],
and Sotirios A. Tsaftaris[2]

[1] IMT School for Advanced Studies Lucca, Piazza S. Francesco,
55100 Lucca, LU, Italy
`gabriele.valvano@imtlucca.it`
[2] School of Engineering, University of Edinburgh, West Mains Rd,
Edinburgh EH9 3FB, UK

Abstract. There has been an increasing focus in learning interpretable feature representations, particularly in applications such as medical image analysis that require explainability, whilst relying less on annotated data (since annotations can be tedious and costly). Here we build on recent innovations in style-content representations to learn anatomy, imaging characteristics (appearance) and temporal correlations. By introducing a self-supervised objective of predicting future cardiac phases we improve disentanglement. We propose a temporal transformer architecture that given an image conditioned on phase difference, it predicts a future frame. This forces the anatomical decomposition to be consistent with the temporal cardiac contraction in cine MRI and to have semantic meaning with less need for annotations. We demonstrate that using this regularization, we achieve competitive results and improve semi-supervised segmentation, especially when very few labelled data are available. Specifically, we show Dice increase of up to 19% and 7% compared to supervised and semi-supervised approaches respectively on the ACDC dataset. Code is available at: https://github.com/gvalvano/sdtnet.

Keywords: Disentangled representations · Semi-supervised learning · Cardiac segmentation

1 Introduction

Recent years have seen significant progress in the field of machine learning and, in particular, supervised learning. However, the success and generalization of such algorithms heavily depends learning suitable representations [2]. Unfortunately,

Electronic supplementary material The online version of this chapter (https://doi.org/10.1007/978-3-030-33391-1_2) contains supplementary material, which is available to authorized users.

© Springer Nature Switzerland AG 2019
Q. Wang et al. (Eds.): DART 2019/MIL3ID 2019, LNCS 11795, pp. 11–19, 2019.
https://doi.org/10.1007/978-3-030-33391-1_2

obtaining them usually requires large quantities of labelled data, which need expertise and in many cases are expensive to obtain.

It has been argued [3] that good data representations are those separating out (disentangling) the underlying explanatory factors into disjoint subsets. As a result, latent variables become sensitive only to changes in single generating factors, while being relatively insensitive to other changes [2]. Disentangled representations have been reported to be less sensitive to nuisance variables and to produce better generalization [16]. In the context of medical imaging, such representations offer: (i) better interpretability of the extracted features; (ii) better generalization on unseen data; (iii) and the potential for semi-supervised learning [5]. Moreover, disentanglement allows interpretable latent code manipulation, which is desirable in a variety of applications, such as modality transfer and multi-modal registration [5,10,13].

Medical images typically present the spatial information about the patient's anatomy (shapes) modulated by modality-specific characteristics (appearance). The SDNet framework [5] is an attempt to decouple anatomical factors from their appearance towards more explainable representations. Building on this concept, we introduce a new architecture that drives the model to learn anatomical factors that are both spatially and temporally consistent. We propose a new model, namely: Spatial Decomposition and Transformation Network (SDTNet).

The main **contributions** of this paper are: (**1**) we introduce a modality invariant transformer that, conditioned on the temporal information, predicts future anatomical factors from the current ones; (**2**) we show that the transformer provides a self-supervised signal useful to improve the generalization capabilities of the model; (**3**) we achieve state of the art performance compared to SDNet for semi-supervised segmentation at several proportions of labelled data available; (**4**) and show for the first time preliminary results of cardiac temporal synthesis.

2   Related Works

2.1   Learning Good Representations with Temporal Conditioning

The world surrounding us is typically affected by smooth temporal variations and is known that temporal consistency plays a key role for the development of invariant representations in biological vision [17]. However, despite that temporal correlations have been used to learn/propagate segmentations in medical imaging [1,12], their use as a learning signal to improve representations remains unexplored. To the best of our knowledge, this is the first work to use spatiotemporal dynamics to improve disentangled representations in cardiac imaging.

Outside the medical imaging community, we find some commonalities of our work with Hsieh et al. [7], who address the challenge of video frame prediction decomposing a video representation in a time-invariant *content* vector and a time-dependent *pose* vector. Assuming that the content vector is fixed for all frames, the network aims to learn the dynamics of the low-dimensional pose vector. The predicted pose vector can be decoded together with the fixed content features to generate a future video frame in pixel space. Similarly, we decompose the features space in a fixed and a time-dependent subset (*modality* and *anatomy*). However, our objective is not merely predicting a future temporal frame, but we use the temporal prediction as a self-supervised signal to ameliorate the quality of the representation: i.e. we constrain its temporal transformation to be smooth. By doing so, we demonstrate that we can consistently improve the segmentation capabilities of the considered baselines.

2.2   Spatial Decomposition Network (SDNet)

Here, we briefly review a recent approach for learning disentangled anatomy-modality representations in cardiac imaging, upon which we build our model.

The SDNet [5] can be seen as an autoencoder taking as input a 2D image $x \sim X$ and decomposing it into its anatomical components $s = f_A(x)$ and modality components $z = f_M(x)$. The vector z is modelled as a probability distribution $Q(z|X)$ that is encouraged to follow a multivariate Gaussian, as in the VAE framework [9]. s is a multi-channel output composed of binary discrete maps. A decoder $g(\cdot)$ uses both s and z to reconstruct the input image $\tilde{x} = g(s, z) \approx x$. An additional network $h(\cdot)$ is supervisedly trained to extract the heart segmentation $\tilde{y} = h(s)$ from s, while an adversarial signal forces $\tilde{y}$ to be realistic even when few pairs of labelled data are available, enabling semi-supervised learning.

While SDNet was shown to achieve impressive results in semi-supervised learning, it still requires human annotations to learn to decouple the cardiac anatomy from other anatomical factors. Furthermore, it doesn't take advantage of any temporal information to learn better anatomical factors: as a result they are not guaranteed to be temporally correlated.

3   Proposed Approach

Herein, we address the above limitations, by a simple hypothesis: components s of different cardiac phases should be similar within the same cardiac cycle and their differences, if any, should be consistent across different subjects. To achieve this we introduce a new neural network $T(\cdot)$ in the SDNet framework that, conditioned on temporal information, regularizes the anatomical factors such that they can be consistent (e.g. have smooth transformations) across time. Obtaining better representations will ultimately allow improved performance in the segmentation task, too. $T(\cdot)$ is a modality-invariant transformer that 'warps' the s factors learnt by the SDNet according to the cardiac phase. Furthermore, by combining the current z factors with the predicted s factors for future time points, one can reconstruct the future frames in a cardiac sequence: e.g., given time $t_1 < t_2$, we have $\tilde{x}_{t_2} = g(T(s_{t_1}), z_{t_1}) \approx x_{t_2}$. Our model is shown in Fig. 1. Below we focus our discussion on the design of the transformer and the training costs, all other network architectures follow that of SDNet [5]. In the following, t, dt are scalars, while remaining variables are considered as tensors.

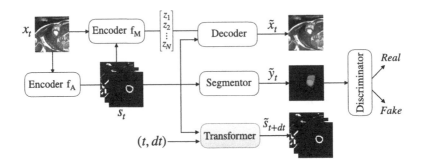

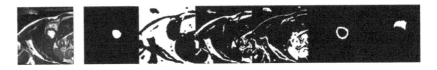

Fig. 1. SDTNet block diagram. The transformer (in yellow) predicts the future anatomical factors conditioned on the temporal information. The future frame can be generated by the decoder using $\tilde{s}_{t+dt}$ and the current z factor. (Color figure online)

Fig. 2. Anatomical factors extracted by the SDTNet from the image on the left.

3.1 Spatial Decomposition and Transformation Network (SDTNet)

The transformer $T(\cdot)$ takes as input the binary anatomical factors s (Fig. 2) and their associated temporal information t. Under the assumption that the modality factors remain constant throughout the temporal dimension (e.g. the heart contracting from extra-diastole to extra-systole), the transformer must deform the current anatomy s_t such that, given a temporal change dt, it estimates s_{t+dt}, i.e. the anatomy of image x_{t+dt} when given as input. Using this prediction $\tilde{s}_{t+dt} = T(s_t, t, dt)$ together with the fixed modality factors z_t, we should be able to correctly reconstruct the image at the future time point $\tilde{x}_{t+dt}$. By capturing the temporal dynamics of the anatomical factors, the transformer guides their generation to be temporally coherent, resulting in a self-supervised training signal, that is the prediction error of future anatomical factors.

3.2 Transformer Design

After testing several architecture designs for the transformer, we found that the best results could be obtained by adapting a UNet [14] to work with binary input/output conditioned on temporal information on the bottleneck.

Temporal information, the tuple (t, dt), is encoded via an MLP consisting of 3 fully connected layers, arranged as 128-128-4096, with the output reshaped to $16 \times 16 \times 16$. This information is concatenated at the bottleneck of the UNet where features maps have resolution $16 \times 16 \times 64$, to condition the transformer and control the required deformation. To encourage the use of the temporal features and retain the notion of the binary inputs, the features at the bottleneck and of the MLP are bounded in [0, 1], using a sigmoid activation function.

We hypothesised that it would be easier to model differential changes to anatomy factors. Thus, we added a long residual connection between the UNet input and its output. We motivate this by observing that the anatomical structure that mostly changes in time is the heart: thus learning the spatial transformation should be similar to learning to segment the cardiac structure in the binary tensor s: a task that the UNet is known to be effective at solving. The output of the transformer is binarized again (key for disentanglement), as in [5].

3.3   Cost Function and Training

The overall cost function is the following weighted sum:

$$Loss = \lambda_0 \cdot L_S + \lambda_1 \cdot L_{US} + \lambda_2 \cdot L_{ADV} + \lambda_3 \cdot L_{TR} , \qquad (1)$$

where $\lambda_0 = 10$, $\lambda_1 = 1$ and $\lambda_2 = 10$ as in [5], and $\lambda_3 = 1$ found experimentally.

L_S is the cost associated to the supervised task (segmentation) and can be written as $L_S = L_{DICE}(y, \tilde{y}) + 0.1 \cdot L_{CE}(y, \tilde{y})$, where y and $\tilde{y}$ are the ground truth and predicted segmentation masks, respectively; L_{DICE} is the differentiable Dice loss evaluated on left ventricle, right ventricle and myocardium, while L_{CE} is the weighted cross-entropy on these three classes plus the background (with class weights inversely proportional to the number of pixels for the class).

L_{US} is the cost associated to the unsupervised task and can be decomposed as $L_{US} = |\tilde{x} - x| + \lambda_{KL} \cdot D_{KL}[Q(z|X)||N(0, I)] - MI(\tilde{x}, z)$. The first term is the mean absolute error between the input and the reconstruction, while the second term is the KL divergence between $Q(z|X)$ and a Normal Gaussian (with $\lambda_{KL} = 0.1$). The last term is the mutual information between the reconstruction $\tilde{x}$ and the latent code z and is approximated by an additional neural network, as in the InfoGAN framework [6]. By maximizing the mutual information between the reconstruction and z, we prevented posterior collapse and constrained the decoder $g(\cdot)$ to effectively use the modality factors.

L_{ADV} is the adversarial loss of a Least-Squares GAN [11], used to discriminate ground truth from predicted segmentations in the unsupervised setting.

L_{TR} is the loss associated to the self-supervised signal, computed as the differentiable Dice loss between $\tilde{s}_{t+dt}$ and s_{t+dt}. This error serves as a proxy for the reconstruction error of future cardiac phases $|x_{t+dt} - g(T(s_t), z_t)|$. In practice, we find it much easier to train $T(\cdot)$ with a loss defined in the anatomy space rather than one on the final reconstruction: in fact, the gradients used to update the network parameters can flow into $T(\cdot)$ directly from its output layer, rather than from that of the decoder $g(\cdot)$.

The model was optimized using the Exponential Moving Average (EMA): we maintained a moving average of the parameters during training, and employed their average for testing. The learning rate was scheduled to follow a triangular wave [15] in the range 10^{-4} to 10^{-5} with a period of 20 epochs. Both EMA and the learning rate scheduling facilitated comparisons, allowing to detect wider and more generalizable minima (hence, reducing loss fluctuations). We used Adam [8] with an early stopping criterion on the segmentation loss of a validation set.

4   Experiments and Discussion

4.1   Data and Preprocessing

Data. We used ACDC data from the 2017 Automatic Cardiac Diagnosis Challenge [4]. These are 2-dimensional cine-MR images acquired using 1.5T and 3T MR scanners from 100 patients, for which manual segmentations for the left ventricular cavity (LV), the myocardium (MYO) and the right ventricle (RV) are provided in correspondence to the end-systolic (ES) and end-diastolic (ED) cardiac phases. ES and ED phase instants are also provided. We used a 3-fold cross validation and randomly divided the data to obtain 70 MRI scans for training, 15 for validation and 15 for the test sets.

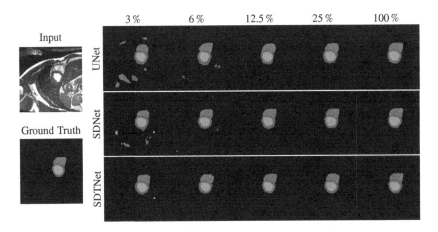

Fig. 3. Comparison of predicted segmentations obtained from the UNet, SDNet, SDT-Net after being trained with different percentages of the labelled data.

Preprocessing. After removing outliers outside 5th and 95th percentiles of the pixel values, we removed the median and normalized the images on the interquartile range, centering each volume approximately around zero.

Training. Since our objective was to introduce temporal consistency in the anatomical factors rather then predicting the whole cardiac cycle, we split the cine MRI sequences in two halves: (i) temporal frames in the ED-ES interval; (ii) temporal frames from ES to the end of the cardiac cycle. The latter frames were reversed in their temporal order, to mimic once again the cardiac contraction: as a result, we avoided the inherent uncertainty associated to the transformations of frames in the middle of the cardiac cycle. Finally, we applied data augmentation at run-time, consisting of rotations, translations and scaling of each 2D slice.

4.2   Results

Semi-supervised Segmentation. We compared SDTNet to the fully supervised training of a UNet and to the semi-supervised training of SDNet in a segmentation task, varying the percentage of labelled training samples. As Fig. 3 and Table 1 show, the SDTNet consistently outperforms the others, especially at lower percentages of labelled pairs in the training set. Furthermore, SDT-Net exhibits lower variance in its predictions, so it's more consistent. A paired Wilcoxon test demonstrated most of these improvements to be statistically significant. We find that the transformer forces the anatomical decomposition to follow more "semantic" disentanglement even with little human annotations. This translates to better segmentation results. While secondary to the thesis of the paper, both the SDNet and the SDTNet outperform the UNet.

Cardiac Synthesis. Figure 4 shows that it is possible to predict future cardiac phases from ED through ES by using the predicted anatomical factors $\tilde{s}_{t>0}$ together with the modality factors $z_{t=0}$. We note that this is the first attempt of deep learning-based temporal synthesis in cardiac albeit preliminary. Note that we train the transformer with both pathological and healthy subjects and

Table 1. DICE scores comparing SDTNet and other baselines at various proportions of available labeled data. The last column shows the average improvement of SDTNet over SDNet. Asterisks denote statistical significance ($p < 0.01$).

Labels	UNet	SDNet	SDTNet	Improvement
100%	80.03 ± 0.38	85.11 ± 0.73	85.83 ± 0.40	0.72
25%	77.55 ± 1.02	81.64 ± 0.96	83.69 ± 0.37	2.05*
12.5%	71.04 ± 1.71	78.07 ± 1.52	79.48 ± 0.82	1.41*
6%	59.20 ± 1.38	72.18 ± 1.91	74.22 ± 0.57	2.04*
3%	44.89 ± 9.52	56.89 ± 2.48	63.74 ± 1.59	6.85*

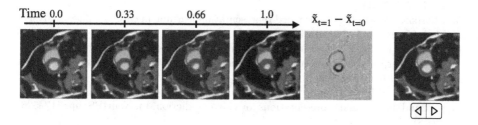

Fig. 4. Interpolation on the temporal axis between ED and ES phases. The images are obtained by fixing the modality-dependent factors $z_{t=0}$ and using the anatomical factors $\tilde{s}_{t>0}$ predicted for future time points. In Acrobat, clicking on the rightmost image frames animates frames showing the predicted cardiac contraction. (See Supplementary material)

it thus predicts average temporal transformations. Conditioning also with prior pathology information and validation of synthesis are left as future work.

5   Conclusion

We introduced a self-supervised objective for learning disentangled anatomy-modality representations in cardiac imaging. By leveraging the temporal information contained in cine MRI, we introduced a spatiotemporal model in SDNet [5], improving its generalization capabilities in the semi-supervised setting at several proportions of labelled data available. Also, the resulting approach considerably outperforms the fully-supervised baseline, confirming the potential for semi-supervised and self-supervised training in medical imaging.

Acknowledgements. This work was supported by the Erasmus+ programme of the European Union, during an exchange between IMT School for Advanced Studies Lucca and the School of Engineering, University of Edinburgh. S.A. Tsaftaris acknowledges the support of the Royal Academy of Engineering and the Research Chairs and Senior Research Fellowships scheme. We thank NVIDIA Corporation for donating the Titan Xp GPU used for this research.

References

1. Bai, W., et al.: Recurrent neural networks for aortic image sequence segmentation with sparse annotations. In: Frangi, A.F., Schnabel, J.A., Davatzikos, C., Alberola-López, C., Fichtinger, G. (eds.) MICCAI 2018. LNCS, vol. 11073, pp. 586–594. Springer, Cham (2018). https://doi.org/10.1007/978-3-030-00937-3_67
2. Bengio, Y., Courville, A., Vincent, P.: Representation learning: a review and new perspectives. IEEE PAMI **35**(8), 1798–1828 (2013)
3. Bengio, Y., et al.: Learning deep architectures for AI. Found. Trends Mach. Learn. **2**(1), 1–127 (2009)
4. Bernard, O., et al.: Deep learning techniques for automatic MRI cardiac multi-structures segmentation and diagnosis: is the problem solved? IEEE TMI **37**(11), 2514–2525 (2018)
5. Chartsias, A., et al.: Disentangled representation learning in cardiac image analysis. Med. Image Anal. **58**, 101535 (2019)
6. Chen, X., Duan, Y., Houthooft, R., Schulman, J., Sutskever, I., Abbeel, P.: Info-GAN: Interpretable representation learning by information maximizing generative adversarial nets. In: NeurIPS, pp. 2172–2180 (2016)
7. Hsieh, J.T., Liu, B., Huang, D.A., Fei-Fei, L.F., Niebles, J.C.: Learning to decompose and disentangle representations for video prediction. In: NeurIPS, pp. 517–526 (2018)
8. Kingma, D.P., Ba, J.: Adam: a method for stochastic optimization. In: ICLR (2015)
9. Kingma, D.P., Welling, M.: Auto-encoding variational bayes. In: ICLR (2014)
10. Lee, H.Y., Tseng, H.Y., Huang, J.B., Singh, M., Yang, M.H.: Diverse image-to-image translation via disentangled representations. In: ECCV, pp. 35–51 (2018)
11. Mao, X., Li, Q., Xie, H., Lau, R.Y.K., Wang, Z., Smolley, S.P.: On the effectiveness of least squares generative adversarial networks. IEEE PAMI **PP**(99), 1–13 (2018)

12. Qin, C., et al.: Joint Learning of motion estimation and segmentation for cardiac MR image sequences. In: Frangi, A.F., Schnabel, J.A., Davatzikos, C., Alberola-López, C., Fichtinger, G. (eds.) MICCAI 2018. LNCS, vol. 11071, pp. 472–480. Springer, Cham (2018). https://doi.org/10.1007/978-3-030-00934-2_53

13. Qin, C., Shi, B., Liao, R., Mansi, T., Rueckert, D., Kamen, A.: Unsupervised deformable registration for multi-modal images via disentangled representations. arXiv preprint arXiv:1903.09331 (2019)

14. Ronneberger, O., Fischer, P., Brox, T.: U-Net: convolutional networks for biomedical image segmentation. In: Navab, N., Hornegger, J., Wells, W.M., Frangi, A.F. (eds.) MICCAI 2015. LNCS, vol. 9351, pp. 234–241. Springer, Cham (2015). https://doi.org/10.1007/978-3-319-24574-4_28

15. Smith, L.N.: Cyclical learning rates for training neural networks. In: 2017 IEEE WACV, pp. 464–472. IEEE (2017)

16. Van Steenkiste, S., Locatello, F., Schmidhuber, J., Bachem, O.: Are disentangled representations helpful for abstract visual reasoning? arXiv preprint arXiv:1905.12506 (2019)

17. Wood, J.N.: A smoothness constraint on the development of object recognition. Cognition **153**, 140–145 (2016)

Multi-layer Domain Adaptation for Deep Convolutional Networks

Ozan Ciga$^{(\boxtimes)}$, Jianan Chen, and Anne Martel

Medical Biophysics, University of Toronto, Toronto, Canada
`ozan.ciga@mail.utoronto.ca`

Abstract. Despite their success in many computer vision tasks, convolutional networks tend to require large amounts of labeled data to achieve generalization. Furthermore, the performance is not guaranteed on a sample from an unseen domain at test time, if the network was not exposed to similar samples from that domain at training time. This hinders the adoption of these techniques in clinical setting where the imaging data is scarce, and where the intra- and inter-domain variance of the data can be substantial. We propose a domain adaptation technique that is especially suitable for deep networks to alleviate this requirement of labeled data. Our method utilizes gradient reversal layers [4] and Squeeze-and-Excite modules [6] to stabilize the training in deep networks. The proposed method was applied to publicly available histopathology and chest X-ray databases and achieved superior performance to existing state-of-the-art networks with and without domain adaptation. Depending on the application, our method can improve multi-class classification accuracy by 5–20% compared to DANN introduced in [4].

1 Introduction

Deep learning models have achieved great success in recent years on computer vision tasks. Fully convolutional networks (FCNs) consistently achieve the state-of-the-art performance in various tasks such as segmentation, classification and detection. Despite their success, however, FCNs usually require large amounts of labeled data from the domain in which the network will be deployed. As network architectures become deeper with more trainable parameters, the requirement for large amounts of data is further exacerbated as the networks are more prone to overfitting. This leads to a need for even larger amounts of data to achieve generalization. Furthermore, regardless of the size or the domain diversity of the training set, there is no performance guarantee on an unseen dataset from a domain that the network was not exposed to at training time. These issues are especially problematic in medical image analysis, as the labeled data is scarce due to the tedious and expensive data annotation process, and a large distributional shift can be observed even if data comes from the same source.

Several methods, including network weight regularization, semi-supervised approaches [3], meta-learning [8], and domain adaptation [4] have been proposed to improve generalization performance on unseen datasets. In the present

Q. Wang et al. (Eds.): DART 2019/MIL3ID 2019, LNCS 11795, pp. 20–27, 2019.
https://doi.org/10.1007/978-3-030-33391-1_3

work, we will focus on the domain adaptation. These methods aim to leverage large amounts of cheap unlabeled data from a target domain to improve generalization performance using small amounts of labeled data. In past work, [11] proposed correcting covariate shift between domains by reweighting samples from source domain to minimize the discrepancy between source and the target. This approach was later improved by minimizing distances between feature mappings of source and target domains instead of the samples itself [4]. Further modifications were proposed later that improved the benchmark performances such as tri-learning, which assumes high confidence predictions are correct [10], or leveraging the cluster assumption, in which the decision boundaries based on the modified feature representations should not cross the high density data regions [12].

In the present article we propose a simple, robust method that requires minimal modifications to an existing deep network to achieve domain adaptation. Our model repurposes Squeeze-and-Excite blocks, introduced by [6] for feature selection, to perform domain classification in the intermediate layers of a large network. We use the "squeeze" operation to get a summary statistic at the end of each convolutional block, and use a domain adaptation technique [4] to extract domain-independent features at each layer. The "excitation network" is repurposed to perform domain classification. We extend this method by matching distributions of source and target features at each layer via minimizing the Wasserstein distance.

2   Methods

Due to its conceptual simplicity, we will build our model on top of the gradient reversal layer (GRL) based domain adaptation, which was first introduced in [4]. In an FCN, convolutional layers extract salient features layer by layer as the feature maps shrink in spatial size and expand in semantic (depthwise) information. Once enough abstraction on the image is achieved, features $\mathbf{f}$ are flattened and typically fed into a few fully connected layers to perform the task objective, e.g., classification. As the network usually optimizes a minimization objective, extracted features may (and are likely to) overfit to the domain-specific noise. Domain adaptation via gradient reversal aims to alleviate this by attaching another classifier to the input $\mathbf{f}$, which simultaneously optimizes an adversarial objective: Given $\mathbf{f}$, it tries to minimize the domain classification loss L_d between N samples of the domain classifier with parameters θ_d while trying to maximize this loss with respect to the feature extractor (with parameters θ_f) of the original FCN. In effect, this procedure aims to remove the learned features which are domain-specific, while forcing the network to retain the domain-independent features with error gradient signals $\frac{\partial L_y}{\partial \theta_y}$ and $\frac{\partial L_y}{\partial \theta_f}$, where θ_y are the parameters of the label classifier.

In [4], domain adaptation is achieved by backpropagating the negative binomial cross-entropy loss of the domain classifier network. Features from the last layer prior to the fully connected classification layers are used as inputs to the domain classifier network. We note several problems with this approach: (1) as the network depth increases, the error signal from the domain classifier will tend to vanish, or will be insufficient to remove domain specific features in the earlier layers, (2) given feature maps $\mathbf{X}^i$ and $\mathbf{X}^j$ where $i < j$, it becomes more challenging for the network to extract domain-independent features for $\mathbf{X}^j$ if the features from $\mathbf{X}^i$ are domain dependent, (3) even if domain specific features in map $\mathbf{X}^i$ somehow are discarded in the later layers, the encoding of these features into map $\mathbf{X}^i$ results in capacity underuse of the network, (4) even with the adversarial training objective which forces the preservation of salient features, it is likely for a high capacity network to employ arbitrary transformations on the target samples to match source and target distributions (for a formal derivation, see Appendix E of [12]). For simple tasks that do not require deep networks, vanishing gradients or accumulation of domain dependent features across layers do not affect the performance as much. However, in more complex medical imaging analysis tasks, larger networks tend to perform better; hence, the domain adaptation techniques are more likely to suffer from aforementioned issues. We aim to alleviate this by regulating extracted features at each layer simultaneously by attaching a domain classifier at the end of the layer (see Fig. 1), or by performing unsupervised matching of distributions at each layer.

Given a feature map $\mathbf{X} \in \mathbb{R}^{H' \times W' \times C'}$, we transform $\mathbf{X}$ into $\mathbf{z} \in \mathbb{R}^{C'}$ by average pooling, i.e., $z_k = \frac{1}{H' \times W'} \sum_{i=1}^{H'} \sum_{j=1}^{W'} u_k(i,j)$, where $u_k(i,j)$ indexes the $(i,j)^{th}$ element of the response to the kth kernel of the map $\mathbf{X}$, and z_k is the kth element of the vector $\mathbf{z}$. We will use the shorthand $\mathbf{f}_{tr}(\mathbf{X}_i) = \mathbf{z}_i$ for the transformation of map $\mathbf{X}_i$ (feature maps of layer i) into $\mathbf{z}_i$, which is coined as the "squeeze" operation by [6]. Although $\mathbf{z}_i$ itself is not enough for downstream tasks such as classification or segmentation, it may contain enough information to differentiate between two samples at a given layer. Given this information, we aim to be able to perform domain adaptation at each layer, rather than just the final feature map representation at the end of the network.

2.1   Gradient Reversal Layer Based Domain Adaptation

Analogous to [4], we add domain classifiers at the end of each feature map $\mathbf{X}_i$. By interfering at the intermediate layers, we aim to extract robust features that are invariant to the training domain using the supervision signal. The network is then trained simultaneously for the domain adaptation along with the original objective. We denote this as layer-wise domain-adversarial neural network, or *L-DANN*, as our model is based on DANN [4].

The mini domain classifier network for each layer has the same structure for each layer C', but with varying number of parameters (see Table 1, r indicates the reduction ratio). As the earlier layers in convolutional networks tend to extract more high level information such as texture patterns and edges, we increase the complexity of the domain classifier network progressively, proportional to the depth of the feature map $\mathbf{X}_i$. Given N domains, the domain classifier network maximizes the N-class cross entropy loss via backpropagation to obscure domain information by removing the features from the map $\mathbf{X}_i$.

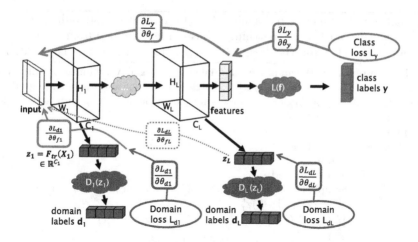

Fig. 1. Proposed modification to the DANN architecture.

2.2 Wasserstein Distance Based Domain Adaptation

Instead of using the domain labels directly, we can also achieve domain adaptation by interpreting z_i as samples drawn from different distributions. Given two domains $\mathcal{X}^s$, $\mathcal{X}^t$, with z_s and z_t are samples drawn from $\mathcal{X}^s$ and $\mathcal{X}^t$, respectively, our objective is $\min_{z_s, z_t} d(z_s, z_t)$ where $d(\cdot, \cdot)$ is an arbitrary distribution divergence. For our experiments, we use the Wasserstein-1 distance, also known as the Earth mover's distance, due to its stability in training [2]. In order to stabilize the training further, we will use the method described in [5] to ensure Lipschitz constraint on the critic, as opposed to the gradient clipping method suggested in [2]. We use the term "critic" as opposed to discriminator/classifier, to be consistent with [2,5]. The procedure is summarized in Algorithm 1, we omit the details for brevity, and refer the interested reader to [5]. In the upcoming sections, we will refer to this method as *L-WASS*, or layer-wise Wasserstein.

3 Experimental Results

3.1 Implementation Details

We do not use any padding or bias in the convolutional layers described in Table 1, and use the reduction ratio $r = 16$ for all the layers. We use ResNet architecture enhanced with Squeeze-and-Excite blocks as our task objective network with varying number of layers depending on the task. Contrary to [4], we do not use a constant λ to scale $\frac{\partial L_d}{\partial \theta}$, nor do we use annealing to stabilize the training. We use stochastic gradient descent (SGD) optimizer in all domain classifier, critic, and the objective network with the learning rate 0.001, momentum 0.9 and weight decay of 0.0001. We have tried updating the domain classifier and critic parameters with and without freezing the preceding layers and observed simultaneous training achieves superior performance. We perform 10 runs per

---

Algorithm 1. Unsupervised domain adaptation via Wasserstein distance with gradient penalty for feature matching. Squeezed feature map from layer l is $\mathbf{z}_l^k$, given input x^k. The objective loss is $\mathcal{L}_{obj}$ (e.g., cross-entropy for classification).

Require: source X^s with samples x^s and labels y^s, target X^t, number of critic iterations n_{critic} per generator iteration, batch size m, learning rates $\alpha_{1,2}$, gradient penalty coefficient λ, initial parameters for the critic and the neural network for the objective, θ_d, θ_f

1: **repeat**
2: **for** each layer j **do**
3:   **for** t=1 to n_{critic} **do**
4:    **for** i=1 to m **do**
5:     Sample $(x_i^s, y_i^s) \sim X^s$, $x_i^t \sim X^t$, a random number $\epsilon \sim U[0,1]$
6:     $\mathbf{z}_j^b \leftarrow \epsilon \mathbf{z}_j^s + (1-\epsilon)\mathbf{z}_j^t$
7:     $L^{(i)} \leftarrow D_j(\mathbf{z}_j^s) - D_j(\mathbf{z}_j^t) - \lambda(\|\nabla_{\mathbf{z}_j^b} D_j(\mathbf{z}_j^b)\|_2 - 1)^2$
8:     $L_{obj}^{(i)} \leftarrow \mathcal{L}_{obj}(x_i^s, y_i^s) - \lambda(\|\nabla_{\mathbf{z}_j^b} D_j(\mathbf{z}_j^b)\|_2 - 1)^2$
9:    **end for**
10:    $\theta_d \leftarrow SGD(\nabla_d \frac{1}{m}\sum_{i=1}^m L^{(i)}, \theta_d, \alpha_1)$
11:   **end for**
12: **end for**
13: $\theta_f \leftarrow SGD(\nabla_f \frac{1}{m}\sum_{i=1}^m L_{obj}^{(i)}, \theta_f, \alpha_2)$
14: **until** θ_f converges

---

experiment, and report the mean accuracy $\pm$ the standard deviation. All experiments are run for 100 epochs regardless of the network architecture or the data, and we use the model with the highest validation accuracy achieved in the last 30 epochs for testing, to avoid selecting a model that achieved high accuracy randomly, and has actually converged.

Table 1. Domain classifier/critic $D(\mathbf{f}_{tr}(\mathbf{X}_i))$. The final output shape N' depends on the architecture used: For L-DANN, we use $N' = N$, or number of classes, and for L-WASS, we use $N' = C'$, number of input channels to perform distribution matching.

	Input shape	Kernel size	Output shape
$\mathbf{f}_{tr}(\mathbf{X}_i)$	$[1 \times 1] \times C'$	–	–
Conv	$[1 \times 1] \times C'$	$[1 \times 1] \times C'/r$	$[1 \times 1] \times C'/r$
ReLU	$[1 \times 1] \times C'/r$	–	$[1 \times 1] \times C'/r$
Conv	$[1 \times 1] \times C'/r$	$[1 \times 1] \times N'$	N'

3.2   Effect of Layer-Wise Domain Adaptation on Small Networks

In order to determine whether layer-wise domain adaptation improves results on networks with a small number of layers, we use the MNIST handwritten digits,

MNIST-M (MNIST blended with random RGB color patches from the BSDS500 dataset), and the SVHN (street view house numbers) to perform digit classification given an image which contains a single digit. SVHN has more variation within the dataset; hence classifying SVHN digits is considered to be more challenging than MNIST or MNIST-M. For all experiments, we use ~60000 images per dataset for training, and ~10000 for testing. We use a single 2-layer neural network, *MNIST architecture* defined in [4], enhanced with batch normalization prior to ReLU layers. As we do not optimize the architecture depending on the dataset, or the direction of the adaptation, our results should only be interpreted within the context of Table 2, and not to the results reported in [4]. As the MNIST architecture is not convolutional, we use the domain classifier given in MNIST architecture for each layer. For L-WASS, the classifier remains the same, with the exception that the number of output elements are 100, to achieve more meaningful matching of distributions. Although the performance of L-DANN remains comparable to DANN, L-WASS fails to converge for the simplest experiment, hinting that for simple distributions, layer-wise Wasserstein distribution matching is not suitable.

Table 2. Comparison between DANN, L-DANN and L-WASS for smaller networks. N/C: Network did not converge.

Method	MNIST→MNIST-M	MNIST→SVHN	SVHN→MNIST
No adaptation	58 ± 2	27.9 ± 5.41	77 ± 0.96
DANN	90.8 ± 1.06	27.7 ± 1.43	46.1 ± 2.27
L-DANN	90.5 ± 0.12	22.8 ± 1.72	53.8 ± 2.22
L-WASS	N/C	21.0 ± 2.11	71.2 ± 0.91

3.3 Effect of Model Complexity on Domain Adaptation

We test our method on another modality, namely on chest X-ray images acquired from two separate institutions in USA, and in China that are classified into normal patients as well as patients with manifestations of tuberculosis [9]. The datasets vary in resolution, quality, contrast, positive to negative samples ratio, and the number of samples. In addition, each dataset has separate watermarks and descriptive texts in different parts of the X-rays, which are known to degrade performance in neural networks. The first dataset consists of 138 images, which we refer to as S, or small, and the second dataset consists of 662 image, which we refer to as L, or large. In order to show that our method performs better with deeper architectures, we compare two architectures: SE-ResNet-101 (49.6 million trainable parameters) and SENET 154 (116.3M). Results are shown in Table 3. Note that although DANN slightly outperforms L-WASS in one of the experiments, its performance is not consistent. In some settings, it performs worse than networks without any domain adaptation, and even fails to converge for the deepest setting. In contrast, both L-DANN and L-WASS consistently perform better than the no domain adaptation baseline. The utility of using a deeper architecture can be observed in the $S \rightarrow L$ direction, where we gain up to ~7% in accuracy, for $L - DANN$ setting. In other words, deeper networks can help better generalize to larger datasets given a small labeled dataset, which is often the case in the clinical setting.

Table 3. Comparison between DANN, L-DANN and L-WASS for deeper networks.

Architecture	Source→Target	Method	Precision	Recall	F1-score	Accuracy
SE-ResNet-101	L→S	No adaptation	100	18.9	31.8	65.9
		DANN	80.9	65.5	72.4	79
		L-DANN	88.1	63.8	74	81.2
		L-WASS	91.1	53.4	67.3	78.3
	S→L	No adaptation	68.7	72.6	70.6	69.3
		DANN	71.8	67.6	69.6	70.1
		L-DANN	72.6	73.7	73.1	73.9
		L-WASS	70.9	76.1	73.4	72.1
SENET 154	L→S	No adaptation	100	3.4	6.6	59.4
		DANN	90.9	51.7	65.9	77.5
		L-DANN	100	43.1	60.3	76.1
		L-WASS	90.9	68.9	78.4	84.1
	S→L	No adaptation	79.3	65.1	71.5	73.7
		DANN	N/C	N/C	N/C	N/C
		L-DANN	75.1	84.5	79.5	80.9
		L-WASS	88.8	75.1	81.6	81.3

3.4   Domain Adaptation for Feature Regularization

We also test our method on the BACH (BreAst Cancer Histopathology) challenge [7]. This challenge is composed of classification of patches extracted from whole-slide images (WSI) into 4 classes (normal, benign, in-situ, and invasive cancer) and segmentation of the WSI into these classes. As it is not uncommon to achieve ~90% accuracy on the classification part, we turn our attention to the segmentation. There are 10 labeled + 20 unlabeled WSI for training, and 10 for testing. Given the stain variation among WSI, we are using the unlabeled 20 images for stain normalization, and for source (i.e., the institution, scanner or the hospital) agnostic feature extraction. In this respect, the domain adaptation acts as a regularizer on extracted features, retaining only the features which are common in both domains. We train the same network, SE-ResNet-50, without domain adaptation, with *L-DANN* module, with *L-WASS*, and with *DANN*, and achieve scores (as defined in [1], which penalizes false negatives, or incorrect "normal" class, more than false positives, or any of the remaining three classes) **0.63**, **0.68**, **0.66**, **0.65**, respectively. Note that the 2nd best score on the public leaderboard is **0.63**.

4 Conclusions

We presented a novel domain adaptation method for fully convolutional networks that can alleviate the requirements for large amounts of data, especially in deep networks. Our method is simple, requires minimal amount of modification to the original network architecture, adds small overhead to the training cost, and is cost-free in test time. We tested our method with multiple public medical imaging datasets and showed promising gains on multiple baseline networks.

Acknowledgments. This work was funded by Canadian Cancer Society (grant #705772) and NSERC RGPIN-2016-06283.

References

1. Aresta, G., et al.: Bach: grand challenge on breast cancer histology images. Med. Image Anal. **56**, 122–139 (2019)
2. Arjovsky, M., Chintala, S., Bottou, L.: Wasserstein GAN. arXiv preprint arXiv:1701.07875 (2017)
3. Baur, C., Albarqouni, S., Navab, N.: Semi-supervised deep learning for fully convolutional networks. In: Descoteaux, M., Maier-Hein, L., Franz, A., Jannin, P., Collins, D.L., Duchesne, S. (eds.) MICCAI 2017. LNCS, vol. 10435, pp. 311–319. Springer, Cham (2017). https://doi.org/10.1007/978-3-319-66179-7_36
4. Ganin, Y., Lempitsky, V.: Unsupervised domain adaptation by backpropagation. arXiv preprint arXiv:1409.7495 (2014)
5. Gulrajani, I., Ahmed, F., Arjovsky, M., Dumoulin, V., Courville, A.C.: Improved training of Wasserstein GANs. In: Advances in neural information processing systems, pp. 5767–5777 (2017)
6. Hu, J., Shen, L., Sun, G.: Squeeze-and-excitation networks. In: Proceedings of the IEEE conference on computer vision and pattern recognition, pp. 7132–7141 (2018)
7. ICIAR: Iciar 2018-challenge - home (2018). https://iciar2018-challenge.grand-challenge.org/. Accessed 16 Aug 2019
8. Maicas, G., Bradley, A.P., Nascimento, J.C., Reid, I., Carneiro, G.: Training medical image analysis systems like radiologists. In: Frangi, A.F., Schnabel, J.A., Davatzikos, C., Alberola-López, C., Fichtinger, G. (eds.) MICCAI 2018. LNCS, vol. 11070, pp. 546–554. Springer, Cham (2018). https://doi.org/10.1007/978-3-030-00928-1_62
9. Openi: what is open-i ? (2018). https://openi.nlm.nih.gov/faq/. Accessed 16 Aug 2019
10. Saito, K., Ushiku, Y., Harada, T.: Asymmetric tri-training for unsupervised domain adaptation. In: Proceedings of the 34th International Conference on Machine Learning-Volume 70, pp. 2988–2997 (2017). JMLR.org
11. Shimodaira, H.: Improving predictive inference under covariate shift by weighting the log-likelihood function. J. Stat. Plann. Infer. **90**(2), 227–244 (2000)
12. Shu, R., Bui, H.H., Narui, H., Ermon, S.: A dirt-t approach to unsupervised domain adaptation. arXiv preprint arXiv:1802.08735 (2018)

Intramodality Domain Adaptation Using Self Ensembling and Adversarial Training

Zahil Shanis[1,2], Samuel Gerber[1], Mingchen Gao[2], and Andinet Enquobahrie[1(✉)]

[1] Kitware Inc., Carrboro, NC 27510, USA
andinet.enqu@kitware.com
[2] SUNY at Buffalo, Buffalo, NY 14260, USA

Abstract. Advances in deep learning techniques have led to compelling achievements in medical image analysis. However, performance of neural network models degrades drastically if the test data is from a domain different from training data. In this paper, we present and evaluate a novel unsupervised domain adaptation (DA) framework for semantic segmentation which uses self ensembling and adversarial training methods to effectively tackle domain shift between MR images. We evaluate our method on two publicly available MRI dataset to address two different types of domain shifts: On the BraTS dataset [11] to mitigate domain shift between high grade and low grade gliomas and on the SCGM dataset [13] to tackle cross institutional domain shift. Through extensive evaluation, we show that our method achieves favorable results on both datasets.

1 Introduction

Existence of domain shift between related datasets pose a serious challenge for CNN based tasks like segmentation which require a large amount of annotated data for training. Unlike in the natural images, the problem of domain shift is ubiquitous in biomedical image analysis as images acquired by various institutions belong to different domains due to difference in image acquisition parameters used for capturing data. In addition, tumors and cancers of different grades and severity may belong to different distributions, limiting the ability of single segmentation model in labeling cancerous tumors of varying severity and growth (Fig. 1). To tackle this issue, unsupervised domain adaptation has been extensively studied to enable CNN to achieve competitive performance in a domain different than the training domain [19].

In this paper, we study intramodality domain adaptation where both source and target domains belong to same modality, but have different distributions due to difference in image acquisition parameters or tumor severity. Intramodality domain shift is often neglected in biomedical image analysis as most of the deep learning based networks are trained and tested on a mixture of data collected from different institutions and devices, disregarding the associated domain shift.

© Springer Nature Switzerland AG 2019
Q. Wang et al. (Eds.): DART 2019/MIL3ID 2019, LNCS 11795, pp. 28–36, 2019.
https://doi.org/10.1007/978-3-030-33391-1_4

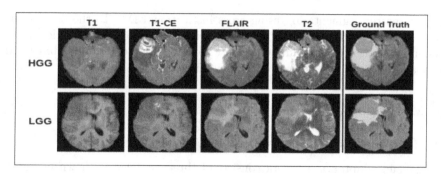

Fig. 1. Tumor size variability in BraTS dataset. Top row: Axial slices of high grade (HGG) tumors, bottom row: low grade (LGG) tumors. In Ground Truth (GT), union of all colors = whole tumor, green = enhanced tumor and blue = core tumor. HGG and LGG have different size and distributions for tumor regions. (Color figure online)

This often results in unpredictable performance if test set is from a data source different than training.

Numerous unsupervised domain adaptation methods have been proposed in the literature, with a growing emphasis on learning domain invariant representation to implicitly learn the feature mapping between domains [19]. These methods can be broadly classified as divergence minimising methods [3,10,17] which propose to minimise the distribution statistics between domains and adversarial methods [5,16,20] which use discriminators for aligning feature spaces. In contrast, French et al. [4] employed self-ensembling for domain adaptation and achieved state-of-the-art results on VisDA-2017 domain adaptation challenge. This technique is based on the Mean-Teacher Network [18] introduced for semi-supervised learning and requires extensive task-specific data augmentation. Additionally, pixel space translation [2] and modulating batchnorm statistics [9] are also explored in detail for domain adaptation and achieved promising results [19].

In biomedical imaging, Kamnitsas et al's [7] work on brain lesion MRI domain adaptation using adversarial training demonstrated the effectiveness of adversarial loss for unsupervised domain adaptation on medical datasets. The latest study on medical data that is closely related to our work is [12], which performed unsupervised domain adaptation using self ensembling techniques for spinal cord grey matter segmentation and achieved promising results.

Current research trends in domain adaptation are directed towards combining multiple techniques to achieve superior performance in various computer vision tasks [6,15]. Following this direction, we propose a combined network which uses domain invariant feature training with self ensembling technique for MRI domain adaptation in the context of semantic segmentation. We demonstrate the performance of our method on two publicly available MRI datasets: (1) On BraTS [1,11] dataset for multiclass tumor segmentation using high grade to low grade glioma domain adaptation, (2) On SCGM [13] Segmentation dataset for grey matter segmentation using cross institutional DA. To the best of our knowledge, our work here is the first to perform high grade to low grade glioma domain adaptation and the first one to use a combination of self-ensembling and adversarial training for medical image domain adaptation.

2   Methodology

2.1   Overview of the Proposed Model

Our domain adaptation network consists of three modules as shown in Fig. 2: A student segmentation network G, a teacher segmentation network $\overline{G}$ and a discriminator D. First, we forward source images with labels through segmentation network G and update its weights. Then we pass unlabeled target images through G and obtain its pre-softmax layer predictions. Predictions from both the domains are passed through discriminator D to distinguish whether the input belongs to source or target domain. Adversarial loss from D is then back-propagated through G to update network weights to learn domain invariant feature representation. Teacher network $\overline{G}$ weights are then updated as the exponential moving average (EMA) of student network (G) weights. Finally, we compute consistency loss between student and teacher networks predictions for target images and back-propagate through student network (G). Figure 2 illustrates the proposed algorithm.

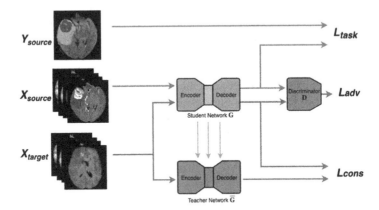

Fig. 2. Our proposed architecture. Green arrows correspond to source data and red arrows correspond to target data. Teacher Network weights are updated via EMA.

2.2   Adversarial Training

The objective behind adversarial training is to adapt the segmentation network invariant to variations between source and target. This is achieved by using a fully convolutional discriminator network (D) to distinguish the domain of input data. D is trained with a cross entropy loss using source and target domain predictions. For target images predictions, we compute an adversarial loss($\mathcal{L}_{adv}$) and back-propagate it to segmentation network (G) to fool the discriminator by pushing the feature representation to a domain invariant space.

2.3   Self Ensembling and Mean Teacher

We combine adversarial training with self ensembling using Mean-Teacher in our network. Although initial self ensembling papers [8, 18] were specifically designed for semi-supervised learning, French et al. extended mean-teacher algorithm for UDA in his seminal paper [4]. Their proposed architecture consists of a student network and a teacher network where the student network is trained with back-propagation while the teacher network weights are an exponential moving average of student network weights. We use self ensembling as a regularizer to smoothen the weights of our feature space domain adaptation network. Student network weights are updated by task loss and adversarial loss which is then exponentially averaged over time to update teacher network weights. We finally use teacher network for making predictions. For our mean teacher self ensembling model, we use the same architecture proposed by [4].

Perone et al. [12] has adapted and implemented this network for domain adaptation for medical imaging segmentation and achieved favorable results. A key difference between their work and ours is that their model uses only self ensembling for domain adaptation while we combine it with adversarial training as a regularizer for feature-space domain adaptation.

2.4   Objective Function

With the proposed network, we formulate the final loss function for domain adaptation as follows:

$$\mathcal{L} = \mathcal{L}_{task}(I_s) + \lambda_{adv}\mathcal{L}_{adv}(I_t) + \lambda_{cons}\mathcal{L}_{cons}(I_t) \tag{1}$$

where I_s, and I_t are inputs from source and target domains respectively. $\mathcal{L}_{task}(I_s)$ is the segmentation task loss computed on the paired input data. We use dice loss for segmentation which is commonly employed in biomedical image segmentation due to its low sensitivity to class imbalance. Adversarial loss $\mathcal{L}_{adv}(I_t)$ is computed as a cross entropy loss on target images to adversarially align feature representation of both domains. Consistency loss $\mathcal{L}_{cons}(I_t)$ measures the difference between predictions from teacher and student networks for distilling the knowledge on the student model for self ensembling. We use mean squared error (MSE) for $\mathcal{L}_{cons}(I_t)$ as suggested by [12]. Additionally, discriminator network is trained using source and target feature representations using a standard cross-entropy discriminator loss ($\mathcal{L}_{disc}(I_s, I_t)$).

2.5 Model Architecture

Discriminator Network : For Discriminator, we use a fully convolutional neural network consisting of four convolutional layers with 4×4 kernels and stride of 2. Except for the last layer, each convolution layer is followed by a leaky ReLU parameterized by 0.2. Discriminator is trained with Adam as optimizer with default set of parameters and a polynomial decay function for learning rate.

Segmentation Network : We use UNet [14] as our segmentation network with 15 layers, batch normalization and dropout. Network is trained using Adam as optimizer with $\beta_1 = 0.9$ and $\beta_2 = 0.99$. Both student and teacher networks have identical UNet architecture and only student network weights are updated by back-propagation. Performance of the model is validated using teacher network on validation data from both domains.

3 Datasets

We used two publicly available MRI datasets to evaluate our methodology. We performed HGG to LGG domain adaptation on BraTS dataset [1,11] and cross institutional domain adaptation on SCGM segmentation challenge dataset [13].

BraTS 2018 [1,11] dataset consists of 285 MRI samples (210 HGG and 75 LGG) each with T1, T1-contrast enhanced, T2-weighted and FLAIR volumes with ground truth voxel-wise labels for enhancing tumor, peritumoral edema and necrotic and non-enhancing tumor core. Both HGG and LGG volumes are splitted into train and test and we use train HGG as source and train LGG as target for domain adaptation experiments. Since we are using 2D-Unet for segmentation, we slice 3D voxels into 2D axial slices of 128×128 and concatenated all four MRI modalities to get a 4-channel input. More information about dataset can be found at [11].

Spinal Cord Gray Matter Challenge(SCGM) [13] dataset contains single channel Spinal Cord MRI data with grey matter labels from 4 different centers. Data is collected from four centers (UCL, Montreal, Zurich, Vanderbilt) using three different MRI systems (Philips Acheiva, Siemens Trio, Siemens Skyra) with institution specific acquisition parameters. From each center, 10 MRI volumes are publicly available which we center cropped 2D axial slices of 200×200 for our experiment. We use our network to perform cross institutional domain adaptation on this dataset with centers 3 and 1 as source and center 2 as target and validate the performance on all four centers.

4 Experiments and Results

In this section, we present experimental results to validate the proposed domain adaptation method for semantic segmentation on both datasets. First we evaluate model performance on SCGM dataset for cross institutional domain adaptation. Second, we carry out experiments for HGG to LGG domain adaptation on BraTS dataset. We also conduct extensive experiments and ablation studies on both dataset to substantiate the efficacy of our proposed architecture. For a fair comparison and analysis, all experiments are run for the same number of epochs with the same set of parameters for optimizers and learning rate decay. Model performance is evaluated using the dice coefficient. For each dataset we conduct the following experiments:

1. Training the segmenter network (with no DA) on combined source and target data and test separately on heldout sets (*super-all*).
2. Training the segmenter network (with no DA) on source data alone and test separately on source and target (*super-source*).
3. Domain adaptation using only adversarial training (*da-adv*).
4. Domain adaptation using only self ensembling (*da-ensemble*).
5. Proposed domain adaptation algorithm with both adversarial training and self-ensembling(*da-combined*).

4.1   Spinal Cord Cross Institutional Domain Adaptation

All networks for cross institutional DA are trained for 350 epochs with centers 3 and 1 as source and center 2 as target. Weights for adversarial and consistency losses($\lambda_{adv}, \lambda_{cons}$) are optimized separately using *da-adv* and *da-ensemble* models. We found $\lambda_{adv} = 0.001$ and $\lambda_{cons} = 2$ to have best performance on individual domain adaptation models and used them for the combined DA model as well.

Table 1. Dice score for cross institutional domain adaptation.

Experiment	Center1	Center2	Center3	Center4
super-all	87.5	87.9	87.8	87.96
super-source	87.48	77.11	87.19	85.25
da-adv	87.27	79.43	87.49	87.2
da-ensemble	87.7	84.76	**87.59**	87.33
da-combined	**87.93**	**85.75**	87.56	**87.43**

We present experimental results for cross-institutional domain adaptation in Table 1. Combined supervised model achieved similar dice scores on all heldout sets while source-only supervised model produced poor results for center 2. This substantiates the existence of intramodality domain shift among multi institutional MRI data and validates the importance of medical image domain adaptation. In contrast, all domain adaptation networks achieved improved results on center2, showing the effectiveness of DA techniques in mitigating domain shift. Our proposed model achieved highest dice score on 3 out of 4 centers and produced results on par with supervised training using combined data. Figure 3 presents some example results for adapted segmentation using combined model. Although domain adaptation models are adversarially trained against center2, model performance has improved for all centers. This suggests that DA with the proposed architecture can be used for domain generalisation as well.

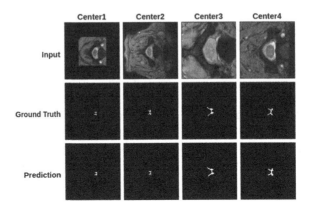

Fig. 3. Example results of adapted segmentation for SCGM Dataset. Model is trained using combined adversarial and self ensembling domain adaptation.

4.2 Brain Tumor Segmentation Using Domain Adaptation

We trained all experiments for 150 epochs with HGG as source and LGG as target. Networks are trained with 4-channel sliced 2D axial MRI images to perform 4-class segmentation (background, enhanced tumor, whole tumor and core tumor). Performance scores for all experiments with class wise dice scores are presented in Table 2. Supervised model results clearly show the domain shift between high grade and low grade gliomas in BraTS dataset. LGG heldout set produced inferior results when the network is trained only using HGG volumes. Our proposed domain adaptation method mitigated this domain shift to an extent and achieved noticeable improvement in segmenting whole and core tumor regions in LGG dataset.

Table 2. Dice scores for BraTS domain adaptation.

Experiment	HGG				LGG			
	Whole	Enh	Core	Overall	Whole	Enh	Core	Overall
super-all	85.51	67.84	67.13	78.47	85.23	38.22	55.14	64.34
super-source	85.66	66.84	66.59	77.34	79.29	33.09	44.11	58.44
da-adv	85.47	59.01	64.63	73.44	80.09	30.35	44.90	60.07
da-ensemble	85.90	66.84	66.59	77.61	82.97	**33.84**	46.87	60.97
da-combined	85.80	66.43	67.11	78.23	**84.11**	32.67	**47.11**	**62.17**

5   Conclusion

In this paper, we presented a novel approach to intra-modality domain adaptation using adversarial training and self ensembling. We evaluated our model on two publicly available MRI datasets to address cross institutional domain shift and tumor severity domain shift. The results showed improved segmentation performance on both datasets. Superior performance on two different datasets validates the generalisability of our proposed model which can be extended to other intra-modality DA applications for biomedical image segmentation. Future work includes extensive hyperparameter tuning for improved segmentation for unsupervised domain adaptation.

References

1. Bakas, S., et al.: Advancing the cancer genome atlas glioma MRI collections with expert segmentation labels and radiomic features. Sci. Data **4**, 170117 (2017)
2. Bousmalis, K., Silberman, N., Dohan, D., Erhan, D., Krishnan, D.: Unsupervised pixel-level domain adaptation with generative adversarial networks. In: IEEE Conference on Computer Vision and Pattern Recognition (CVPR), pp. 95–104 (2017)
3. Eric, T., Judy Hoffman, N.Z., Darrell., T.: Deep domain confusion: maximizing for domain invariance. arXiv preprint arXiv:1412.3474 (2014)
4. French, G., Mackiewicz, M., Fisher, M.H.: Self-ensembling for domain adaptation. CoRR abs/1706.05208 (2017)
5. Ganin, Y., Lempitsky, V.: Unsupervised domain adaptation by backpropagation. In: ICML (2016)
6. Hoffman, J., et al.: Cycada: cycle-consistent adversarial domain adaptation. CoRR abs/1711.03213 (2017)
7. Kamnitsas, K., et al.: Unsupervised domain adaptation in brain lesion segmentation with adversarial networks. CoRR abs/1612.08894 (2016). http://arxiv.org/abs/1612.08894
8. Laine, S., Aila, T.: Temporal ensembling for semi-supervised learning. CoRR abs/1610.02242 (2016). http://arxiv.org/abs/1610.02242
9. Li, Y., Wang, N., Shi, J., Liu, J., Hou, X.: Revisiting batch normalization for practical domain adaptation. CoRR abs/1603.04779 (2016)
10. Long, M., Cao, Y., Wang, J., Jordan, M.I.: Learning transferable features with deep adaptation networks. In: On ICML, ICML 2015, vol. 37, pp. 97–105 (2015)
11. Menze, B., et al.: The multimodal brain tumor image segmentation benchmark (brats). IEEE Trans. Med. Imaging **34**(10), 1993–2024 (2014)
12. Perone, C.S., Ballester, P., Barros, R.C., Cohen-Adad, J.: Unsupervised domain adaptation for medical imaging segmentation with self-ensembling. CoRR abs/1811.06042 (2018). http://arxiv.org/abs/1811.06042
13. Prados, F., et al.: Spinal cord grey matter segmentation challenge. NeuroImage **152**, 312–329 (2017)
14. Ronneberger, O., Fischer, P., Brox, T.: U-Net: convolutional networks for biomedical image segmentation. In: Navab, N., Hornegger, J., Wells, W.M., Frangi, A.F. (eds.) MICCAI 2015. LNCS, vol. 9351, pp. 234–241. Springer, Cham (2015). https://doi.org/10.1007/978-3-319-24574-4_28
15. Saito, K., Watanabe, K., Ushiku, Y., Harada, T.: Maximum classifier discrepancy for unsupervised domain adaptation. arXiv preprint arXiv:1712.02560 (2017)

16. Sankaranarayanan, S., Balaji, Y., Castillo, C.D., Chellappa, R.: Generate to adapt: aligning domains using generative adversarial networks. CoRR 1704.01705 (2017)
17. Sun, B., Saenko, K.: Deep CORAL: correlation alignment for deep domain adaptation. CoRR abs/1607.01719 (2016). http://arxiv.org/abs/1607.01719
18. Tarvainen, A., Valpola, H.: Mean teachers are better role models: weight-averaged consistency targets improve semi-supervised deep learning results. In: Advances in Neural Information Processing Systems, vol. 30, pp. 1195–1204 (2017)
19. Wilson, G., Cook, D.J.: Adversarial transfer learning. arXiv, vol. 1812, p. 02849 (2018)
20. Ganin, Y., et al.: Domain-adversarial training of neural networks. J. Mach. Learn. Res. **17**(59), 1–35 (2016)

Learning Interpretable Disentangled Representations Using Adversarial VAEs

Mhd Hasan Sarhan[1,2](✉) ⓘ, Abouzar Eslami[2] ⓘ, Nassir Navab[1,3],
and Shadi Albarqouni[1] ⓘ

[1] Computer Aided Medical Procedures, Technical University of Munich,
Munich, Germany
`hasan.sarhan@tum.de`
[2] Carl Zeiss Meditec AG, Munich, Germany
[3] Computer Aided Medical Procedures, Johns Hopkins University, Baltimore, USA

Abstract. Learning Interpretable representation in medical applications is becoming essential for adopting data-driven models into clinical practice. It has been recently shown that learning a disentangled feature representation is important for a more compact and explainable representation of the data. In this paper, we introduce a novel adversarial variational autoencoder with a total correlation constraint to enforce independence on the latent representation while preserving the reconstruction fidelity. Our proposed method is validated on a publicly available dataset showing that the learned disentangled representation is not only interpretable, but also superior to the state-of-the-art methods. We report a relative improvement of 81.50% in terms of disentanglement, 11.60% in clustering, and 2% in supervised classification with a few amount of labeled data.

Keywords: Deep learning · Disentangled representation · Interpretability

1 Introduction

Data-driven models with the help of Deep Learning (DL) are affecting wide areas of scientific research and the medical domain is no exception in this matter. However, in healthcare, developing a machine learning algorithm with expert level performance is important but not enough for the adoption of the algorithm when the issues of trust and explainability are not taken into consideration [14]. Explainability of a model is approached either by (1) explicitly learning it by model design or (2) after model design such as using gradient-based localization [15].

Approaching explainability by model design could be facilitated in a supervised manner as in decision trees and rule-based systems or in an unsupervised manner as in Variational Autoencoder (VAE) [9] or β-Variational Autoencoder (β-VAE) [6]. In the latter, a lower dimensional representation of the data is learned and utilized for analyzing the data. The rest of the paper discusses this

© Springer Nature Switzerland AG 2019
Q. Wang et al. (Eds.): DART 2019/MIL3ID 2019, LNCS 11795, pp. 37–44, 2019.
https://doi.org/10.1007/978-3-030-33391-1_5

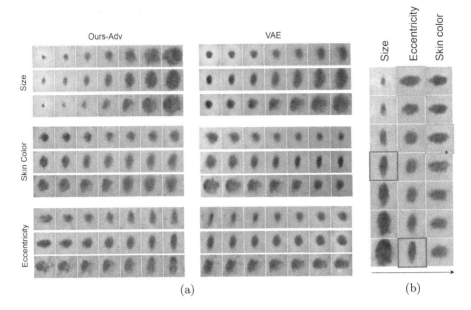

Fig. 1. Comparison of our model to VAE on examples for traversal over the representation components. Traversal is done between $[-3, 3]$ (a) Examples of traversal for three images form ISIC 2018. Each row shows reconstructions of latent traversals across one latent dimension; (b) Example of a smooth transition over the manifold by changing multiple latent dimensions to go from small lesion on pale skin (top left image) to bigger horizontal lesion on red skin (bottom right image). Each column represents one dimension of change. The colored squares represent the image of the previous column from which the traversal has started on the current dimension.

type of explainability. Deep learning models extract features from data in order to represent it in a compressed high-level representation that suits the application. The quality of this representation is crucial for the model performance and it is argued that disentangled representations would be helpful for having better control and interpretability over the data [1,6]. A disentangled representation can be defined as a representation where one latent unit represents one generative factor of variation in the data while being invariant to other generative factors [1]. For example, a model trained on a dataset of faces would learn disentangled latent units that represent independent ground truth generative factors such as hair color, pose, lighting or skin color. Disentangling as many explanatory factors as possible is important for a more compact, explainable, transferable, abstract representation of the data [1].

Most of the previous work regarding disentanglement relied on information about the number or nature of the ground truth generative factors [7,10]. In medical applications, the data is complex and a priori knowledge about the generative factors is mostly unavailable. Recently, multiple models for unsupervised disentangled feature learning were proposed [2,3,6,8]. β-VAE [6] is proposed as a modification on VAE [9] where the parameter β is used to introduce more emphasis on the KL-Divergence part of the VAE objective. This enforces the posterior to match the factorized Gaussian prior which constraints the bottleneck representation to be factorized while still reconstructing the data. Higher β values encourage more disentangled representations with a trade-off on the reconstruction error. In β-Total Correlation VAE (β-TCVAE) [2], the training is focused on the total correlation part of KL term which is responsible for the factorized representation. This lowers the trade-off on the reconstruction fidelity proposed by β-VAE. β-TCVAE is validated on examples from a controlled environment with clear factors of generation. This does not represent the complexity of medical data and should be addressed.

Contributions: In this work, we propose a framework for learning disentangled representations in medical imaging in an unsupervised manner. To our knowledge, this is the first work that analyzes the strength of unsupervised disentangled feature representations in medical imaging and proposes a framework that is well suited to medical applications. We propose a novel residual adversarial VAE with total correlation constraint. This enhances the fidelity of the reconstruction and captures more details that describe better the underlying generative factors.

2   Methodology

We utilize deep generative disentangled representation learning to learn the distribution of a medical imaging dataset. We then use the learned representation to generate images while controlling some generative factors. We first show how disentanglement is approached with β-VAE as a motivation for incorporating β-TCVAE. We then present our contributions to the disentanglement framework by utilizing adversarial loss with residual blocks to enhance the disentanglement and reduce the compromise on the reconstruction. We hypothesize that using adversarial loss with residual blocks in a disentanglement framework would result in higher quality representations with more disentanglement in the feature space.

Background: Let $x_n \in \mathcal{X}, n = 1, ..., N$ be a set of images generated by combinations of K ground-truth generative factors $V = (v_1, ..., v_K)$. Our aim is to build an unsupervised generative model that utilizes only the images in $\mathcal{X}$ to learn the joint distribution of the images and the set of latent generative factors $z \sim q_\phi(z|x) \in \mathbb{R}^d$ allowing us to have better control and interpretability of the latent space. It is worth mentioning the latent generative factors capture both disentangled and entangled factors. To realize our aim, we follow the concept of β-VAE in learning a posterior distribution that could be used to generate images from $\mathcal{X}$. The posterior representation is approximated by $q_\phi(z|x)$. The model is built such that the generative factors V are represented by the posterior bottleneck in a disentangled fashion.

In β-VAE, implicit independence is enforced on the posterior to encourage a disentangled representation. This is done by constraining the posterior to match a prior $q(z)$. The prior is set to be an isotropic unit Gaussian $(p(z) = \mathcal{N}(0, I))$. Adding extra pressure on the posterior to match $p(z)$ constraints the capacity of the bottleneck and pushes it to be factorized [6]. Thus, the objective function for β-VAE is as follows

$$arg \min_{\phi, \theta} \Big[\underbrace{-\mathbb{E}_{q_\phi(z|x)}[logp_\theta(x|z)] + \beta D_{KL}(q_\phi(z|x)||p(z))}_{\text{reconstruction loss } \mathcal{L}_{rec}} \Big] \qquad (1)$$

where θ and ϕ are trainable weights of encoder and decoder respectively, D_{KL} is the Kullback-Leibler divergence. For enforcing disentanglement, values of $\beta > 1$ are typically chosen. Using this formula enhances the disentanglement at the cost of reconstruction fidelity. It is suggested by [2] that the total correlation term within D_{KL} is responsible for the factorized disentangled representation. Hence, focusing the training on the total correlation would result in better disentanglement while having less effect on the reconstruction. The objective function changes such as D_{KL} is decomposed and β is multiplied by the total correlation term as follows

$$arg \min_{\phi, \theta} \Big[- \mathbb{E}_{q_\phi(z|x)}[logp_\theta(x|z)] +$$
$$\underbrace{I_q(z, x) + \beta D_{KL}\big(q_\phi(z) || \prod_j q_\phi(z_j)\big) + \sum_j D_{KL}\big(q_\phi(z_j)||p(z_j)\big)}_{D_{KL}(q_\phi(z|x)||p(z)) \text{ decomposition } (\mathcal{L}_{prior})} \Big] \qquad (2)$$

The term $D_{KL}(q(z)|| \prod_j q(z_j))$ is the total correlation (TC) which is a generalization of mutual information to more than two variables. Penalizing TC forces independence in the represented factors. We use β-TCVAE for its good results on disentanglement on various datasets while having better reconstruction that other disentanglement models and for the parameter-less approximation of $q(z)$. For more details about the D_{KL} decomposition and the approximation of $q(z)$ the reader is referred to [2].

Proposed Approach: To enhance the fidelity of the reconstructions and improve the generative factors captured by z, we propose using a discriminator network with β-TCVAE disentanglement model. The discriminator is trained to decide whether an input image is generated synthetically or sampled from the real data distribution. We employ adversarial loss scheme for the training. The discriminator in this scenario has to learn implicitly a rich similarity metric based on features extracted from the images rather than relying only on pixel-wise similarity. This does not only improve generated images visually, but also learns a richer representation in the code z [11]. This is because the pixel-wise loss acts as a *content* loss while the discriminator loss acts as a *style* loss [4]. Moreover, we incorporate residual blocks rather than convolutional layers applied in [2]. This is because residual blocks have shown a better flow of the gradients. This limits the problems related to vanishing/exploding gradients [5] and is being used in state-of-the-art Generative Adversarial Nets (GANs) literature [17] for more stable training. We denote $Dis(.;\psi)$ to the discriminator network described by trainable parameters ψ, x is a real image sampled from $p(x)$ and $\hat{x}$ is the reconstructed image from $p_\theta(x|z)$. The final objective is

$$\arg\min_{\phi,\theta}[\mathcal{L}_{gen}] = \arg\min_{\phi,\theta}[\mathcal{L}_{rec} + \mathcal{L}_{prior} - log(Dis(\hat{x}))]$$
$$\arg\min_{\psi}[\mathcal{L}_{disc}] = \arg\min_{\psi}[-log(Dis(x)) - log(1 - Dis(\hat{x}))] \qquad (3)$$

The model is trained by alternating between $\mathcal{L}_{gen}$ and $\mathcal{L}_{disc}$ optimization. We use pixel-wise l_2-distance between x and $\hat{x}$ as $\mathcal{L}_{rec}$.

3 Experiments

Experimental validation evaluates the proposed framework in two main experiments: First, we compare our proposed method disentanglement performance to state-of-the-art methods in learning both entangled and disentangled representations. We also utilize the learned representations in two use-cases, namely, unsupervised clustering and supervised classification with a few amounts of labels. In the second experiment, we evaluate the results visually and analyze the interpretable learned representation.

Dataset: We opt for the publicly available Skin Lesion dataset from ISIC 2018 Challenge [16] to perform our validations. To train our model, we utilize the dataset of Task 3 which consists of $10k$ RGB images with 7 types of skin lesions capturing 7 pathological generative factors. To evaluate the model against ground-truth generative factors, i.e. *eccentricity, orientation, and size*, we utilize the dataset of Task 2 which consists of $2k$ images with pixel-wise segmentation. Note that all images are down-sampled to $64 \times 64px$.

Evaluation Metrics: To quantitatively evaluate the disentanglement quality, we report the Mutual Information Gap (MIG) metric as proposed and suggested in [2]. As opposed to the disentanglement metric in [6], MIG takes axis-alignment (one v_k is captured by one z_j) into consideration, and it is unbiased to hyper-parameters opposite to [6,8]. MIG measures the mutual information (MI) between z_j and the known generative factor v_k, then the difference between the two highest MIs of a generative factor is calculated, and normalized then by the entropy of v_k. The average MIG is then reported as the final MIG score. The generative factors are set as follows:

1. **MIG Pathologies** (MIG_p): The ground truth classes are used as generative factors in one vs. all fashion. For instance, $K = 7$ for the Skin Lesion dataset. Each generative factor has two possible values in this scenario.
2. **MIG Handcrafted Factors** (MIG_{hf}): In addition, we handcrafted a few generative factors which are easily visible in the image space, e.g. geometric and morphological changes. To do so, the segmentation masks given in Task 2 are utilized. The handcrafted factors are *eccentricity, orientation, and size* (i.e $K = 3$). Each generative factor has two possible values.

In addition, we report the Peak signal-to-noise ratio (PSNR), Normalized Mutual Information (NMI), and Accuracy (ACC) to evaluate the reconstruction error, clustering, and classification, respectively.

Baselines: We compare the proposed model to two representation learning models. The first is VAE [9] model which does not take disentanglement into account explicitly. The second model is β-TCVAE [2] which adds constraints on the representation to disentangle the components. Further, We employ two variations of our proposed method with bottleneck residual blocks [5]; (1) without the adversarial loss in Eq. 3 denoted as *Ours-resnet*; and (2) with the adversarial loss denoted as *Ours-adv*.

Implementation Details: We implement the same architecture appeared in the CelebA experiments in [2] for both VAE and β-TCVAE. For our proposed method, we replace the convolutional layers with bottleneck residual blocks for both *Ours-resnet* and *Ours-adv*, while the additional discriminator network in *Ours-adv* has the same architecture of the encoder except for the last layer which has a single output. All models are trained using Adam optimizer for $100K$ iterations with a minibatch size of 256, and a learning rate of $1e-4$. β and d are set to 6 and 32, respectively. Note that we employ leakyReLU in our *Ours-adv* which has been successfully applied in the adversarial training literature.

Comparison with State-of-the-Art: We compare our method with the recent state-of-the-art methods by reporting the evaluation metrics (*cf.* Table 1). We notice improvements over the β-TCVAE in terms of disentanglement with a relative improvement of 81.6% and 161.8% on MIG_p and MIG_{hf}, respectively. For reconstruction error, it is expected that VAE would be superior to other models because there is no extra focus on the prior constraining part of the loss function which allows reconstruction error to optimize better. However, we notice an improvement on PSNR compared to β-TCVAE model which compromises reconstruction error for disentanglement. This experiment shows that adding the bottleneck residual blocks together with adversarial training not only improves the disentanglement, but also improves the reconstruction quality.

Use-Cases: In order to show that the disentangled representation is rather capturing some meaningful generative factors, which might be relevant to the task at hand. We design two use-cases in both unsupervised and supervised paradigms. For the clustering use-case, we utilize the learned representations to fit a Gaussian Mixture Model (GMM) with 7 components and assign a label to each data point. NMI is then calculated between assigned labels and ground-truth labels. We report an average of 10 realizations. Regarding the classification use-case, we utilize the learned representations of a few amounts of labeled data to train a multi-layer perceptron (MLP) on 10% of the data and evaluate it on the remaining 90% of the data. 10-fold stratified cross-validation is performed.

The model gives a relative improvement of 11.6% and 2% on the NMI and ACC, respectively. This could be attributed to the quality of the learned representation where features responsible for the pathologies are captured by disentanglement models as generative factors.

Table 1. Comparison of various representation learning models.

	$MIG_p\%$	$MIG_{hf}\%$	PSNR	NMI%	ACC%
VAE	5.23	2.74	**22.91**	9.12	67.88
β-TCVAE	6.92	3.53	20.79	10.66	68.61
Ours-resnet	11.61	5.89	19.42	9.89	69.19
Ours-Adv	**12.57**	**9.24**	21.18	**11.86**	**70.02**

Interpretability: We qualitatively examine the interpretability of the learned representations by manipulating the latent code. For instance, Fig. 1a shows a comparison of the traversal between the proposed model and VAE. We notice that the dimension responsible for changing skin color has some entanglement with eccentricity and size in the case of VAE. In contrast, we can see in our proposed model that the size and eccentricity are barely changed when the skin color dimension is changed. For eccentricity, we notice in the case of VAE that fewer variations are captured such as the absence of the horizontal elliptic lesions that are captured with the proposed approach.

In Fig. 1b, we show the possibility of generating images with specific features by smoothly moving over the manifold of the representations. We show the transition of a small lesion on pale skin to a big horizontal lesion on reddish skin by changing multiple latent dimensions responsible for each feature. Having this control over the representation does not only give the ability to generate images with specific known features, but also gives an interpretable representation of the data which can be utilized in many applications.

4 Discussion

In this paper, we introduce a novel adversarial VAE with a total correlation constraint to enforce disentanglement on the latent representation while preserving the reconstruction fidelity. The proposed framework is evaluated on skin lesions dataset and shows improvements over other state-of-the-art methods in terms of disentanglement. The learned representations have shown remarkable performance in both unsupervised clustering and supervised classification. One interesting direction to investigate is the usage of few labels to enhance the disentanglement and allow for better strategies for model selection as suggested in [12,13].

References

1. Bengio, Y., Courville, A., Vincent, P.: Representation learning: a review and new perspectives. IEEE Trans. Pattern Anal. Mach. Intell. **35**(8), 1798–1828 (2013)
2. Chen, T.Q., Li, X., Grosse, R.B., Duvenaud, D.K.: Isolating sources of disentanglement in variational autoencoders. In: Advances in Neural Information Processing Systems, pp. 2615–2625 (2018)
3. Chen, X., Duan, Y., Houthooft, R., Schulman, J., Sutskever, I., Abbeel, P.: Info-GAN: Interpretable representation learning by information maximizing generative adversarial nets. In: Advances in Neural Information Processing Systems, pp. 2172–2180 (2016)
4. Gatys, L.A., Ecker, A.S., Bethge, M.: A neural algorithm of artistic style. arXiv preprint arXiv:1508.06576 (2015)
5. He, K., Zhang, X., Ren, S., Sun, J.: Identity mappings in deep residual networks. In: Leibe, B., Matas, J., Sebe, N., Welling, M. (eds.) ECCV 2016. LNCS, vol. 9908, pp. 630–645. Springer, Cham (2016). https://doi.org/10.1007/978-3-319-46493-0_38
6. Higgins, I., et al.: beta-VAE: Learning basic visual concepts with a constrained variational framework. In: International Conference on Learning Representations (2017)
7. Hinton, G.E., Krizhevsky, A., Wang, S.D.: Transforming auto-encoders. In: Honkela, T., Duch, W., Girolami, M., Kaski, S. (eds.) ICANN 2011. LNCS, vol. 6791, pp. 44–51. Springer, Heidelberg (2011). https://doi.org/10.1007/978-3-642-21735-7_6
8. Kim, H., Mnih, A.: Disentangling by factorising. arXiv preprint arXiv:1802.05983 (2018)
9. Kingma, D.P., Welling, M.: Auto-encoding variational Bayes. arXiv preprint arXiv:1312.6114 (2013)
10. Kulkarni, T.D., Whitney, W.F., Kohli, P., Tenenbaum, J.: Deep convolutional inverse graphics network. In: Advances in Neural Information Processing Systems, pp. 2539–2547 (2015)
11. Larsen, A.B.L., Sønderby, S.K., Larochelle, H., Winther, O.: Autoencoding beyond pixels using a learned similarity metric. arXiv preprint arXiv:1512.09300 (2015)
12. Locatello, F., Bauer, S., Lucic, M., Gelly, S., Schölkopf, B., Bachem, O.: Challenging common assumptions in the unsupervised learning of disentangled representations. arXiv preprint arXiv:1811.12359 (2018)
13. Locatello, F., Tschannen, M., Bauer, S., Rätsch, G., Schölkopf, B., Bachem, O.: Disentangling factors of variation using few labels. arXiv preprint arXiv:1905.01258 (2019)
14. Miotto, R., Wang, F., Wang, S., Jiang, X., Dudley, J.T.: Deep learning for healthcare: review, opportunities and challenges. Briefings Bioinform. **19**(6), 1236–1246 (2017)
15. Selvaraju, R.R., Cogswell, M., Das, A., Vedantam, R., Parikh, D., Batra, D.: Grad-CAM: Visual explanations from deep networks via gradient-based localization. In: Proceedings of the IEEE International Conference on Computer Vision, pp. 618–626 (2017)
16. Tschandl, P., Rosendahl, C., Kittler, H.: The HAM10000 dataset, a large collection of multi-source dermatoscopic images of common pigmented skin lesions. Sci. Data **5**, 180161 (2018)
17. Zhang, H., Goodfellow, I., Metaxas, D., Odena, A.: Self-attention generative adversarial networks. arXiv preprint arXiv:1805.08318 (2018)

Synthesising Images and Labels Between MR Sequence Types with CycleGAN

Eric Kerfoot[1(✉)], Esther Puyol-Antón[1], Bram Ruijsink[1,2], Rina Ariga[3], Ernesto Zacur[3], Pablo Lamata[1], and Julia Schnabel[1]

[1] School of Biomedical Engineering and Imaging Sciences,
King's College London, London, UK
`eric.kerfoot@kcl.ac.uk`
[2] St Thomas' Hospital NHS Foundation Trust, London, UK
[3] University of Oxford, Oxford, UK

Abstract. Real-time (RT) sequences for cardiac magnetic resonance imaging (CMR) have recently been proposed as alternatives to standard cine CMR sequences for subjects unable to hold the breath or suffering from arrhythmia. RT image acquisitions during free breathing produce comparatively poor quality images, a trade-off necessary to achieve the high temporal resolution needed for RT imaging and hence are less suitable in the clinical assessment of cardiac function. We demonstrate the application of a CycleGAN architecture to train autoencoder networks for synthesising cine-like images from RT images and vice versa. Applying this conversion to real-time data produces clearer images with sharper distinctions between myocardial and surrounding tissues, giving clinicians a more precise means of visually inspecting subjects. Furthermore, applying the transformation to segmented cine data to produce pseudo-real-time images allows this label information to be transferred to the real-time image domain. We demonstrate the feasibility of this approach by training a U-net based architecture using these pseudo-real-time images which can effectively segment actual real-time images.

Keywords: Cardiac MR · Cardiac quantification · Convolutional neural networks · Generative adversarial networks · Image synthesis

1 Introduction

Free breathing non-gated real-time cine (RT) is a cardiac magnetic resonance imaging (cMRI) protocol proposed as a solution to restrictions present in the standard short axis cine protocol [12,13]. The latter protocol reconstructs images from multiple cardiac cycles and thus relies on electrocardiogram (ECG) gating, consistent cardiac cycle periods, and breath holds during acquisition. For patients with arrhythmia or who cannot hold their breath, a characteristic often seen in patients with heart diseases, this protocol is not feasible for producing useful CMR images.

© Springer Nature Switzerland AG 2019
Q. Wang et al. (Eds.): DART 2019/MIL3ID 2019, LNCS 11795, pp. 45–53, 2019.
https://doi.org/10.1007/978-3-030-33391-1_6

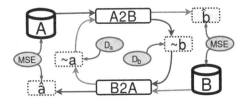

Fig. 1. The CycleGAN network setup. The path for real-time images is in red and that for cine MR images in green. Image data is shown as grey boxes and loss functions in blue. (Color figure online)

Real-time cine by contrast is neither ECG-gated nor breath-held, capturing cardiac motion over multiple cycles which is not directly reconstructed. The drawbacks to this protocol include through-plane motion during respiration impacting quantification of flow, the absence of ECG data informing where in the cardiac cycle each image is placed, and the poor quality of RT images in terms of feature resolution relative to standard acquisitions.

Previous work to address motion issues and identify cardiac cycle position [9,15] can be applied to mitigate these drawbacks, however this does not improve image quality directly. Real-time images suffer from a blurring effect due to fast acquisition, reconstructing a sharper version of these images with clearer delineation of cardiac tissues would potentially aid in visual assessment by clinicians.

In this paper we outline a method for converting between real-time images and short-axis images using a CycleGAN [22] based neural network architecture. We used trained autoencoders to enhance the quality of real-time images by converting them to a pseudo-cine image which present a better delineation between myocardial and surrounding tissues. Since we also can convert cine to pseudo-real-time images, we demonstrate the feasibility of converting segmented cine data to pseudo-real-time to use as training input. Consecutively we trained a U-net [14] based network to segment real-time images and compare its output against clinician labelled data, showing that our approach also allows transfer of training data to improve automation of analysis of this less common used technique lacking rich labelled datasets.

Related Work: Deep learning has recently shown great promise in synthesising medical images across different sequencing types within the same image modality based on conditional generative networks [8] and cycle generative adversarial networks [7,19,20,22]. Huo *et al.* [7] proposed an end-to-end synthetic segmentation network for abdominal images and for intracranial volume synthetic segmentation. A known problem with image synthesis is that of "hallucinating" data [2], where features commonly found in a target domain, but absent in the source image, are added to synthesised images. We address this problem in this work by using images representing roughly the same cardiac geometry and excluding cases having pathological geometric variation from the datasets, thus no image feature is expected to coincide with one image domain.

Several non-gated RT imaging techniques have been proposed to overcome the limitations with ECG-gated CMR [3,12,13,16]. Despite solving an important problem for patients with severe heart disease (who often have arrhythmia and problems holding breath) feature definition and image quality remains inferior to standard imaging, even using advanced acceleration techniques.

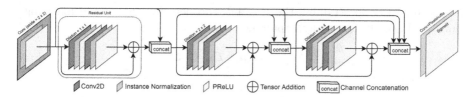

Fig. 2. Autoencoder network topology. Input tensors are first downsamples to half the original dimensions using a strided convolution (yellow). Each subsequent residual block (first one marked with dotted box) is composed of convolution layers with strides of 1 and dilation factors given above. All convolutions are 2D with 3×3 kernels. (Color figure online)

2   Method

To train our image synthesis autoencoders we employed a CycleGAN approach outlined in Fig. 1. Given two image distributions A and B (in our case real-time and cine images respectively), we train one autoencoder $A2B$ to convert an image from distribution A to appear like one from distribution B (labelled $\sim b$), and another autoencoder $B2A$ to perform the opposite translation ($\sim a$). Discriminator networks D_A and D_B are used to discriminate between real and synthetic images from each distribution.

These are then passed through the other network to produce reconstructed images $\hat{a}$ and $\hat{b}$ which are then compared against the original images using mean squared error. The discriminator networks are trained subsequently using the generated batches $\sim a$ and $\sim b$, plus images from A and B, as input.

The input data consists of ~20000 real-time CMRI images [15] acquired on a 1.5T Philips Ingenia MR scanner (Philips, Best, Netherlands) from 10 healthy participants as dataset A, plus ~5000 short-axis cine images acquired from the same participants as dataset B. Having an unbalanced ratio between the size of A and B was found to produce poor results during training, and so ~15000 cine images from the ACDC challenge dataset [1] were added to B. The selected ACDC images were acquired from Siemens 1.5T and 3T scanners (Siemens Medical Solutions, Germany) and include healthy subjects as well as those with myocardial infarction.

Binary cross entropy is used as the loss function to discriminate between real and synthetic images, given that 1 labels real images and 0 synthetic:

$$\mathcal{L}_{D_A} = \mathbb{E}_{a \sim A}[log(D_A(a))] + \mathbb{E}_{b \sim B}[log(1 - D_A(B2A(b)))]$$

$$\mathcal{L}_{D_B} = \mathbb{E}_{b \sim B}[log(D_B(b))] + \mathbb{E}_{a \sim A}[log(1 - D_B(A2B(a)))]$$

Mean squared error is used as the loss between real and synthetic images:

$$\mathcal{L}_A = \mathbb{E}_{a \sim A}[\|B2A(A2B(a)) - a\|_2], \quad \mathcal{L}_B = \mathbb{E}_{b \sim B}[\|A2B(B2A(b)) - b\|_2]$$

The final loss for training the two autoencoders together is the following, using a value of 10 for the hyperparameter λ:

$$\mathcal{L} = \lambda\mathcal{L}_A + \lambda\mathcal{L}_B + \mathcal{L}_{D_A} + \mathcal{L}_{D_B}$$

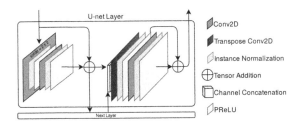

Fig. 3. The U-net segmentation network is built as a stack of these layers. The "Next Layer" is either another such layer or the bottom layer consisting of only a convolution/instance-norm/PReLU sequence. In this way each layer represents both the encoding and decoding pathway where input data flows through the left-hand residual block, through next layer, up through the right-hand residual block which also upsamples and concatenates, and then the layer above.

Figure 2 illustrates the architecture of the two autoencoders. As a memory efficiency measure the input image is downsampled by a factor of 2 using a convolution with a stride of 2 in both dimensions, followed by instance normalisation and PReLU [4] activation. The network then consists of three residual blocks [5] containing two sets of convolution-normalisation-activation layers. The final layer is a convolution with 1×1 kernels to adjust the number of channels to 4, followed by a pixel shuffle layer [17] to output an image with the same dimensions as the original input, to which sigmoid activation is applied.

To increase the perceptive field of the residual blocks, the convolutions of the second and third block are dilated by factors of 2 and 4. Input to each block is the concatenated image volume of the outputs from the original set of convolutions plus the outputs of previous blocks. This implements a dense block similar to [6] which permits data from convolutions with smaller dilations to be passed directly to those with larger dilations.

It was found in this experiment that dilated convolutions are an effective alternative to downsampling as a means of expanding the perceptive area of convolutions. The more common autoencoder architecture involves multiple downsampling layers (the encode step) following by upsampling layers (the decode step). Using dilated kernels it was possible to define an alternative autoencoder model which operated on near-full resolution data but was still feasible to train and produced good quality output. Another factor contributing to good results was the dense block architecture which allowed information from convolutions with smaller perceptive fields to be passed directly to those with larger, thus feeding information about smaller scale features down the encoder pipeline to be integrated with information about larger scale features.

3   Segmentation

Using synthetic data we have trained a segmentation network based on the residual U-net [14, 21] architecture to label the left ventricle. Our U-net architecture (Fig. 3) is defined as a stack of downstream/upstream layers, and uses residual blocks throughout the encoding and decoding path. Our network consists of four such blocks with encoding paths producing output volumes with 16, 32, 64, and 128 channels respectively. Strided convolutions and strided transpose convolutions are used to downsample and upsample data, which are followed by instance normalisation and PReLU layers.

Input data was acquired from multiple datasets of cine images defined with three label segmentations (left-ventricle chamber, left ventricle myocardium, right ventricle chamber). These datasets are the ACDC challenge dataset [1] of 100 cases, 175 healthy cases from the UK Biobank segmented by a clinician, 116 cases captured on Siemens Trio 3T scanners (Siemens Medical Solutions, Germany), and 215 cases captured on 1.5T Philips Ingenia scanners. The total number of images used for training is 9095. With the images converted to pseudo-real-time with unaltered segmentations, the network was trained to transfer the amalgamated label information from one form of MR to another.

During training, random batches of image/segmentation pairs are drawn from this training dataset and a random set of operations are applied to each. This follows [10] in its use of data augmentation [11,18] as so is not suitable to be trained with the generator networks as in [7]. These augmentations include simple array transforms (flip, rotate, transpose, etc.) but more importantly also include randomised free-form deformations. The previous work has shown that this combination of network architecture and training process results in robust and accurate segmentation networks.

4   Results

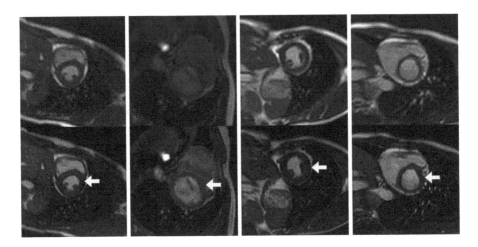

Fig. 4. Examples of image synthesis, arrows pointing to cardiac area of interest. For each image pair the original real-time image is above and the generated pseudo-cine image below.

Image Comparison. Figure 4 gives examples of the translation from real-time images to pseudo-cine images. The generated images exhibit greater contrast than the originals and the myocardium (specifically the left ventricle) is better defined with a more distinct boundary between myocardial tissue and pool or surrounding tissue. The peak signal-to-noise ratio between the generated images the ~20000 original images is -54.22 dB ($\sigma = 1.42$), and the structural similarity index between them is 0.77 ($\sigma = 0.08$).

Temporal information is not used in the transformation process so the relative motion between images is preserved in the pseudo-real-time images. This allows arrhythmia to be observed in the translated images as the cardiac cycle time is not affected. Typically arrhythmia excludes the use of cine MR thus our approach is an effective means of analysing such patients with high quality imagery.

Wall motion abnormalities are difficult to visualise in cine MR images as the wall position will vary from cycle to cycle, when multiple cycles are combined the resulting image is less distinct in this area. These abnormalities are thus more clearly identified with the sharper imaging produced by our method which does not reconstruct images based on the assumption of uniform geometry across cycles.

Segmentation Comparison. To assess the segmentation network, we use our set of manually-segmented real-time images as a ground truth comparison with generated segmentations. The manual segmentations were drawn by clinicians on images where they were confident the left ventricle was sufficiently distinct to define a reasonable boundary for the segmentation. This data is composed of binary segmentations of the LV myocardium only, thus our comparison study will use only these labels from the generated label set.

The segmentation network was applied to the 3194 expert-segmented real-time images in our dataset. Of these we were able to predict 2747 correct annular segmentations after extracting the largest element from each segmentation image. The mean dice score between these segmentations and the clinician-defined ground truth is 0.783 with a standard deviation of 0.083. Figure 5 illustrates examples of generated segmentations as compared to their ground truths.

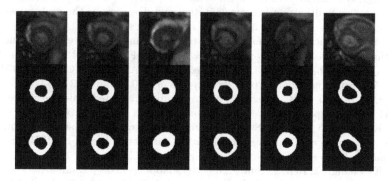

Fig. 5. Segmentation examples with original real-time image (top of each column), ground truth segmentation (middle), and predicted segmenation (bottom).

5   Conclusion

We have in this work defined a methodology for overcoming some of the deficiencies with real-time MR sequences by using a CycleGAN deep learning architecture to improve image quality. By training autoencoders to produce cine-like images from real-time images, we can produce a processed version of a real-time image sequence where the myocardial tissue is better differentiated from its surroundings and the ventricular cavities. This can serve as an aid to clinicians when assessing cardiac function by providing a sharper and more distinct image with improved contrast levels.

Using the second autoencoder to convert cine MR images to pseudo-real-time images allows a segmentation network to be trained using existing labelled cine data but which can be applied to real-time images. We have demonstrated the feasibility of this approach to reusing data between MR image types, which is especially important for real-time images as very little labelled data exists for the left ventricle and none for the right ventricle. In the future we intend to use this combined data to train networks capable of segmenting both ventricles despite current real-time datasets only having left ventricle labels.

Acknowledgements. This research was supported by the National Institute for Health Research (NIHR) Biomedical Research Centre (BRC) at Guy's and St Thomas' NHS Foundation Trust, and by the Wellcome EPSRC Centre for Medical Engineering at the School of Biomedical Engineering and Imaging Sciences, King's College London (WT 203148/Z/16/Z). This research has been conducted using the UK Biobank Resource under Application Number 17806.

References

1. Bernard, O., Lalande, A., Zotti, C., et al.: Deep learning techniques for automatic MRI cardiac multi-structures segmentation and diagnosis: is the problem solved? IEEE Trans. Med. Imaging **37**(11), 2514–2525 (2018)

2. Cohen, J.P., Luck, M., Honari, S.: Distribution matching losses can hallucinate features in medical image translation. In: Frangi, A.F., Schnabel, J.A., Davatzikos, C., Alberola-López, C., Fichtinger, G. (eds.) MICCAI 2018. LNCS, vol. 11070, pp. 529–536. Springer, Cham (2018). https://doi.org/10.1007/978-3-030-00928-1_60

3. Feng, L., Srichai, M.B., Lim, R.P., et al.: Highly accelerated real-time cardiac cine MRI using k-t sparse-sense. Magn. Reson. Med. **70**(1), 64–74 (2013)

4. He, K., Zhang, X., Ren, S., Sun, J.: Delving deep into rectifiers: surpassing human-level performance on imagenet classification. In: Proceedings of the IEEE International Conference on Computer Vision, pp. 1026–1034 (2015)

5. He, K., Zhang, X., Ren, S., Sun, J.: Identity mappings in deep residual networks. In: Leibe, B., Matas, J., Sebe, N., Welling, M. (eds.) ECCV 2016. LNCS, vol. 9908, pp. 630–645. Springer, Cham (2016). https://doi.org/10.1007/978-3-319-46493-0_38

6. Huang, G., Liu, Z., Weinberger, K.Q.: Densely connected convolutional networks. CoRR abs/1608.06993 (2016)

7. Huo, Y., Xu, Z., Moon, H., et al.: Synseg-net: synthetic segmentation without target modality ground truth. IEEE Trans. Med. Imaging **38**(4), 1016–1025 (2018)

8. Isola, P., Zhu, J.Y., Zhou, T., Efros, A.A.: Image-to-image translation with conditional adversarial networks. In: Proceedings of the IEEE Conference on Computer Vision and Pattern Recognition, pp. 1125–1134 (2017)

9. Kerfoot, E., Puyol Anton, E., Ruijsink, B., Clough, J., King, A.P., Schnabel, J.A.: Automated CNN-based reconstruction of short-axis cardiac MR sequence from real-time image data. In: Stoyanov, D., et al. (eds.) RAMBO/BIA/TIA -2018. LNCS, vol. 11040, pp. 32–41. Springer, Cham (2018). https://doi.org/10.1007/978-3-030-00946-5_4

10. Kerfoot, E., Clough, J., Oksuz, I., Lee, J., King, A.P., Schnabel, J.A.: Left-ventricle quantification using residual U-net. In: Pop, M., et al. (eds.) STACOM 2018. LNCS, vol. 11395, pp. 371–380. Springer, Cham (2019). https://doi.org/10.1007/978-3-030-12029-0_40

11. Krizhevsky, A., Sutskever, I., Hinton, G.E.: Imagenet classification with deep convolutional neural networks. In: Advances in Neural Information Processing Systems, pp. 1097–1105 (2012)

12. La Gerche, A., Claessen, G., Van de Bruaene, A., et al.: Cardiac MRI: a new gold standard for ventricular volume quantification during high-intensity exercise. Circ. Cardiovasc. imaging **6**(2), 329–38 (2013)

13. Lurz, P., Muthurangu, V., Schievano, S., et al.: Feasibility and reproducibility of biventricular volumetric assessment of cardiac function during exercise using real-time radial k-t SENSE magnetic resonance imaging. J. Magn. Reson. Imaging **29**(5), 1062–1070 (2009)

14. Ronneberger, O., Fischer, P., Brox, T.: U-Net: convolutional networks for biomedical image segmentation. In: Navab, N., Hornegger, J., Wells, W.M., Frangi, A.F. (eds.) MICCAI 2015. LNCS, vol. 9351, pp. 234–241. Springer, Cham (2015). https://doi.org/10.1007/978-3-319-24574-4_28

15. Ruijsink, B., et al.: Semi-automatic cardiac and respiratory gated MRI for cardiac assessment during exercise. In: Cardoso, M.J., et al. (eds.) CMMI/SWITCH/RAMBO -2017. LNCS, vol. 10555, pp. 86–95. Springer, Cham (2017). https://doi.org/10.1007/978-3-319-67564-0_9

16. Setser, R.M., Fischer, S.E., Lorenz, C.H.: Quantification of left ventricular function with magnetic resonance images acquired in real time. J. Magn. Reson. Imaging **12**(3), 430–438 (2000)

17. Shi, W., et al.: Real-time single image and video super-resolution using an efficient sub-pixel convolutional neural network. In: Proceedings of the IEEE Conference on Computer Vision and Pattern Recognition, pp. 1874–1883 (2016)

18. Simard, P.Y., Steinkraus, D., Platt, J.C., et al.: Best practices for convolutional neural networks applied to visual document analysis. In: ICDAR, vol. 3 (2003)

19. Welander, P., Karlsson, S., Eklund, A.: Generative adversarial networks for image-to-image translation on multi-contrast MR images-a comparison of cyclegan and unit. arXiv preprint arXiv:1806.07777 (2018)

20. Wolterink, J.M., Dinkla, A.M., Savenije, M.H.F., Seevinck, P.R., van den Berg, C.A.T., Išgum, I.: Deep MR to CT synthesis using unpaired data. In: Tsaftaris, S.A., Gooya, A., Frangi, A.F., Prince, J.L. (eds.) SASHIMI 2017. LNCS, vol. 10557, pp. 14–23. Springer, Cham (2017). https://doi.org/10.1007/978-3-319-68127-6_2

21. Zhang, Z., Liu, Q., Wang, Y.: Road extraction by deep residual u-net. IEEE Geosci. Remote Sens. Lett. **15**(5), 749–753 (2018)

22. Zhu, J.Y., Park, T., Isola, P., Efros, A.A.: Unpaired image-to-image translation using cycle-consistent adversarial networks. In: 2017 IEEE International Conference on Computer Vision (ICCV) (2017)

Multi-domain Adaptation in Brain MRI Through Paired Consistency and Adversarial Learning

Mauricio Orbes-Arteaga[1,2]($\boxtimes$), Thomas Varsavsky[1,3], Carole H. Sudre[1,3,4],
Zach Eaton-Rosen[1,3], Lewis J. Haddow[5], Lauge Sørensen[2,6,7],
Mads Nielsen[2,6,7], Akshay Pai[2,6,7], Sébastien Ourselin[1], Marc Modat[1],
Parashkev Nachev[4], and M. Jorge Cardoso[1]

[1] Biomedical Engineering and Imaging Sciences, King's College London, London, UK
henry.m.orbes_arteaga@kcl.ac.uk
[2] Biomediq A/S, Copenhagen, Denmark
[3] Department of Medical Physics and Biomedical Engineering, UCL, London, UK
[4] Institute of Neurology, University College London, London, UK
[5] Chelsea and Westminster Hospital NHS Foundation Trust, London, UK
[6] Cereriu A/S, Copenhagen, Denmark
[7] Department of Computer Science, University of Copenhagen,
Copenhagen, Denmark

Abstract. Supervised learning algorithms trained on medical images will often fail to generalize across changes in acquisition parameters. Recent work in domain adaptation addresses this challenge and successfully leverages labeled data in a source domain to perform well on an unlabeled target domain. Inspired by recent work in semi-supervised learning we introduce a novel method to adapt from one source domain to n target domains (as long as there is paired data covering all domains). Our multi-domain adaptation method utilises a consistency loss combined with adversarial learning. We provide results on white matter lesion hyperintensity segmentation from brain MRIs using the MICCAI 2017 challenge data as the source domain and two target domains. The proposed method significantly outperforms other domain adaptation baselines.

Keywords: Domain adaptation · Adversarial learning · Brain MR

1 Introduction

In medical imaging, fully automated tools using deep learning techniques are increasing in popularity for numerous clinical tasks, including image segmentation, image classification and instance counting [8]. Among these tools, deep

---

M. Orbes-Arteaga and T. Varsavsky—Equal contribution

Q. Wang et al. (Eds.): DART 2019/MIL3ID 2019, LNCS 11795, pp. 54–62, 2019.
https://doi.org/10.1007/978-3-030-33391-1_7

learning frameworks exhibit excellent performance (often described as 'superhu-man') when applied on images drawn from the same distribution (scanner type, parameters, patient pool etc.) as the one used in training the model. However, the performance may deteriorate drastically when the algorithm is applied in previously unseen domains. This performance gap is a critical barrier to the safe implementation and widespread adoption of these techniques in clinical practice.

The process of adapting a model from a 'source' domain to a target domain is called 'domain adaptation'. Successful methods have included:

1. Training with a small number of labeled examples from the target domain. While this solution is theoretically straightforward, its practical use is limited as it requires additional labelling on the target domain.
2. Embedding the imaging data in a latent space. This latent space is learnt so as to ignore domain-specific features (e.g. contrast), while retaining domain-invariant features (pathology). Adversarial approaches have been proposed to address this angle in the context of lesion segmentation [5]and heart structure segmentation between MR and CT [2]. In both cases, the adversarial training is used to make the latent space as uninformative as possible about the domain the images come from.
3. Semi-supervised methods use a model trained on a small number of labeled examples to provide pseudo-labels for unlabeled data, which is then trained on. The model-fitting and updating semi-supervised labels can be seen as a form of expectation maximisation and has been used in medical imaging [1].
4. Enforcing output robustness to input perturbation. Recent methods have exploited the property that the distribution of predictions should be invariant to small perturbations on the input data. This observation can be expressed as $p(y|x) \approx p(y|\tilde{x})$, where $\tilde{x}$ is an augmented/perturbed version of x. The enforcement of this property has the additional advantage of limiting the unwanted behaviour of drastic output change for minimal input perturbations, which can be seen as improving robustness. For instance Perone et al. [9] proposed a teacher-student framework ensuring consistency between the outputs when passing to the student an augmented version of the unlabeled input of the teacher, that is similarly augmented afterwards.

Methods 2 to 4 fall under the purview of 'Unsupervised Domain Adaptation' (UDA), as does the presented work. In general, UDA does not rely on labeled training examples from the desired target domain. This is especially desirable in medical imaging, where labelling is time-consuming and highly variable, and the 'domain' depends on scanner manufacturer, acquisition protocol and reconstruction strategy. The augmentations required to create the perturbed input data can either be generic (geometric or contrast operations) or application-specific. In the context of medical imaging, the latter includes physics-based image augmentation, synthetic bias field addition or registration-based approaches [14]. These methods lean on domain-specific knowledge to generate plausible transformations.

We propose a UDA pipeline applied to the segmentation of white matter hyperintensities (WMH) which introduces a paired consistency (PC) loss which guides the adaptation. The proposed (PC) method enforces the output consistency between the results obtained on two separate acquisitions per subject: an in-plane and a volumetric FLAIR sequence. We aim to (1) segment WMH lesions on completely unlabeled examples and (2) to make these predictions similar between the in-plane and volumetric cases. In other words, we regularize the fitting by explicitly promoting similarity in the labels generated by each FLAIR acquisition. This adaptation method was supplemented with an adversarial loss in order to prevent the model from getting stuck in bad local minima. After an overview of the proposed approach and its variants in Sect. 2, we present the experiments which show that our proposed method leverages the unlabeled data to produce more consistent lesion segmentations across all domains.

2   Methods

The proposed training strategy for domain adaptation occurs in two phases. In the first phase the network is trained only on labeled data until convergence. During the second phase of the training, the paired unlabeled data is presented in addition to the labeled data and a consistency term is added to the loss function. This consistency term is inspired from the loss proposed by Xie et al. [13] that aims at minimizing the Kullback-Leibler divergence $\mathcal{D}_{KL}$ between the output probability distribution y when conditioned on the unlabeled input x from the set U or its augmented countrapart $\hat{x}$ drawn from $q(\hat{x}|x)$.

$$\min_{\theta} \mathcal{L}_{PC} = \mathop{\mathbb{E}}_{x \in U} \mathop{\mathbb{E}}_{\hat{x} \sim q(\hat{x}|x)} [\mathcal{D}_{KL}(p_{\tilde{\theta}}(y|x)||p_{\theta}(y|\hat{x}))] \tag{1}$$

We adapt this method to the segmentation task by using the dice loss [7] instead of the KL divergence. In the following, we denote as y_l the labeled ground truth, $\hat{y}_l$ the prediction over labeled images, $\hat{y}_u$ the prediction over unlabeled input and $\hat{y}_{\hat{u}}$ the prediction over its augmented/paired counterpart. The losses used in our framework are thus expressed as follows:

$$\mathcal{L}_S = dice(\hat{y}_l, y), \quad \mathcal{L}_{PC} = dice(\hat{y}_u, \hat{y}_{\hat{u}}), \quad \mathcal{L}_{tot} = \mathcal{L}_S + \alpha \mathcal{L}_{PC} \tag{2}$$

We trained networks using $\mathcal{L}_{tot}$ as specified in (2) and denote them as PC. These networks $f_{\theta}(h|x)$ produce a feature representation h from which $\hat{y}$ is calculated.

Preventing Trivial Solutions: Early in our experiments, we encountered a specific degenerate solution: our network was able to produce one solution for source images (a good lesion mask) while producing a trivial result on the target domain (in this case, a mask of the foreground). This meant that there was good agreement between in-plane and volumetric FLAIRs because they simply segmented foreground—ignoring the lesions altogether. This means that the network was identifying the domain of the images and using this to inform its solution: undesirable behaviour. We introduced an additional adversarial term to avoid these 'solutions'. Inspired by the domain adversarial literature (methods 2 in Sect. 1) we propose an adversarial loss to minimize the amount of information about domain contained in h. We introduce a discriminator d_Ω which takes h as input and outputs a domain prediction $\hat{d}$. The adversarial loss, $\mathcal{L}_{adv}$ is given by the cross-entropy, $\mathcal{L}_{adv} = -\sum_{i=1}^{n} \mathcal{L}_{ce}^i(d_i, \hat{d}_i)$ where n is the number of domains, $\mathcal{L}_{ce}^i$ is the multi-class cross entropy loss, d is a one-hot encoded vector of the domain label and $\hat{d}$ is the model's domain prediction as in [11]. We use a gradient reversal layer as in [5] in order to minimize L_{tot} whilst maximizing L_{adv}. Figure 1 presents the diagram of the proposed method with the combination of different losses, where β controls the strength with which the model is adapting its features whereas α controls the weights the consistency effect.

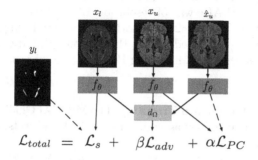

$$\mathcal{L}_{total} = \mathcal{L}_s + \beta\mathcal{L}_{adv} + \alpha\mathcal{L}_{PC}$$

Fig. 1. Diagram of proposed method. At training time, x_u, x_l and y_l are supplied to the network. x_u is an image from the unlabeled target domain and $\hat{x}_u$ is the result of applying some augmentation function to x_u. A labeled image, x_l, is passed through the network, f_θ before combining with a label y_l to form the segmentation loss, $\mathcal{L}_s$. The image representations are fed to a domain discriminator d_Ω which attempts to maximise the cross-entropy between predicted domain and actual domain, $\mathcal{L}_{adv}$. Finally, similarity is promoted between the network predictions on x_u and $\hat{x}_u$ using $\mathcal{L}_{PC}$.

Augmentation: In [13] the authors suggest various properties of augmented samples necessary for performing Unsupervised Data Augmentation. Samples should be realistic, valid (meaning they should not alter the underlying label), smooth, diverse and make use of targeted inductive biases (domain knowledge). In the absence of sufficiently realistic augmentation functions we use paired scans which are considered as augmented samples. However, taking them as they are makes for a discrete augmentation function with discontinuous jumps. In order to encourage continuity we used a large range of augmentations on the paired data, including generic geometric transformations and MR specific non-geometric transformations. Geometric augmentations were sampled independently and combined as one affine transform, using random rotations (all axis ranging from -10 to $10°$), random shears ($[0.5, 0.5]$) and random scaling ($[0.75, 1.5]$). For the non-geometric augmentations we applied k-space motion artefact augmentation as described in [12] and bias field augmentation as implemented in [3]. We measure how useful these additional augmentations are in our experiments.

3   Experiments and Results

Data: In this work we focus on white matter hyperintensity segmentation. The data comes from two separate studies. As a source domain we use the White Matter Hyperintensity challenge data presented in MICCAI 2017 [6]. The other dataset was used as target domain and comes from a sub-study within the Pharmacokinetic and Clinical Observations in PeoPle over fiftY (POPPY) [4]. In this study two different FLAIR sequences were acquired during the same MR session for all 72 subjects on a Philips 3 T scanner. The in-plane FLAIR was an axial acquisition with 3 mm slice thickness and $1\,mm^2$ planar resolution (Repetition time (TR) 8000 ms, Inversion time (TI) 2400 ms and echo time (TE) 125 ms) while the volumetric FLAIR was of resolution $1.04 \times 1.04 \times 0.56\,mm^3$ (TR = 8000ms TI = 1650 ms TE = 282 ms). Both images were rigidly coregistered to the $1\,mm^3$ T1 sequence acquired during the session. All individuals were male with mean age of 59.1 ± 6.9 yrs, including HIV-positive subjects and population-matched controls.

Implementation Details and Training: The MICCAI Challenge dataset was split with a train:validation:test assignment of 40:10:10 subjects. For the POPPY dataset, the split was 38:15:20.

Training was done using 2d axial slices of size 256×256 with inference carried out by concatenating the predictions across all slices to form a 3d volume. The segmentation network uses the U-Net architecture [10] with depth of 4 and a maximum number of filters of 256 at the deepest layer, with ReLU as the activation function. Initial training on the MICCAI dataset only was performed using the Adam optimizer with an initial learning rate 10^{-3} and a learning rate decay schedule decaying with $\gamma = 0.1$ (γ is a multiplicative factor of learning rate decay) at epoch 300 and 350. The validation set is used for early stopping, thus the baseline model takes the network configuration at the epoch where it showed the highest accuracy on the validation set. All adaptation models and adversarial models were initialized with the weights of this trained baseline model.

The choice of α parameter balancing the segmentation and the consistency loss in the domain adaptation runs proved to be important. Generally, high values of α led to degenerate solutions, where predictions on the target dataset were no longer capturing lesions. Since scheduling a slowly increasing α did not help, α was fixed at 0.2 in all experiments.

In case of an adversarial setting, empirical assessment of the best choice of architecture for the discriminator led to the following choice: four 2D convolutional layers with a kernel size of 3×3 and a stride of 2 followed by batch normalisation and leaky ReLU activation. The number of output channels is 4 to begin with and doubles at each layer to a total of 32. Finally, there are three fully connected layers with output sizes of 64, 32, and 2 with relu activations and dropout applied ($p = 0.5$).

Points of Comparison: In order to assess the relevance of the proposed paired consistency, we compared the proposed PC with adversarial setting and augmentation (PC+Adv+Aug) to the version without adversarial setting (PC+Aug) and the simplest version removing also the augmentation (PC). In addition, we trained classical UDA methods with a mean-teacher framework (MT) as well as the adversarial setting without PC with (Adv+Aug) and without augmentation (Adv). Finally we compared to the baseline U-Net model trained only on the MICCAI dataset with (Baseline+Aug) and without (Baseline) augmentation.

For the final results table checkpoints were chosen for each of the experiments by looking at the performance across the validation set.

Table 1. Performance of different methods on the target (POPPY) and the source domain (MICCAI 2017 WMH Challenge). We report the dice between our models' predictions and the ground truth annotations in the source domain as well as the HD95. The evaluation on target domains is done with the Dice, the HD95, the volume difference (VD) and the recall. A significative rank measure is calculated across all metrics. Results are reported with the format median (IQR) in percentages for all metrics except the HD95 in mm. Best results are in bold andunderlined when significantly better than all others ($p < 0.05$ paired Wilcoxon tests).

	POPPY				MICCAI		
	Dice	HD	VD	Recall	Dice	HD	Rank
PC+Adv+Aug	__54.5__ **(10.6)**	32.7 (9.8)	__15.2__ **(22.8)**	__52.4__ **(14.4)**	81.4 (9.6)	28.5 (8.6)	2.5
PC+Aug	53.2 (15.1)	39.2 (15.5)	25.4 (15.6)	43.5 (12.5)	81.6 (15.5)	18.6 (4.8)	3.3
PC	50.7 (17.0)	35.1 (11.9)	16.6 (21.4)	43.6 (11.0)	81.4 (22.6)	**17.2 (3.6)**	3.4
MT	48.6 (12.3)	33.6 (14.8)	33.7 (19.0)	40.9 (5.0)	80.0 (18.2)	20.0 (7.3)	4.3
Baseline+Aug	42.8 (14.6)	34.9 (11.1)	39.3 (22.3)	33.5 (12.6)	80.6 (14.8)	17.8 (4.9)	4.9
Baseline	43.0 (16.2)	33.3 (15.1)	40.3 (24.8)	33.3 (14.8)	81.1 (16.9)	17.5 (3.3)	5.6
Adv	41.8 (15.4)	**32.6 (6.1)**	25.2 (24.0)	33.5 (12.7)	**82.5 (12.0)**	17.6 (5.2)	5.7
Adv+Aug	41.4 (16.4)	36.6 (9.0)	38.0 (16.0)	33.6 (13.9)	81.9 (11.1)	19.7 (11.0)	6.3

Reported Metrics: As a first metric of consistency, we compute the Dice score overlap between the two volumes. However, high dice agreement may arise without predicting lesions, for instance with the segmentation of foreground or of another anatomical structure. Such degenerate solutions can indeed occur as the consistency term in the loss can be minimized for any consistent prediction between volumes.

As there are no lesion segmentations for the POPPY dataset, we use the known association between age and white matter hyperintensity load reported for this dataset [4] as surrogate evaluation that the segmented elements are lesions. The effect size is a useful metric for determining whether the lesion loads predicted by the various models agree with the reported literature. For the eight compared models, the effect size ranged from 1.2-fold to 1.5-fold increase in lesion load normalized by total intracranial volume per decade. This compares well with the reported effect size on the POPPY dataset of 1.4-fold with a 95th confidence interval of $[1.0; 2.0]$. Predictions from in-plane POPPY and volumetric POPPY were compared using the dice overlap, the 95th percentile Hausdorff distance measured in mm (HD95), the recall (or sensitivity), the ratio of difference in volume between the two predictions (VD) as was used in [6].

The results, gathered in Table 1, reporting median and interquartile range are ordered according to the average significance ranking, follows the guidelines of the MICCAI Decathlon challenge 2018[1].

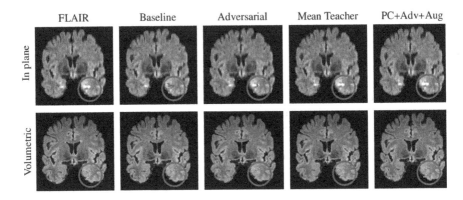

Fig. 2. Qualitative results on a single slice from a single subject in the POPPY dataset. The top row shows a slice from the in-plane FLAIR acquisition whilst the bottom row shows a slice from the volumetric FLAIR acquisition. Each column shows a model's predictions on that row's image. This slice is used to highlight an example of an artefact (shown in the red circle) introduced by the in-plane acquisition. The baseline method introduces a false positive in this region whilst the domain adaptation methods perform better at ignoring it. Our approach shows the best in-plane to volumetric agreement.

4   Discussion

In this work, we presented a novel method of performing unsupervised multi-domain adaptation. A pretrained model from one domain is retrained on paired unlabeled data from two target domains, encouraging consistent predictions. The proposed approach was evaluated against existing UDA strategies including representation learning approaches using domain adversarial training [5], and the 'Mean Teacher' algorithm for unsupervised domain adaptation [13] as well as an unsupervised baseline for WMH segmentation. Overall, our method was able to produce more consistent predictions across two target domains while retaining similar performance on its original training domain. More specifically, adaptation techniques optimizing pairwise consistency not only outperformed baseline models not benefitting from any adaptation but also adversarial strategies. Furthermore, it appeared that the PC method while closest to the mean teacher algorithm, outperformed this approach potentially thanks to differences

---

[1] http://medicaldecathlon.com/files/MSD-Ranking-scheme.pdf.

in the optimisation strategies. Understanding the reasons for these differences also reported by [13] could be an interesting avenue of future investigation. Regarding the adversarial results, the observed inferior performance suggests that depending on the adaptation problem, the learning of a latent space invariant to domain (as enforced in the adversarial approach) may cause an information loss detrimental to the segmentation task. Additionally, the effects of data augmentation (which normally impacts performance positively) did not provide any benefit in the pure adversarial setting. Specific investigation of the effect of each type of augmentation would be needed to better understand this behaviour. While a pure adversarial setting proved ineffective, best performance across all models was obtained when combining it with our proposed PC strategy as it promoted a good label distribution in our target images. Future work will focus on removing the need for paired data by finding sufficiently realistic augmentation functions.

In conclusion, PC is a promising method to adapt automated image segmentation tools to different scanner manufacturers, MR sequences and other confounds. This adaptation is critical to the clinical translation of these tools notably in the context of scanner upgrades and multicentre trials.

Acknowledgements. We gratefully acknowledge the support of NVIDIA Corporation with the donation of one Titan Xp. This project has received funding from the EU H2020 under the Marie Skłodowska-Curie grant agreement No 721820, Wellcome Flagship Programme (WT213038/Z/18/Z) and Wellcome EPSRC CME (WT203148/Z/16/Z). Carole H. Sudre is supported by AS-JF-17-011 Alzheimer's Society Junior Fellowship.

References

1. Bai, W., et al.: Semi-supervised learning for network-based cardiac MR image segmentation. In: Descoteaux, M., Maier-Hein, L., Franz, A., Jannin, P., Collins, D.L., Duchesne, S. (eds.) MICCAI 2017. LNCS, vol. 10434, pp. 253–260. Springer, Cham (2017). https://doi.org/10.1007/978-3-319-66185-8_29
2. Dou, Q., et al.: Unsupervised cross-modality domain adaptation of convnets for biomedical image segmentations with adversarial loss. In: Proceedings of the 27th International Joint Conference on Artificial Intelligence, pp. 691–697. AAAI Press (2018)
3. Gibson, E., et al.: NiftyNet: a deep-learning platform for medical imaging. arXiv preprint arXiv:1709.03485 (2017)
4. Haddow, L.J., et al.: Magnetic resonance imaging of cerebral small vessel disease in men living with HIV and HIV-negative men aged 50 and above. AIDS Res. Hum. Retroviruses **35**(5), 453–460 (2019)
5. Kamnitsas, K., et al.: Unsupervised domain adaptation in brain lesion segmentation with adversarial networks. In: Niethammer, M., et al. (eds.) IPMI 2017. LNCS, vol. 10265, pp. 597–609. Springer, Cham (2017). https://doi.org/10.1007/978-3-319-59050-9_47
6. Kuijf, H.J., et al.: Standardized assessment of automatic segmentation of white matter hyperintensities; results of the WMH segmentation challenge. IEEE Trans. Med. Imaging **99**, 1 (2019)

7. Milletari, F., et al.: V-net: fully convolutional neural networks for volumetric medical image segmentation. In: 3DV, pp. 565–571. IEEE (2016)

8. Miotto, R., et al.: Deep learning for healthcare: review, opportunities and challenges. Briefings bioinform. **19**(6), 1236–1246 (2017)

9. Perone, C.S., et al.: Unsupervised domain adaptation for medical imaging segmentation with self-ensembling. NeuroImage **194**, 1–11 (2019)

10. Ronneberger, O., Fischer, P., Brox, T.: U-Net: convolutional networks for biomedical image segmentation. In: Navab, N., Hornegger, J., Wells, W.M., Frangi, A.F. (eds.) MICCAI 2015. LNCS, vol. 9351, pp. 234–241. Springer, Cham (2015). https://doi.org/10.1007/978-3-319-24574-4_28

11. Schoenauer-Sebag, A., et al.: Multi-domain adversarial learning. arXiv preprint arXiv:1903.09239 (2019)

12. Shaw, R., et al.: MRI k-space motion artefact augmentation: model robustness and task-specific uncertainty. In: MIDL, pp. 427–436 (2019)

13. Xie, Q., et al.: Unsupervised data augmentation. arXiv:1904.12848 (2019)

14. Zhao, A., et al.: Data augmentation using learned transforms for one-shot medical image segmentation. CoRR abs/1902.09383 (2019). http://arxiv.org/abs/1902.09383

Cross-Modality Knowledge Transfer for Prostate Segmentation from CT Scans

Yucheng Liu[1]([✉]), Naji Khosravan[2], Yulin Liu[1,3], Joseph Stember[1], Jonathan Shoag[4], Ulas Bagci[2], and Sachin Jambawalikar[1]

[1] Department of Radiology, Columbia University Irving Medical Center, New York, NY, USA
yl3830@cumc.columbia.edu
[2] Center for Research in Computer Vision, University of Central Florida, Orlando, FL, USA
[3] Department of Information and Computer Engineering, Chung Yuan Christian University, Taoyuan City, Taiwan
[4] Urologic Oncology, Weill Cornell Medicine, New York, NY, USA

Abstract. Creating large scale high-quality annotations is a known challenge in medical imaging. In this work, based on the CycleGAN algorithm, we propose leveraging annotations from one modality to be useful in other modalities. More specifically, the proposed algorithm creates highly realistic synthetic CT images (SynCT) from prostate MR images using unpaired data sets. By using SynCT images (without segmentation labels) and MR images (with segmentation labels available), we have trained a deep segmentation network for precise delineation of prostate from real CT scans. For the generator in our CycleGAN, the cycle consistency term is used to guarantee that SynCT shares the identical manually-drawn, high-quality masks originally delineated on MR images. Further, we introduce a cost function based on structural similarity index (SSIM) to improve the anatomical similarity between real and synthetic images. For segmentation followed by the SynCT generation from CycleGAN, automatic delineation is achieved through a 2.5D Residual U-Net. Quantitative evaluation demonstrates comparable segmentation results between our SynCT and radiologist drawn masks for real CT images, solving an important problem in medical image segmentation field when ground truth annotations are not available for the modality of interest.

Keywords: Domain adaptation · Deep learning · CT synthesis · Prostate segmentation · 2.5D · Generative Adversarial Networks

1 Introduction

Prostate segmentation from radiology scans is often necessary for radiotherapy, prostatectomy, and calculation of prostate-specific antigen (PSA) density [1]. Among imaging modalities, magnetic resonance imaging (MRI) provides the

Q. Wang et al. (Eds.): DART 2019/MIL3ID 2019, LNCS 11795, pp. 63–71, 2019.
https://doi.org/10.1007/978-3-030-33391-1_8

best soft tissue contrast and yields the most accurate estimation on prostate volume, consistent with prostatectomy specimen volumes [2]. Unlike MRI, computed tomographic (CT) scans have difficulties to distinguish the boundaries of prostates and other adjacent tissues during segmentation [3]. Despite this, in current clinical practice, prostate radiation therapy dose calculations is primarily based on CT scans as it is the only modality that can derive electron density needed for the dosimetry calculations [4]. Therefore, planning systems generally require anatomical information to be delineated on CT scans.

In this study, we address a practical yet still very challenging issue of prostate segmentation from CT images when there are no ground truth CT annotations to supervise the segmentation algorithm. Instead, we target utilizing segmentation labels from widely available MRI data sets, and propose a two step knowledge transfer algorithm to map the segmentation labels from MRI to CT scans. The correspondence between MRI to CT is established through a CycleGAN algorithm [5] with a structural similarity preserving cost function. Highly realistic synthetic CT scans generated in the first step are then used to supervise a deep segmentation network in the second step. The training for the segmentation network is performed only on the synthetic images while testing is done on both synthetic and real CT scans for evaluation. While our framework does not enforce the use of any specific segmentation network to finalize the delineation process, we choose 2.5D Res-U-Net to accomplish this task with faster convergence, and higher accuracy.

2   Methods

The proposed workflow includes two main steps as demonstrated in Fig. 1. First step is to generate high-quality and reliable CT images (SynCT) from MR images. Previous work [6] has shown that domain adaptation from MR images to CT images is feasible using the CycleGAN architecture. We used a similar CycleGAN approach as baseline to create high-quality knowledge transfer between unpaired MRI and CT.

Second step is to conduct automatic segmentation of prostate. We trained a U-Net based segmentation network to delineate the whole prostate area but with two main differences from the existing literature: (i) we used SynCT in training and real CT scans in testing, and (ii) we modified the U-Net [7] to increase the segmentation performance by adding residual blocks into the segmentation network. For better 3D information fusion, we also modified the segmentation architecture to utilize two additional adjacent slices in its input (i.e., 3-channel input).

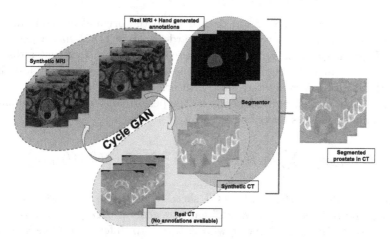

Fig. 1. Workflow of CT image synthesis and automatic segmentation. The red box indicate the first step, CT image synthesis via CycleGAN model. SynCTs with identical anatomical structures as MRI were generated thus shared high-quality segmentation with MRI (labeled red). The blue box indicate the second step, automatic segmentation via 2.5D Res-U-Net train with SynCT. The automatic generated segmentation (labeled pink) on true CT images were compared against manual segmentation from radiologist. (Color figure online)

2.1   Data

We used a total of three different data sets for our experiments and evaluations. For cycleGAN training, 346 T2 weighted MRI scans from publicly available PROSTATEx-challenge data [9] was used. T2-weighted images were acquired using a turbo spin echo sequence with in-plane resolution of 0.4–0.6 mm, slice thickness of 3.6 mm and zero gap. Secondly, the testing data set for Cycle-GAN included 60 prostate MRI cases along with their high-quality delineation obtained from publicly available NCI-ISBI 2013 challenge data [10]. This data was used for generating the synthetic CT scans. We used 6-fold stratified cross validation for evaluation of the algorithms. Third, for real CT scans, as part of retrospective IRB approved study, we acquired prostate CT data from 120 anonymized patients from our institution with resolution $(0.8 \times 0.8 \times 1\,\text{mm}^3)$. CT intensity was clipped to -500HU to 500HU to reveal more soft tissue contrast similar to a soft tissue CT window. Prostate MRI and CT data are completely different from each other, namely unpaired. Among in-house collected CT data, we chose 19 of them to be manually segmented by a board certified radiologist for Dice score (DSC) comparison with our automatic segmentation method.

2.2   Synthetic CT Network: CycleGAN

The synthetic CT images were generated by the CycleGAN model [5], which consisted of two pairs of generative adversarial networks (GAN) and two extra generators that convert generated data back to the original domain enforcing cycle consistency. In our study, the forward-direction GAN has a generator, $G_{CT}(MR)$, that generate synthetic CT as real as possible such that a discriminator, D_{CT} cannot distinguish it from the real CT. The discriminator is to ensure the likeness of generated data with original data, hence, the reliability of the generated data heavily depends on the performance of the discriminator, the discriminator loss is described by Eq. 1.

$$\mathcal{L}_{D(CT)} = \frac{1}{m}\sum_{j=1}^{m}[D_{CT}(I_{CT}^j - 1)]^2 + \frac{1}{n}\sum_{i=1}^{n}[D_{CT}(G_{CT}(I_{MR}^i))]^2 \qquad (1)$$

Where I_{CT}^j denotes the j-th true CT slice; I_{MR}^i represents the i-th MRI slice; $G_{CT}(I_{MR}^i)$ represents the generated image by generator $G_{CT}(MR)$ from I_{MR}^i; D_{CT} represents the discriminator who is trying to differentiate the generated image from CT images, if the discriminator cannot distinguish the generated image, it is labeled 1, which means the discriminator recognized this generated image as true CT image, otherwise a 0 label is given.

The generator $G_{MR}(SynCT)$ is translating the SynCT back to its' original data domain (MR domain). By minimizing the difference between the reconstructed data and the original data (cycle-consistency loss), a powerful constraint has been enforced on the model to prevent generated data deviation from ground-truth. The cycle-consistency loss is express as Eq. 2 here.

$$\mathcal{L}^{SSIM}(P) = \frac{1}{N}\sum_{p=1}^{N}[1 - SSIM(p)] \qquad (2)$$

$$SSIM(p) = (\frac{2\mu_x\mu_y + C_1}{\mu_x^2 + \mu_y^2 + C_1})(\frac{2\sigma_{xy} + C_2}{\sigma_x^2 + \sigma_y^2 + C_2}), \qquad (3)$$

where P is the image patch, N is number of pixels in P, and p is the index of pixel; SSIM, for a pixel p, is defined as in Eq. 3. Where μ_x, μ_y and σ_x, σ_y denotes mean pixel intensity and the standard deviations of pixel intensity in a local image patch centering at either x or y. Also, C_1 and C_1 are small constants being added for stability. The cycle loss compares the reconstructed MRI with the true MRI slices in a pixel by pixel manner. In our new formulation, instead of computing mean-square-error (MSE), we propose to use structural similarity index (SSIM) that takes into account the context of the images at a higher level than pixel-level MSE [11].

2.3   Segmentation Network: 2.5D Res–U-Net

The U-Net architecture [7] has long skip connections to preserve spatial information during down-sampling. Besides long skip connections, short skip connections were also added forming residual blocks to prevent vanishing gradient and increase the convergence speed, the U-Net with short skip connections is called Res-U-Net [8]. Also, the proposed 2.5D input technique loads multiple slices simultaneously, which includes one central slice and its adjacent slices in out-of-plane direction. The number of channels is determined as the sum of central slice and the adjacent slices ($channel\,No. = central\,slice + adjacent\,slices$). The number of adjacent slices is defined through a designated context number which can query adjacent slices in both positive and negative directions ($adjacent\,slices = 2 \times context\,No$). For instance, if the context number is set to be 1, the selected adjacent slices will include +1 and −1 slices adjacent to the central slices. The context number can be adjusted in order to optimized the segmentation results.

3   Results

The CycleGAN model was trained using Adam optimizer for 200 epochs with initial learning rate 0.0002; the 2.5D Res-U-Net model was trained using Adam optimizer for 300 epochs and binary cross entropy loss function was used because there are only two classes, masks and non-masks. Training took about 24 h for CycleGAN to generate SynCT and about 12 h for 2.5D Res-U-Net on a DGX-station with 4x Tesla V100 GPUs each with 32 GB RAM. The segmentation results are displayed in Fig. 2. For data augmentation, rotation, flipping, and random crops from ratio 1 (no crop) to 0.5 (half crop) of original images were performed during training.

Table 1. Segmentation results (DSC) of MRI, SynCT and CT testing dataset.

Training dataset	Testing dataset	Dice score (DSC)
MRI	MRI	0.90 ± 0.05
SynCT	SynCT	0.83 ± 0.13
	CT	0.45 ± 0.29
Soft-tissue SynCT	SynCT	0.82 ± 0.12
	CT	0.62 ± 0.15
Soft-tissue SynCT Data augmented	SynCT	0.65 ± 0.09
	CT	0.68 ± 0.09
Soft-tissue SynCT Data augmentated SSIM loss	SynCT	0.80 ± 0.12
	CT	0.73 ± 0.09

2.5D Res-U-Net trained and tested on MRI data illustrates the upper bounds of performance, network trained on CT/SynCT data will intuitively be lower than 0.9 (Table 1). SynCTs paired with MRI segmentations were used to train the automatic segmentation network. For SynCT generated from default CycleGAN setting (MSE loss, random crop with fix ratio, 284 to 256 pixels) and no intensity clipping, we achieved 0.83 ± 0.13 and 0.45 ± 0.29 DSC for SynCT and CT testing set, respectively; for Soft-tissue SynCT (intensity clipped from −500 HU to 500

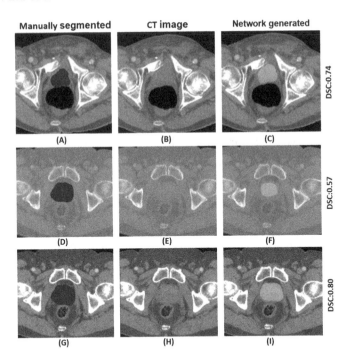

Manually segmented   CT image   Network generated

(A)   (B)   (C)   DSC:0.74

(D)   (E)   (F)   DSC:0.57

(G)   (H)   (I)   DSC:0.80

Fig. 2. Example slices of segmentation results on true CT. (A) Under-segmented prostate by expert radiologists. 2.5D Res-U-Net can generate better segmentation (C) since it adapted the segmentation from MRI, however, resulting a misleadingly lower DSC, 0.74. CT with normal intensity can vary from -1000 HU (air) to 1000 (bone), therefore soft tissues consists of similar HU numbers may not be seen clearly on the images, as demonstrated on the middle part of the figure, where (D) is CT with ground-truth segmentation from radiologist, (E) is CT without any intensity adjustment, and (F) is CT with 2.5D Res-U-Net generated segmentation. Last row demonstrates CT with soft tissue window (-500 HU to 500 HU, we called ST-CT (soft tissue CT)), which is slightly larger than typical soft tissue window, -150 HU to 350 HU, to accommodate more information in the slices. Where (G) is ST-CT with ground-truth segmentation, (H) is the ST-CT, and (I) is the ST-CT with 2.5D Res-U-Net generated segmentation. At the same case, the DSC of CT and ST-CT is 0.57 and 0.80, respectively.

HU), we achieved 0.82 ± 0.12 and 0.62 ± 0.15 DSC for SynCT and CT testing set, respectively. More aggressive data augmentation (random crop with random ratio, rotation, flipping) also adapted to generate higher quality SynCT from CycleGAN, which achieved 0.65 ± 0.09 and 0.68 ± 0.09 DSC for SynCT and CT segmentation testing set, respectively. To increase the structure accuracy, the cycle loss has replaced into structural similarity index (SSIM), the 2.5D Res-U-Net trained with SynCT-SSIM achieved 0.80 ± 0.12 and 0.73 ± 0.09 DSC for SynCT and CT testing set, respectively. Note that the DSC of SynCT decrease and the DSC of CT increase to reach a compatible point with no statistical difference ($p > 0.05$), also the standard deviations are converging. This tendency

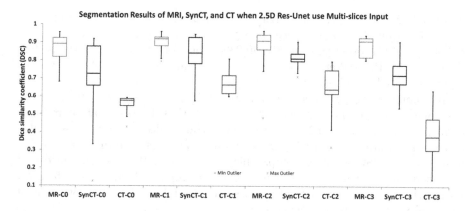

Fig. 3. Boxplots are showing the Dice scores for prostate segmentation from MRI, SynCT, and CT, respectively.

indicated our SynCT gradually reached a point where there was no difference with true CT from 2.5D Res-U-Net network perspective.

4   Discussion and Concluding Remarks

Intensive studies have been made regarding prostate CT automatic segmentation. Recently, the reported highest DSC is 0.88 ± 0.03 by Liu *et al.* [12] using U-Net and 1114 ture CT cases. Our average result is 0.73 ± 0.09 which is compatible with Burgos *et al.* [13] using multi-atlas based SynCT (0.73 DSC). We have shown that the SynCT and the CT testing results have no statistical difference indicating the feasibility of using SynCT to train a neural network for a very challenging segmentation task. In some cases DCS is low but not due to low performance of the proposed network. The low DSC is sometimes due to noise in the contouring in the hand-drawn CT ground-truth segmentation and large anatomical and pathological variations (see Fig. 2).

Data Augmentation: We used MRI and CT scans from different data sources, MRI have smaller field-of-view (FOV) compared to CT. Inconsistent FOV encouraged CycleGAN to shift the anatomy without focusing on anatomical details. To generate high-quality SynCT, we central cropped the CT images by 50% to remove the surrounding air and scanning table. Then augment the data with random ratio (1–0.5) random crop, rotation, and flipping to reduce certain geometry tendency affecting the learning process.

2.5D Technique: 2.5D multi-slices input technique can affect the segmentation network performance as Fig. 3 shows here. For SynCT, from single slice to 3-slices, DSC increases significantly ($p < 0.05$) by 19.11%, from 3-slices to 5-slices no significant difference was found, from 5-slices to 7-slices, DSC decreased 12.5%; for CT, from single slice to 3-slices, DSC increase significantly by 24.17%, from 3-slices to 5-slices no significant difference found, from 5-slices to 7-slices, DSC drop significantly by 40.93%. Therefore, to optimized the performance of 2.5D Res-U-Net and also save training time, context number 1 (3-slices input) was used for all experiments.

In summary, we proposed a novel approach to segment prostate from CT scans when the ground-truth was absent. Synthetic CT scans that share high-quality segmentation with MRI were used to train a deep-learning based automatic segmentation network (2.5D Res-U-Net). The testing results on true CT achieved 0.73 DSC which is comparable with SynCT. We also examined and identified the optimal numbers of multiple slices input, which are 3 or 5 slices. Future steps will include 3D volume assessment and continue improvement of the quality of synthetic CT generation.

References

1. Nordstrm, T., et al.: Prostate-specific antigen (PSA) density in the diagnostic algorithm of prostate cancer. Prostate Cancer Prostatic Dis. **21**(1), 57–63 (2017)
2. Smith, W.L., et al.: Prostate volume contouring: a 3D analysis of segmentation using 3DTRUS, CT, and MR. Int. J. Radiat. Oncol. Biol. Phys. **67**(4), 1238–1247 (2007)
3. Rasch, C., et al.: Definition of the prostate in CT and MRI: a multi-observer study. Int. J. Radiat. Oncol. Biol. Phys. **43**(1), 57–66 (1999)
4. Chowdhury, N., et al.: Concurrent segmentation of the prostate on MRI and CT via linked statistical shape models for radiotherapy planning. Med. Phys. **39**(4), 2214–2228 (2012)
5. Zhu, J.-Y., Park, T., Isola, P., Efros, A.A.: Unpaired image-to-image translation using cycle-consistent adversarial networks. arXiv:1703.10593 (2017)
6. Wolterink, J.M., Dinkla, A.M., Savenije, M.H.F., Seevinck, P.R., van den Berg, C.A.T., Išgum, I.: Deep MR to CT synthesis using unpaired data. In: Tsaftaris, S.A., Gooya, A., Frangi, A.F., Prince, J.L. (eds.) SASHIMI 2017. LNCS, vol. 10557, pp. 14–23. Springer, Cham (2017). https://doi.org/10.1007/978-3-319-68127-6_2. https://arxiv.org/abs/1708.01155
7. Ronneberger, O., Fischer, P., Brox, T.: U-Net: convolutional networks for biomedical image segmentation. In: Navab, N., Hornegger, J., Wells, W.M., Frangi, A.F. (eds.) MICCAI 2015. LNCS, vol. 9351, pp. 234–241. Springer, Cham (2015). https://doi.org/10.1007/978-3-319-24574-4_28. arXiv:1505.04597
8. Drozdzal, M., Vorontsov, E., Chartrand, G., Kadoury, S., Pal, C.: The importance of skip connections in biomedical image segmentation. In: Carneiro, G., et al. (eds.) LABELS/DLMIA -2016. LNCS, vol. 10008, pp. 179–187. Springer, Cham (2016). https://doi.org/10.1007/978-3-319-46976-8_19
9. Litjens, G., Debats, O., Barentsz, J., Karssemeijer, N., Huisman, H.: SPIE-AAPM PROSTATEx Challenge Data (2017). https://doi.org/10.7937/K9TCIA.2017.MURS5CL
10. Bloch, N., et al.: NCI-ISBI 2013 Challenge: Automated Segmentation of Prostate Structures. The Cancer Imaging Archive (2015). https://doi.org/10.7937/K9/TCIA.2015.zF0vlOPv

11. Zhao, H., et al.: Loss functions for image restoration with neural networks. IEEE Trans. Comput. Imaging **3**(1), 47–57 (2017)
12. Liu, C., et al.: Automatic segmentation of the prostate on CT images using deep neural networks (DNN). Int. J. Radiat. Oncol. Biol. Phys. **104**(4), 924–932 (2019)
13. Burgos, N., et al.: Iterative framework for the joint segmentation and CT synthesis of MR images: application to MRI-only radiotherapy treatment planning. Phys. Med. Biol. **62**, 4237–4253 (2017)

A Pulmonary Nodule Detection Method Based on Residual Learning and Dense Connection

Feng Zhang[1,2], Yutong Xie[2], Yong Xia[1,2(✉)], and Yanning Zhang[2]

[1] Research & Development Institute of Northwestern Polytechnical University in Shenzhen, Shenzhen 518057, China
`yxia@nwpu.edu.cn`
[2] National Engineering Laboratory for Integrated Aero-Space-Ground-Ocean Big Data Application Technology, School of Computer Science and Engineering, Northwestern Polytechnical University, Xian 710072, China

Abstract. Pulmonary nodule detection using chest CT scan is an essential but challenging step towards the early diagnosis of lung cancer. Although a number of deep learning-based methods have been published in the literature, these methods still suffer from less accuracy. In this paper, we propose a novel pulmonary module detection method, which uses a 3D residual U-Net (3D RU-Net) for nodule candidate detection and a 3D densely connected CNN (3D DC-Net) for false positive reduction. 3D RU-Net contains residual blocks in both contracting and expansive paths, and 3D DC-Net leverages three dense blocks to facilitate gradients flow. We evaluated our method on the benchmark LUng Nodule Analysis 2016 (LUNA16) dataset and achieved a CPM score of 0.941, which is higher than those achieved by five competing methods. Our results suggest that the proposed method can effectively detect pulmonary nodules on chest CT.

Keywords: Pulmonary nodule detection · Residual learning · Dense connection · Chest CT

1 Introduction

Lung cancer is the leading cause of all cancer-related deaths for both men and women [1]. The average five-year survival rate of lung cancer patients is only about 16%, however it is at least 60% if the diagnosis is made in an early stage of the disease [2]. Since malignant pulmonary nodules may be primary lung tumors or metastases, early detection of pulmonary nodules is critical for best patient care. On chest CT scans, a pulmonary nodule usually refers to a spot of less than 3 cm in diameter on the lung. Radiologists typically read chest CT scans for pulmonary nodules on a slice-by-slice basis, which is time-consuming and can be prone to operator bias. Computer-aided pulmonary nodule detection

© Springer Nature Switzerland AG 2019
Q. Wang et al. (Eds.): DART 2019/MIL3ID 2019, LNCS 11795, pp. 72–80, 2019.
https://doi.org/10.1007/978-3-030-33391-1_9

avoids many of these issues and has being increasingly studied to improve its efficiency and accuracy.

Recently, many pulmonary nodule detection methods based on deep convolutional neural networks (DCNNs) have been proposed in the literature. Most of them consist of two successive steps: nodule candidate detection and false positive reduction. Ding et al. [3] introduced a deconvolutional structure to 2D Fast R-CNN to detect candidates on axial slices, then used a 3D DCNN for false positive reduction. Hamidian et al. [4] first used a 3D fully convolutional network (FCN) to generate a score map for the detection of nodule candidates and then employed another 3D DCNN for nodule and non-nodule classification. Dou et al. [5] proposed an FCN trained with an online sample filtering scheme to detect nodule candidates accurately and rapidly, and also designed a hybrid-loss 3D DCNN for false positive reduction. Wang et al. [6] first trained the feature pyramid network (FPN) to detect nodule candidates, then utilized the conditional 3D non-maximal suppression to remove redundant candidates, and finally proposed an attention 3D DCNN to further distinguish nodules and non-nodules. Although yield promising results, these methods still suffer from less-accuracy, due to the loss of low-level information. Since it has been widely recognized that the residual [7] learning and dense connection [8] are two efficient ways to keep the low-level information via boosting the flow of information within the network, we suggest incorporating both techniques into the nodule detection procedure to improve its performance.

In this paper, we propose a two-stage pulmonary module detection method based on a 3D residual U-Net (3D RU-Net) and a 3D densely connected CNN (3D DC-Net). In the first stage, the 3D RU-Net, in which residual blocks are used in both contracting and expansive paths, is constructed to segment nodule candidates on chest CT scans. In the second stage, the 3D DC-Net, which leverages three dense blocks to facilitate gradients flow, is designed to improve the performance of nodules and non-nodules classification. We have evaluated our method on the LUng Nodule Analysis 2016 (LUNA16) dataset [9] and achieved promising results.

2   Dataset

The LUNA16 [9] dataset was used for this study, which contains 888 chest CT scans and 1186 pulmonary nodules. Each scan, with the slice thickness less than 2.5 mm and slice size of 512 × 512 voxels, was annotated during a two-phase procedure by four experienced radiologists. Each radiologist marked lesions they identified as either non-nodule, nodules <3mm, or nodules >=3 mm. The reference standard of the LUNA16 challenge consists of all nodules >=3 mm accepted by at least 3 out of 4 radiologists. Each nodule is equipped with its center coordinate and diameter.

3   Method

The proposed nodule detection method consists of three main procedures, including pre-processing, nodule candidate detection and for false positive reduction. A diagram that summarizes this method is shown in Fig. 1. We now delve into each procedure.

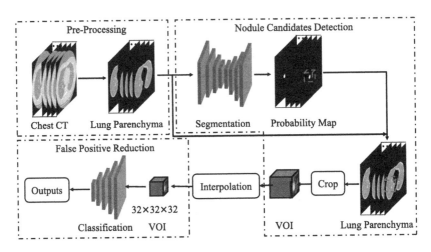

Fig. 1. Diagram of our proposed pulmonary nodule detection method.

3.1   Pre-processing

To normalize the variable spatial resolution of chest CT scans, we re-slice all scans to a unified voxel size of $1.0 \times 1.0 \times 1.0 \, \text{mm}^3$. Meanwhile, since outside-lung organs and tissues such as the sternum may cause an extremely adverse effect on the detection, we need segment lung parenchyma before detecting nodule candidates. The segmentation process include three steps: (a) using the OTSU algorithm to binarize each re-sliced CT scan on a slice-by-slice basis; (b) using the morphology closing and dilation with a disk structure element of radius 5 to fill holes and generate a lung mask that covers all lung parenchyma; and (c) applying the mask to the re-sliced CT scan to remove most outside-lung organs and tissues.

3.2   Nodule Candidate Detection

Architecture of 3D RU-Net. The 3D RU-Net we constructed for nodule candidate detection consists of a contracting path and an expansive path (Fig. 2). The contracting path contains four residual blocks (in green) and three Conv-BN-ReLU layers (in red). Four residual blocks are composed of, subsequently, one, two, three and three cascaded Conv-BN-ReLU layers. The expansive path includes three DeConv-BN-ReLU layers (in blue), three residual blocks (in green), and a Conv-Sigmoid layer (in purple). Three residual blocks are composed of, subsequently, three, two, and one cascaded Conv-BN-ReLU layers. Each Conv/DeConv-BN-ReLU layer contains a convolutional or deconvolutional layer, a bath normalization, and ReLU activation. All hyper-parameters that determine the architecture of 3D RU-Net are shown in Fig. 2. We add residual connections to skip each residual block and skip connections to transfer the feature maps produced by each residual block in the contracting path to the corresponding place in the expansive path.

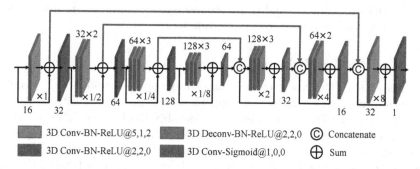

Fig. 2. Architecture of 3D RU-Net. 3D Deconv/Conv-BN-ReLU refers to 3D deconvolutional/convolutional layers with parameters indicating the kernel size, stride and padding size, followed by the batch normalization (BN) and ReLU activation, and 3D Conv-Sigmoid refers to 3D convolutional layers followed by the sigmoid activation (Color figure online)

Training 3D RU-Net. To train 3D RU-Net, we need construct a pseudo segmentation ground truth for each training nodule based on its center coordinate and diameter, which can be done in two steps. First, we define a sphere with the same diameter as the nodule and place it at the center of the nodule. Second, we set the voxel value of sphere center to 1, then calculate the values of voxels inside the sphere according to the Butterworth function, and set all voxels outside the sphere to 0.

We extract partly overlapped patches of size $48 \times 48 \times 48$ on the pre-processed CT scans with a stride of 40, and use them to train 3D RU-Net. Since the volume of pulmonary nodules only occupies a small portion (usually less than 0.5%) of each CT scan, the training suffers from severe class-imbalance. To address this issue, we jointly optimize the combined Dice loss and focal loss [10], which can be formulated as

$$\mathcal{L} = \mathcal{L}_{dice} + \mathcal{L}_{focal} = 1 - \frac{2\sum_{i=1}^{N} P_i G_i}{\sum_{i=1}^{N}(P_i + G_i)}$$
$$+ [-\frac{1}{N}\sum_{i=1}^{N}(1 - P_i)^{\gamma} G_i \ln P_i - \frac{1}{N}\sum_{i=1}^{N} P_i^{\gamma}(1 - G_i)\ln(1 - P_i)], \tag{1}$$

where N is the number of voxels, P_i denotes the predicted probability of the i-th voxel belonging to a nodule, G_i represents the ground truth probability of i-th voxel, L_{dice} and L_{focal} represent the Dice loss and focal loss, respectively, and γ is the tunable focusing parameter, which was empirically set to 2.5.

Testing 3D RU-Net. In the testing stage, we extract $48 \times 48 \times 48$ patches on the pre-processed CT scans in the same way, and feed each patch to the trained 3D RU-Net. The output is a probability map of the same size, which is then binarized by a threshold of 0.5 and smoothed by the morphological dilation with a 3×3 structure element. Finally, each connected volume on the post-processed output is regarded as a detected nodule candidate.

3.3 False Positive Reduction

We construct a 3D DC-Net to classify pulmonary nodule candidates into genuine nodules and non-nodule tissues, aiming to reduce the false positive rate. As shown in Fig. 3, 3D DC-Net consists of a Conv-BN-ReLU layer (in cyan), three dense blocks (in blue), two transition layers (in red), a Conv-BN-ReLU layer (in pink), and a fully connected layer with the sigmoid activation (in purple). Each dense block is composed of 16 modules, each containing two BN-ReLU-Conv layers. The transition layer, which connects two dense blocks, is composed of a BN-ReLU-Conv layer and an average pooling layer. 3D DC-Net is optimized by minimizing the cross-entropy loss. In the testing stage, we cropped concentric patches on the pre-processed CT scans according to the centers of the detected nodule candidates, and fed them to the trained 3D DC-Net for false positive reduction.

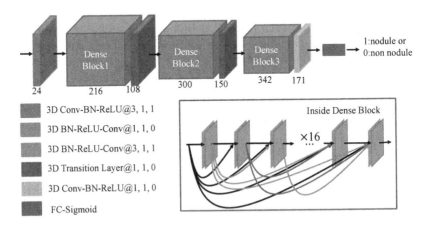

Fig. 3. Architecture of 3D DC-Net: The parameters in each layer indicates the kernel size, stride and padding size, and the growth rate of dense blocks is 12. (Color figure online)

3.4   Implementation

To alleviate the issues of over-fitting and class imbalance, we employed the data argumentation operations, including randomly flips and shift (-10 to 10 voxels) along three axes, to enlarge the positive training set 24 times. Consequently, the ratio of positive and negative samples became 1:3 in the training dataset.

We adopted the Adam algorithm with a batch size of 24 and 12 to optimize the 3D RU-Net and 3D DC-Net, respectively. For both networks, we initialized the parameters via sampling from a standard normal distribution, set the initial bias to 0, set the initial learning rate to 0.001, and decayed it to a half after 10 epochs. Moreover, we randomly chose 20% of the training samples to form a validation set and would terminate the training process if the error on the other 80% of training samples continues to decline but the error on the validation set stops decreasing.

We evaluated our nodule detection method using the 10-fold cross-validation, and, as suggested by the LUNA16 Challenge, assessed its performance using the competition performance metric (CPM), which is the average sensitivity at seven operating points of the free-response receiver operating characteristic (FROC) curve: 0.125, 0.25, 0.5, 1, 2, 4, and 8 false positives per scan (FPs/scan).

4   Results and Discussions

Comparative Evaluation. Table 1 gives the sensitivity at seven operating points and CPM scores of our nodule detection method and five competing methods obtained on the LUNA16 dataset. It reveals that our method substantially outperforms other methods if the number of FPs/scan is no greater than 2 and remains among the best performed methods when the number of FPs/scan is 4 or 8. Moreover, our method achieves the highest CPM score of 0.941, which is markedly superior to that of other methods. These results suggest that our nodule detection method is able to provide an improvement performance over other five competing methods.

Table 1. Sensitivity at seven operating points and CPM scores of our nodule detection method and five competing methods obtained on the LUNA16 dataset

Methods	FPs/scan							
	0.125	0.25	0.5	1	2	4	8	CPM
Dou et al. [5]	0.659	0.745	0.819	0.865	0.906	0.933	0.946	0.839
Wang et al. [6]	0.676	0.776	0.879	0.949	0.958	0.958	0.958	0.878
Ding et al. [3]	0.748	0.853	0.887	0.922	0.938	0.944	0.946	0.891
Khosravan et al. [11]	0.709	0.836	0.921	0.953	0.953	0.953	0.953	0.897
Cao et al. [12]	0.848	0.900	0.925	0.936	0.949	0.957	**0.960**	0.925
Ours	**0.876**	**0.916**	**0.959**	**0.959**	**0.959**	**0.959**	0.959	**0.941**

Effectiveness of 3D RU-Net. To detect nodule candidates, we constructed 3D RU-Net, which uses residual blocks in both contracting and expansive paths. To validate the effectiveness of this design, we compared 3D RU-Net to three of its variants. The first one (denoted by 3D U-Net) does not contain any residual blocks, the second one (denoted by 3D CRSU-Net) contains residual blocks only in the contracting path, and the third one (denoted by 3D DSU-Net) replaces all residual blocks with dense blocks. Figure 4 shows the sensitivity of these networks on validation set of LUNA16 dataset for nodule candidate detection. It reveals that our 3D RU-Net achieves the highest sensitivity than other networks. The results also suggest that our 3D RU-Net can detect more true positives than other networks in the candidate detection stage.

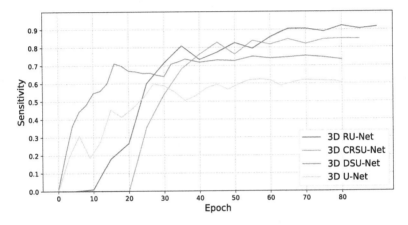

Fig. 4. Sensitivity of 3D RU-Net and its variants on the validation set (176 CT scans) recorded during the training process.

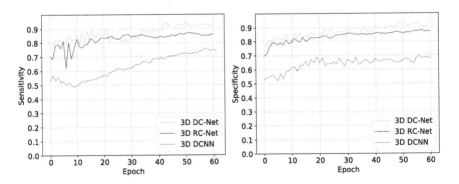

Fig. 5. Sensitivity (left) and specificity (right) of 3D DC-Net and its variants on the validation set (176 CT scans) recorded during the training process.

Effectiveness of 3D DC-Net. With the aim of reducing false positive samples, we constructed 3D DC-Net to classify nodule candidates into genuine nodule and non-nodule tissues. To validate the effectiveness of this network, we compared it to two of its variants. One (denoted by 3D CNN) does not use any skip connections, the other (denoted by 3D RC-Net) replaces all dense blocks with residual blocks. Figure 5 gives the sensitivity and specificity of these networks on validation set recorded during the training process. It shows that our 3D DC-Net outperforms other two networks.

5   Conclusion

This paper proposes a novel method for pulmonary nodule detection using chest CT. Our experiments on the LUNA16 dataset not only demonstrate the effectiveness of 3D RU-Net and 3D DC-Net in nodule candidate detection and false positive reduction, respectively, but also indicate that our method outperforms five existing approaches. In the future, we will exploit multiscale techniques to enable the method to detect both small and large nodules adaptively.

Acknowledgement. This work was supported in part by the Science and Technology Innovation Committee of Shenzhen Municipality, China, under Grants JCYJ20180306171334997, in part by the National Natural Science Foundation of China under Grants 61771397, in part by Synergy Innovation Foundation of the University and Enterprise for Graduate Students in Northwestern Polytechnical University (NPU) under Grants XQ201911, in part by the Seed Foundation of Innovation and Creation for Graduate Students in NPU under Grants ZZ2019029, and in part by the Project for Graduate Innovation team of NPU. We appreciate the efforts devoted by LUNA16 challenge organizers to collect and share the data.

References

1. Bray, F., Ferlay, J., Soerjomataram, I., Siegel, R.L., Torre, L.A., Jemal, A.: Global cancer statistics 2018: GLOBOCAN estimates of incidence and mortality worldwide for 36 cancers in 185 countries. CA Cancer J. Clin. **68**(6), 394–424 (2018)
2. Baldwin, D.R.: Prediction of risk of lung cancer in populations and in pulmonary nodules: significant progress to drive changes in paradigms. Lung Cancer **89**(1), 1–3 (2015)
3. Ding, J., Li, A., Hu, Z., Wang, L.: Accurate pulmonary nodule detection in computed tomography images using deep convolutional neural networks. In: Descoteaux, M., Maier-Hein, L., Franz, A., Jannin, P., Collins, D.L., Duchesne, S. (eds.) MICCAI 2017. LNCS, vol. 10435, pp. 559–567. Springer, Cham (2017). https://doi.org/10.1007/978-3-319-66179-7_64
4. Hamidian, S., Sahiner, B., Petrick, N., Pezeshk, A.: 3D convolutional neural network for automatic detection of lung nodules in chest CT. In: Medical Imaging 2017: Computer-Aided Diagnosis, vol. 10134, p. 1013409. International Society for Optics and Photonics (2017)

5. Dou, Q., Chen, H., Jin, Y., Lin, H., Qin, J., Heng, P.-A.: Automated pulmonary nodule detection via 3D convnets with online sample filtering and hybrid-loss residual learning. In: Descoteaux, M., Maier-Hein, L., Franz, A., Jannin, P., Collins, D.L., Duchesne, S. (eds.) MICCAI 2017. LNCS, vol. 10435, pp. 630–638. Springer, Cham (2017). https://doi.org/10.1007/978-3-319-66179-7_72
6. Wang, B., Qi, G., Tang, S., Zhang, L., Deng, L., Zhang, Y.: Automated pulmonary nodule detection: high sensitivity with few candidates. In: Frangi, A.F., Schnabel, J.A., Davatzikos, C., Alberola-López, C., Fichtinger, G. (eds.) MICCAI 2018. LNCS, vol. 11071, pp. 759–767. Springer, Cham (2018). https://doi.org/10.1007/978-3-030-00934-2_84
7. He, K., Zhang, X., Ren, S., Sun, J.: Deep residual learning for image recognition. In: Proceedings of the IEEE Conference on Computer Vision and Pattern Recognition, pp. 770–778 (2016)
8. Huang, G., Liu, Z., Van Der Maaten, L., Weinberger, K.Q.: Densely connected convolutional networks. In: Proceedings of the IEEE Conference on Computer Vision and Pattern Recognition, pp. 4700–4708 (2017)
9. Setio, A.A.A., et al.: Validation, comparison, and combination of algorithms for automatic detection of pulmonary nodules in computed tomography images: the LUNA16 challenge. Med. Image Anal. **42**, 1–13 (2017)
10. Lin, T.Y., Goyal, P., Girshick, R., He, K., Dollár, P.: Focal loss for dense object detection. In: Proceedings of the IEEE International Conference on Computer Vision, pp. 2980–2988 (2017)
11. Khosravan, N., Bagci, U.: *S4ND*: single-shot single-scale lung nodule detection. In: Frangi, A.F., Schnabel, J.A., Davatzikos, C., Alberola-López, C., Fichtinger, G. (eds.) MICCAI 2018. LNCS, vol. 11071, pp. 794–802. Springer, Cham (2018). https://doi.org/10.1007/978-3-030-00934-2_88
12. Cao, H., et al.: Two-stage convolutional neural network architecture for lung nodule detection. arXiv preprint arXiv:1905.03445 (2019)

Harmonization and Targeted Feature Dropout for Generalized Segmentation: Application to Multi-site Traumatic Brain Injury Images

Yilin Liu[1], Gregory R. Kirk[1], Brendon M. Nacewicz[1], Martin A. Styner[2,4], Mingren Shen[3], Dong Nie[4], Nagesh Adluru[1], Benjamin Yeske[1], Peter A. Ferrazzano[1], and Andrew L. Alexander[1(✉)]

[1] Waisman Laboratory for Brain Imaging and Behavior, University of Wisconsin-Madison, Madison, WI, USA
andy.alexander@wisc.edu
[2] Department of Psychiatry, University of North Carolina at Chapel Hill, Chapel Hill, USA
[3] Department of Materials Science and Engineering, University of Wisconsin-Madison, Madison, WI, USA
[4] Department of Computer Science, University of North Carolina at Chapel Chill, Chapel Hill, USA

Abstract. While learning based methods have brought extremely promising results in medical imaging, a major bottleneck is the lack of generalizability. Medical images are often collected from multiple sites and/or protocols for increasing statistical power, while CNN trained on one site typically cannot be well-transferred to others. Further, expert-defined manual labels for medical images are typically rare, making training a dedicated CNN for each site unpractical, so it is important to make best use of the limited labeled source data. To address this problem, we harmonize the target data using adversarial learning, and propose targeted feature dropout (TFD) to enhance the robustness of the model to variations in target images. Specifically, TFD is guided by attention to stochastically remove some of the most discriminative features. Essentially, this technique combines the benefits of attention mechanism and dropout, while it does not increase parameters and computational costs, making it well-suited for small neuroimaging datasets. We evaluated our method on a challenging Traumatic Brain Injury (TBI) dataset collected from 13 sites, using labeled source data of only 14 *healthy* subjects. Experimental results confirmed the feasibility of using the Cycle-consistent adversarial network for harmonizing multi-site MR images, and demonstrated that TFD further improved the generalization of the vanilla segmentation model on TBI data, reaching comparable accuracy with that of the supervised learning. The code is available at https://github.com/YilinLiu97/Targeted-Feature-Dropout.git.

© Springer Nature Switzerland AG 2019
Q. Wang et al. (Eds.): DART 2019/MIL3ID 2019, LNCS 11795, pp. 81–89, 2019.
https://doi.org/10.1007/978-3-030-33391-1_10

1 Introduction

Traumatic brain injury (TBI) is the leading cause of death or disability in children. For understanding the progression of TBI diseases, it is critical to accurately quantify the alterations in brain structures occurring after TBI. Although convolutional neural network (CNN) based methods have brought extremely promising results in various medical segmentation tasks, its application to TBI neuroimaging studies remains relatively less explored, probably due to two major challenges. First, TBI scans are typically acquired in multiple centers due to the heterogeneity of the injuries, while CNNs often fail to generalize well to out-of-distribution data from unseen sites due to image acquisition/protocol differences [2]. Second, the variations in brain change following a moderate or severe TBI make the segmentation task more challenging, and thus larger labeled training data is desired, which is often unfeasible in medical fields where expert-defined labels are rare. Therefore, re-using labels even from a different domain and making best use of them would be extremely useful. In this study, we focus on segmenting the amygdala which is mainly involved in emotional processing and has been identified as a potentially effective biomarker for symptoms in TBI, and present two strategies to address the above challenges respectively.

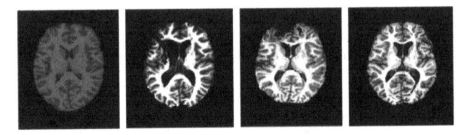

Fig. 1. Representative images from the source domain (a healthy subject, the leftmost) and target domains (TBI patients, the 3 rightmost)

Among the few studies explicitly on generalized segmentation in medical imaging, [2] retrains the model directly on multi-site data and [6] fine-tunes the batch normalization parameters of the model, both requiring additional labelled target images from the new sites. Another line of efforts aims to extract common feature representations of the source and target domain [5]. Nevertheless, the success of such models relies on an assumption that the domains are highly related [9], e.g., both domains consist of TBI subjects, which might limit its applicability to multiple distinct domains. This is particularly crucial in our application where the labeled source data came from *healthy* subjects instead of TBI patients. Thus, we instead harmonize the distribution of multi-site target data into source-like distribution using the cycle-consistent generative adversarial network (CycleGAN) [12]. Our method is among the first approaches to harmonize *multi-site* data using CycleGAN. This makes it possible to flexibly apply a pre-trained segmentation model directly to the adapted target images without prior assumptions on scanner/protocol deviations. In addition, most prior studies usually already have abundant labeled source data (N > 60) while we only have access to a very limited number of labeled images of *healthy* subjects (N ≈ 14). Therefore, besides adaptation, we also aim to enhance the robustness of the segmentation model to the structural changes of typical TBI subjects.

In a label-constraint setting, it is paramount to learn the most effective features that are transferable across different target domains. This is even more challenging in our application where images of TBI patients (target) usually contain abnormal structural characteristics compared to those of healthy subjects (source). Even though many of these abnormal features are not necessarily related to the ROIs to be segmented (e.g., amygdala, in our case), they could severely distract a trained model (Figs. 1 and 4(b)). An intuitive solution is to enhance the discriminative power of the segmentation model by emphasizing the most informative features and suppressing the irrelevant ones during training. Attention mechanism such as the Squeeze & Excitation (SE) blocks [4,8] have been proposed to reweight the features for this purpose. Furthermore, the ROIs themselves tend to vary more or less due to brain pathology. Although SE can generally improve the classification power, the features reweighted by such attention mechanisms alone are inherently source data-dependent and may not necessarily be robust to novel data with different characteristics as in our case. Moreover, these methods bring non-negligible parameters and computational overhead, increasing the risk of overfitting, which is not optimal for small datasets.

Therefore, we propose Targeted Feature Dropout (TFD) that can bias the segmentation model towards more discriminative and robust features at nearly *no cost*. Specifically, we first prioritize the most discriminative features by softly pruning the unimportant ones, which is similar in function to SE [4]. We then apply dropout primarily to features with *higher* importance to further enhance their robustness, based on an intuition that the same brain structures of different images may differ due to injuries, and thus features that are *critical* to model prediction in source images may be absent or vary in target images. Differs from random unit-wise dropout, TFD selectively erases some of the most discriminative features, guided by attention; it also highlights informative features, but unlike SE, it does not require extra trainable parameters to reweight the features but enforces sparsity in the parameter space by pruning unimportant features, which inherently helps generalization. Hence, TFD combines the advantages of attention mechanism and dropout, which makes it appealing especially to small datasets.

Overall, the contribution of this paper is two-fold: (1) the feasibility of applying CycleGAN to harmonize *multi-site* MRI data is evaluated, which enables the re-use of a pre-trained model on target images without the corresponding target labels. (2) we maximized the utility of the small labeled source dataset by exploiting the most effective features via TFD, further enhancing the robustness of the segmentation model more efficiently.

2   Method

2.1   Harmonization

Since the performance of deep learning models can be severely degraded due to data distribution shift, to bridge the distribution gap, we resort to CycleGAN to remap the distributions of targets to that of the source while preserving the original contents of the target images. Specifically, CycleGAN consists of two generators that learn two mappings respectively, $G_1 : S \rightarrow T$ and $G_2 : T \rightarrow S$, and two discriminators D_1, D_2 that distinguish the generated images from the real ones for each domain. In particular, we are interested in the generator G_2 that transforms the target images into realistic source-like images, i.e., $G_2(x^t) = x^{t \rightarrow s}$. The distribution of the target and source images are aligned by applying adversarial losses where G tries to confuse D by producing images that look realistic. Cycle-consistency losses [12] computated by l_1 distance are also applied to ensure the generated target images are similar to the original ones in contents. Thus, the transformed target images eventually obtained from the CycleGAN will be rendered as if they are drawn from the source domain, with the contents preserved. The total loss is defined as:

$$\mathcal{L}_{total}(G_1, G_2, D_1, D_2) = \mathcal{L}_{adv}(G_1, D_2) + \mathcal{L}_{adv}(G_2, D_1) + \lambda \mathcal{L}_{cyc}(G_1, G_2), \quad (1)$$

where λ is used to modulate the strength of the cycle consistency. In our experiments, we set λ to 10. We closely follow CycleGAN's setting for the choice of generators and discriminators (Fig. 2).

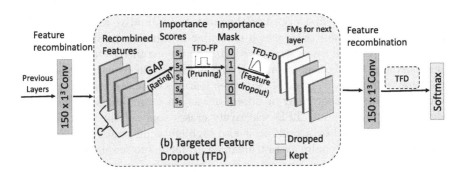

Fig. 2. Illustration of the proposed targeted feature dropout module. In order to remove the discriminative features more effectively, TFD is inserted at higher-level layers where features are class-specific, following feature recombination via $1 \times 1 \times 1$ convolutions.

2.2   Targeted Feature Dropout

Regular dropout drops random units, which has been shown to work well with fully-connected layers, but can be less effective in convolutional layers where units are spatially correlated within feature maps (FMs). That is, due to the correlated nature, features with randomly dropped pixels are very likely to be recovered by contextual information and still propagated to the subsequent layers, which diminishes the regularizing effects. Structural forms of dropout such as Spatial Dropout [10] and Dropblock [1] are therefore proposed, which drops either the entire or contiguous regions of the FMs randomly.

We extend this strategy by dropping the whole FM (i.e., feature-wise), but in a *selective* manner based on the importance of the FMs. In particular, dropout is guided by importance scores to stochastically remove some of the most discriminative features for enhancing robustness of the model to the variants of the same brain structures, hence the name Targeted Feature Dropout. Specifically, it consists of the following three steps:

Feature Rating. In order to guide the feature selection and dropout afterwards, we first assign each feature a score that indicates its importance. In particular, we only consider features in higher-level layers as they are generally more class-specific. Furthermore, we argue that instead of rating each individual FM, rating the *recombinations* of them may be more effective. Therefore, we insert TFD into the last two 1^3 convolutions which performs cross-channel expansion [7] to mix the information of FMs, $x = Conv_{1 \times 1 \times 1}(u)$, and then perform a 3D global average pooling over each 3D channel x_c, obtaining a score vector $z \in \mathbb{R}^{1 \times 1 \times 1 \times C}$,

$$z_c = \frac{1}{D \times W \times H} \sum_{i=1}^{D} \sum_{j=1}^{W} \sum_{k=1}^{H} x_c(i, j, k). \tag{2}$$

Each score describes the magnitude of each channel activation, which can approximate the discriminative power of each feature [11].

Pruning-Based Feature Prioritization. A binary importance mask is then generated to indicate which features to be highlighted/suppressed. This step is similar to the attention mechanisms which improves the classification power of the model by emphasizing the more discriminative features and ignoring features that are not directly related to the ROIs. Since it is likely that the low-valued FMs become important later during training, we select the FMs based on the probabilities $p_c = \frac{z_c}{\sum_{i=1}^{C} z_i}$: FMs with higher scores are more likely to be kept, i.e., masked as 1, and the others are temporarily masked to 0 but could still be updated in the next iteration, so-called soft pruning [3]. Specifically, the k FMs were drawn from a multinomial distribution, i.e., $X \sim Multi(M, P)$, where $X = (x_1, x_2, .., x_c)$ and $P = (p_1, p_2, ..., p_c)$. $k = N * keep\_ratio$, where N denotes the number of FMs and $keep\_ratio$ is a hyperparameter that indicates the targeted proportion of FMs that are considered to be important and used for dropout afterwards.

Feature Dropout. Now features have been filtered and the remaining ones with higher activations typically contain more important information. Since in our case, even features that are highly related to ROIs may vary in images of patients due to brain pathology, a drop mask is further applied specifically to these discriminative features with a drop_rate p to force the model to learn even without *some* important features, i.e., x_i that was masked as 1 now still has the probability p to be 0 (dropped).

Dynamic Hyperparameters. There are two main hyperparameters in TFD: targeted proportion *keep_ratio* and drop_rate p. We draw their values from certain distributions, which not only simplifies the choices of the hyperparameters but also encourages the model to be robust to different levels of noise. Specifically, *keep_ratio* is drawn from a uniform distribution with range [a, b] in each iteration, i.e., *keep_ratio* $\sim U(a, b)$. We empirically set the range to be [0.85, 0.9] in our experiments; p is drawn from a uniform distribution, i.e., $p \sim N(\mu, \sigma)$, where μ and σ are set to 0.2 and 0.05, respectively.

3   Experiments and Results

3.1   Datasets

We used 14 labeled local T1-weighted MRI studies (all GE MR750 scanner) with labeled bilateral amygdala as the source training data, and 21 unlabeled TBI data collected from 13 different sites as the target data. 3.0 T MRI scanners were used for all cases. Among the TBI scans, 9 of them came from nine different sites, 6 from three different sites and 6 from the remaining one site. Manual labeling of the TBI data was performed by an expert and are only used for evaluation purpose. All data are skull-stripped, and normalized to zero-mean, unit-variance.

3.2   Configuration Details

For harmonization, we train the CycleGAN on the coronal view of all the images from all domains. In total 3304 slices from the source data and 5900 slices from the TBI data are used for training. Each slice is then randomly cropped to 128×128 before being fed into the CycleGAN. Data augmentation includes random rotation and scaling. For the segmentation network backbone, we choose a 3D dual-path fully dilated convolutional network tailored specifically for segmentation of extremely small brain structures such as the amygdalae. Cross entropy was employed as the loss function, optimized via the Adam solver with a fixed learning rate of 0.001. For comparison only, we also trained a model using the labeled TBI data in a 7-fold cross validation scheme. We implemented our method in PyTorch, using one Titan Xp GPU for training.

3.3   Segmentation Results

We compared our method with both the channel-wise and spatial SE blocks, regular dropout and the supervised training. We further analyzed the proposed Targeted Feature Dropout by exploring the impact of the two components, (1) pruning-based feature prioritization, **denoted as TFD-FP**, (2) feature-wise dropout, **denoted as TFD-FD**, and compared their performance with the SE blocks and random unit-wise dropout, respectively. Results are summarized in Fig. 3 which is divided into block A, B and C for separate illustration of each point. Wilcoxon signed rank was used to compared the performance of different methods.

Harmonization. It can be observed from Table 1 that the harmonization using CycleGAN substantially improved the source model's performance on target data. We further augment the training set with synthetic target-like source images, which brought significant improvement ($p < 10^{-6}$). This then laid the foundation for all the other compared techniques.

Table 1. Dice overlap performance before and after harmonization using CycleGAN with/without texture variation. Results are averaged across 5 runs with random initializations.

	No harmonization	CycleGAN	CycleGAN - Aug
Dice	0.329 (0.123)	0.730 (0.015)	0.749 (0.008)

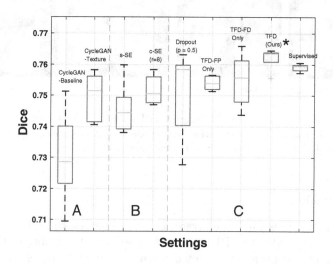

Fig. 3. Results for each technique are averaged across 5 runs with random initializations. * indicates that the proposed method is significant better than all the other settings ($p < 0.005$) and is comparable to the supervised training.

Comparisons with SE Blocks and Regular Dropout. For fair comparison, the spatial (s-SE) and channel-wise (c-SE) SE blocks and regular dropout are also inserted in the same place. As shown below in Fig. 3 (block B, C), TFD outperforms c-SE ($p < 0.005$), s-SE ($p < 10^{-6}$) and dropout ($p < 10^{-3}$), respectively, suggesting the superiority of combined advantages of attention mechanisms and dropout. Further, it is worth noting that TFD achieves the smallest variance in Dice, demonstrating its greater robustness.

Analysis of TFD. Here we evaluate the effectiveness of the two major components in the proposed method: (1) TFD-FP; (2) TFD-FD. From Fig. 3 (block C), we observed the following: (a) TFD-FP alone can generally improve the segmentation accuracy compared with the SE blocks. We believe that this is because softly pruning the unimportant features is similar in function to attention mechanisms which highlights the most informative features; also, (b) TFD-FP achieves much smaller variance, suggesting that keeping only the important features filters the noise, which helps reduce stochasticity during training; (c) TFD-FD performs better than random unit-wise dropout, showing the effectiveness of feature-wise regularization in convolutional layers; (d) when TFD-FP is coupled with TFD-FD, feature-wise dropout is performed selectively (i.e., TFD), yielding even higher accuracy and robustness (smallest variance). Overall, each component of the proposed TFD surpassed the baselines and contributed to the final improvement which is even slightly better than the supervised training directly on target data.

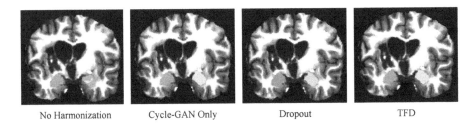

No Harmonization   Cycle-GAN Only   Dropout   TFD

Fig. 4. Qualitative results of a challenging TBI scan. An axial view of this scan is shown in Fig. 1 (the 2nd). Segmentation results are shown in **orange** and **yellow**, and the ground truths are shown in **green**. (Color figure online)

3.4   Conclusion

In this study, we presented two strategies to enable generalized segmentation on a challenging multi-site TBI dataset. To maximize the utility of the source labeled dataset, we proposed targeted feature dropout, a novel method that induces the CNN to learn robust features from healthy subjects as so to generalize well on patients data with different structural characteristics. The proposed method can be seamlessly integrated into any CNN to improve robustness with negligible computational costs. In addition, we confirmed the feasibility of harmonizing MRI scans collected from multiple sites using adversarial learning. The proposed method eventually achieved comparable or even better accuracy than the supervised training in the target domain using less data, suggesting that our method could greatly alleviate the burdensome annotation costs for multi-site data. For future works, we plan to replace CycleGAN with more advanced domain adaptation methods for further improving generalizability.

Acknowledgement. This work was supported by NARSAD: Brain and Behavior grant 24103 (to BN) and National Institutes of Health grant funding NINDS R01 NS092870, NIMH P50 MH100031 and a core grant to the Waisman Center from the National Institute of Child Health and Human Development (U54 HD090256). Disclosure Statement: A Alexander is part owner of Thervoyant, Inc. We gratefully acknowledge the support of NVIDIA Corporation with the donation of the Titan Xp and the Telsa K80 used for this research.

References

1. Ghiasi, G., Lin, T.Y., Le, Q.V.: DropBlock: a regularization method for convolutional networks. In: Advances in Neural Information Processing Systems, pp. 10727–10737 (2018)
2. Gibson, E., et al.: Inter-site variability in prostate segmentation accuracy using deep learning. In: Frangi, A.F., Schnabel, J.A., Davatzikos, C., Alberola-López, C., Fichtinger, G. (eds.) MICCAI 2018. LNCS, vol. 11073, pp. 506–514. Springer, Cham (2018). https://doi.org/10.1007/978-3-030-00937-3_58
3. He, Y., Kang, G., Dong, X., Fu, Y., Yang, Y.: Soft filter pruning for accelerating deep convolutional neural networks. arXiv preprint arXiv:1808.06866 (2018)
4. Hu, J., Shen, L., Sun, G.: Squeeze-and-excitation networks. In: Proceedings of the IEEE Conference on Computer Vision and Pattern Recognition, pp. 7132–7141 (2018)
5. Kamnitsas, K., et al.: Unsupervised domain adaptation in brain lesion segmentation with adversarial networks. In: Niethammer, M., et al. (eds.) IPMI 2017. LNCS, vol. 10265, pp. 597–609. Springer, Cham (2017). https://doi.org/10.1007/978-3-319-59050-9_47
6. Karani, N., Chaitanya, K., Baumgartner, C., Konukoglu, E.: A lifelong learning approach to brain MR segmentation across scanners and protocols. In: Frangi, A.F., Schnabel, J.A., Davatzikos, C., Alberola-López, C., Fichtinger, G. (eds.) MICCAI 2018. LNCS, vol. 11070, pp. 476–484. Springer, Cham (2018). https://doi.org/10.1007/978-3-030-00928-1_54
7. Lin, M., Chen, Q., Yan, S.: Network in network. arXiv preprint arXiv:1312.4400 (2013)
8. Roy, A.G., Navab, N., Wachinger, C.: Concurrent spatial and channel squeeze & excitationin fully convolutional networks. In: Frangi, A., Schnabel, J., Davatzikos, C., Alberola-López, C., Fichtinger, G. (eds.) MICCAI 2018. LNCS, pp. 421–429. Springer, Cham (2018). https://doi.org/10.1007/978-3-030-00928-1_48
9. Shu, R., Bui, H.H., Narui, H., Ermon, S.: A DIRT-T approach to unsupervised domain adaptation. arXiv preprint arXiv:1802.08735 (2018)
10. Tompson, J., Goroshin, R., Jain, A., LeCun, Y., Bregler, C.: Efficient object localization using convolutional networks. In: Proceedings of the IEEE Conference on Computer Vision and Pattern Recognition, pp. 648–656 (2015)
11. Zhou, B., Khosla, A., Lapedriza, A., Oliva, A., Torralba, A.: Learning deep features for discriminative localization. In: Proceedings of the IEEE Conference on Computer Vision and Pattern Recognition, pp. 2921–2929 (2016)
12. Zhu, J.Y., Park, T., Isola, P., Efros, A.A.: Unpaired image-to-image translation using cycle-consistent adversarial networks. In: Proceedings of the IEEE International Conference on Computer Vision, pp. 2223–2232 (2017)

Improving Pathological Structure Segmentation via Transfer Learning Across Diseases

Barleen Kaur[1,2,4]([⊠]), Paul Lemaître[2], Raghav Mehta[2],
Nazanin Mohammadi Sepahvand[2], Doina Precup[1,4], Douglas Arnold[3,5],
and Tal Arbel[2]

[1] School of Computer Science, McGill University, Montreal, Canada
barleen.kaur@mail.mcgill.ca
[2] Centre for Intelligent Machines, McGill University, Montreal, Canada
[3] Montreal Neurological Institute, McGill University, Montreal, Canada
[4] Mila Quebec AI Institute, Montreal, Canada
[5] NeuroRx Research, Montreal, Canada

Abstract. One of the biggest challenges in developing robust machine learning techniques for medical image analysis is the lack of access to large-scale annotated image datasets needed for supervised learning. When the task is to segment pathological structures (e.g. lesions, tumors) from patient images, training on a dataset with few samples is very challenging due to the large class imbalance and inter-subject variability. In this paper, we explore how to best leverage a segmentation model that has been pre-trained on a large dataset of patients images with one disease in order to successfully train a deep learning pathology segmentation model for a different disease, for which only a relatively small patient dataset is available. Specifically, we train a UNet model on a large-scale, proprietary, multi-center, multi-scanner Multiple Sclerosis (MS) clinical trial dataset containing over 3500 multi-modal MRI samples with expert-derived lesion labels. We explore several transfer learning approaches to leverage the learned MS model for the task of multi-class brain tumor segmentation on the BraTS 2018 dataset. Our results indicate that adapting and fine-tuning the encoder and decoder of the network trained on the larger MS dataset leads to improvement in brain tumor segmentation when few instances are available. This type of transfer learning outperforms training and testing the network on the BraTS dataset from scratch as well as several other transfer learning approaches, particularly when only a small subset of the dataset is available.

Keywords: Transfer learning · Brain tumor segmentation · MRI

Electronic supplementary material The online version of this chapter (https://doi.org/10.1007/978-3-030-33391-1_11) contains supplementary material, which is available to authorized users.

Q. Wang et al. (Eds.): DART 2019/MIL3ID 2019, LNCS 11795, pp. 90–98, 2019.
https://doi.org/10.1007/978-3-030-33391-1_11

1   Introduction

An important challenge in developing robust pathology segmentation methods in medical imaging is the lack of access to sufficiently large annotated datasets needed for training. Large datasets are required for a number of reasons. First, many of the state-of-art models are based on deep learning methods, which perform well when trained on large datasets [6,13]. Second, pathological structures (e.g. lesions, tumors) tend to be present in only small parts of an image, leading to large class imbalance, and also presents with high variability between patients, exacerbating the need to have annotations for many patients. Unfortunately, larger proprietary datasets cited in the literature are not always available for public use and public labelled pathology segmentation datasets are often relatively small.

To overcome this problem, transfer learning has recently been explored in various medical imaging applications, including classification [9], detection [10] and segmentation [7] tasks (see [4] for a survey). Investigated tasks include using data acquired from different scanners [7] or detection of different types of abnormality in the same set of data [22]. It has also been shown that knowledge could be transferred from both medical and non-medical datasets to improve results in other medical applications [8,15]. Deep networks trained on a larger source dataset have been used as feature extractors [9] or as a starting point for fine-tuning further on target data [20].

This paper explores the hypothesis that transfer learning for the segmentation of pathological structures can be performed across diseases. Specifically, we leverage a deep learning segmentation network pre-trained on a large pathology segmentation dataset, in order to improve segmentation performance on a small dataset, in a scenario in which: (a) the two image datasets are acquired from patients with different diseases, (b) the pathological structures are different in the two datasets (lesions vs. tumors), and (c) the inference tasks themselves differ (binary vs. multi-class segmentation). We explore several fine-tuning strategies to see how to best leverage the source model and adapt it to the target dataset, including: freezing the network and only retraining the last few layers, fine-tuning only the decoder, or carefully fine-tuning the entire network.

Experimental validation of the methods involves first pre-training a binary classifier for the segmentation of T2 lesions based on a large proprietary, multi-scanner, multi-center, longitudinal clinical trial, MRI dataset of 1385 patients with relapsing-remitting Multiple Sclerosis (RRMS), along with expert-labelled T2 lesions. Next, a series of experiments are performed in order to explore the ability of transfer learning to improve the results of an end-to-end multi-class brain tumor segmentation network trained on subsets of the MICCAI 2018 BraTS dataset [16]. Given that both MRI datasets are acquired from patients with neurological diseases that present with focal pathologies (lesions and tumors), the intuition is that the two dataset share common features. As such, the framework should be able to leverage the representation learned by the lesion segmentation network trained on the bigger MS dataset to improve the segmentation results on the smaller brain tumor dataset.

2   Methodology

We use a 3D deep neural network inspired by UNet [6] for the task of focal pathology segmentation. It consists of an encoder followed by a decoder which combines higher resolution features from the contracting path at different levels, in order to learn multi-scale representations. The architecture is depicted in Fig. 1(a), and the implementation details of the model are described in Sect. 3.2.

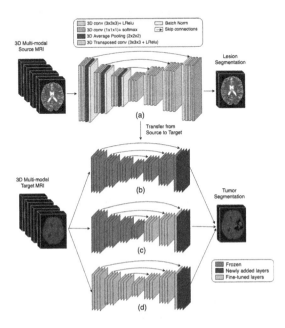

Fig. 1. Transfer learning framework. (a) UNet architecture for pre-trained source network. (b), (c) and (d) depict different methods of adapting the pre-trained source network for the target task. In all three, the last three task-specific layers are replaced with new layers (orange) and the remaining network is fine-tuned such that: (b) only the newly added layers are re-trained (FT-Last Three), (c) only the decoder is fine-tuned (FT-Decoder) and (d) the whole network is fine-tuned (FT-All) with the target data respectively. (Color figure online)

Given a source network trained from scratch on a large source dataset, the objective is to transfer the representation learned by the source network and adapt it to the (smaller) target set in order to improve pathology segmentation performance. A popular strategy for transfer learning consists of fine-tuning the pre-trained source network on the target dataset. In this paper, we explore three different strategies of fine-tuning. The most common way of fine-tuning consists of replacing the last few layers of the source network with new layers, by re-initializing the weights and changing the output dimension of these layers. The remainder of the network is frozen, which prevents the gradient flow. The newly added layers are trained on the target dataset (See Fig. 1(b)). This strategy has been advocated when the amount of target data available is small and the similarity between the two datasets is high [7], as in the context explored in this paper. The intuition behind this approach is that the initial layers of the network tend to learn low level image features (e.g. edges, orientations) that are generic and therefore useful across different datasets and tasks, while the higher layers of the network tend to capture more complex patterns that are specific to a particular task. When the source and target datasets are similar, and/or more target data is available, more layers can be fine-tuned [5, 21]. This leads to the second strategy we explore, which involves freezing the encoder and fine-tuning the entire decoder (See Fig. 1(c)). The third strategy consists of fine-tuning the whole network with target data (See Fig. 1(d)).

3 Experiments and Results

In order to assess the performance of the three different transfer learning approaches in the context of pathology segmentation, we perform experiments using a large source dataset of MS patients, in which the segmentation network is trained to label lesions. The target task is to segment brain tumors and their tissue sub-classes from patient MRI. We compare the performance of the transfer learning approach to training only on the target data, for different dataset sizes. The segmentation performance is assessed using Dice scores.

3.1 Data Description and Preprocessing

Multiple Sclerosis Dataset (Source): The source task involves a binary classification to differentiate T2 hyperintense lesions from healthy tissues in a proprietary, multi-modal MRI dataset acquired from Multiple Sclerosis (MS) patients participating in a multi-site, multi-scanner clinical trial. The dataset consists of 1385 patients, scanned annually for up to a 24-month period, totalling 3630 multi-sequence 3D MRI samples consisting of T1-weighted, T2-weighted, Fluid Attenuated Inverse Recovery (FLAIR), and T1 post-Gadolinium sequences acquired at $1\,\text{mm} \times 1\,\text{mm} \times 3\,\text{mm}$ resolution. They are then interpolated to $1\,\text{mm}^3$ isotropic resolution, which results in MRIs of size $229 \times 193 \times 193$. T2 binary lesion segmentation masks provided with the dataset are obtained through expert manual corrections as a result of a proprietary automatic segmentation method. Preprocessing includes brain extraction [19], N3 bias field in homogeneity correction [18], Nyul image intensity normalization [17], and registration to the MNI-space.

Brain Tumor Dataset (Target): The target datasets are obtained by subsampling datasets of various sizes from the BraTS 2018 MICCAI challenge [2, 3, 16]. The entire training dataset consists of 210 high-grade glioma (HGG) and 75 low-grade glioma (LGG) patients and the validation set consists of 66 patients. Each sample contains T1-w, T1 post contrast (T1c), T2-w, and FLAIR 3D MR sequences. Ground truth segmentation labels are provided for the BraTS Training set (used for training the network) but not for the BraTS Validation set[1] (used for testing). Tumors are segmented into 3 classes: edema, necrotic/non-enhancing core, and enhancing tumor. These three classes combined together are referred to as "whole" tumor. The volumes are co-registered, resampled to $1\,mm^3$ resolution and skull-stripped. Our pre-processing pipeline includes registration of samples to the same space as MS data using ANTs tool [1].

For both MS Dataset and Brain Tumor Dataset, the image intensities are then standardized using mean subtraction, division by standard deviation, and rescaled to range from 0 to 1. The images are standardized to $240 \times 192 \times 192$ using zero-padding and cropping operations.

3.2   Model Implementation Details

The proposed segmentation network takes 3D patient MRI sequences as input and generates a 3D output mask of the same resolution. As is typical of a 3D UNet [6,14], the network consists of an encoder part and a decoder part of 4 resolution steps each. The encoder part consists of two consecutive 3D convolutions of size $3 \times 3 \times 3$ with $k*2^{(n-1)}$ filters, where n is the resolution step and k is the initial number of filters (4 in our case). Each convolution is followed by a leaky rectified linear unit (L-ReLU). Average pooling of size $2 \times 2 \times 2$ and stride of 2 is performed followed by Batch normalization [11]. In the decoder part, each step consists of 3D transposed convolutions of size $3 \times 3 \times 3$ with $2 \times 2 \times 2$ stride and $k*2^{(n-1)}$ filters for upsampling, whose output is concatenated with the corresponding output of the encoder part. Batch normalization is applied again following which, two $3 \times 3 \times 3$ convolutions with L-ReLU activation are applied. The last layer consists of $1 \times 1 \times 1$ convolution with F filters, where F denotes the number of classes for the task, followed by a SoftMax non-linearity. The implementation of the model is done in Pytorch.[2]

Segmenting MS lesions is a binary voxel-wise classification task whereas brain tumor sub-type segmentation is a 4-class voxel-wise classification task [16]. For lesion segmentation, the training objective is weighted binary cross entropy loss (to account for class imbalance). For the multi-class brain tumor segmentation task, the training objective is weighted categorical cross entropy loss. The weight of a class c is calculated as the ratio of the total number of voxels divided by the number of voxels belonging to class c in the training set. The class weights are scheduled to decay [12] with a decay rate lower than 1. As the number of epochs increase, the weight for each class converges to 1, ensuring that every class is given equal importance during the later stages of training.

---

[1] Please note that the predictions made on the BraTS 2018 Validation set must contain all four tumor sub-classes, which are then uploaded onto the BraTS web portal for evaluation.

[2] http://pytorch.org/.

3.3   Experiments

As described in Sect. 2, the baseline experiment consists of training a network from scratch on the brain tumor dataset. The other three experiments use a network trained on the MS dataset from scratch, which is then fine-tuned using the three transfer learning approaches discussed above and denoted as FT-Last Three, FT-Decoder, FT-All in Fig. 1. When pre-training the MS lesion segmentation network, 80% of the MS data (2912 samples) is used for training, and the remaining 20% is left out for validation (718 samples) for 190 epochs. The best validation performance of the pre-trained network is obtained at epoch 186 with an AUC of 0.77.

In order to examine the effect of the size of the target dataset on the transfer learning outcome, the number of patient brain tumor MRI samples extracted from the BraTS 2018 training dataset and used in the target dataset is set to several values: 20, 50, 100, 150. For each case, the fine-tuned networks are compared to the corresponding baseline network. For all experiments, the ratio of high-grade gliomas (HGG) to low-grade gliomas (LGG) is maintained across folds. Four-fold cross validation is performed on the respective training sets to determine the best parameters (see Supplementary Materials[3] document for more information on hyper-parameter tuning). Then, the networks are retrained on the respective complete training sets, using the hyper-parameters that performed best during cross-validation and a local validation set (subset of BraTS 2018 training set) of 50 samples is used to select the operating point. Performance is evaluated on the separate BraTS 2018 Validation set, for which the ground truth is not available.

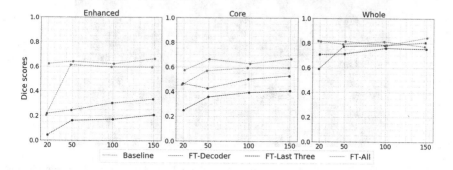

Fig. 2. Comparison of Dice values for baseline method against different fine-tuning methods for enhanced, core and whole tumor segmentation on the Brats 2018 validation set. The x-axis depicts a varying number of brain tumor cases available for training (20, 50, 100, 150).

---

[3] http://cim.mcgill.ca/~barleenk/MICCAI2019_transfer_appendix.pdf.

3.4 Results

Figure 2 summarizes all the Dice scores obtained on the BraTS 2018 validation set for the baseline and various transfer learning methods, as a function of the number of brain tumor cases available for fine-tuning. The epoch for which the sum of the Dice scores is best on the local validation set, is selected as an operating point. The results indicate that FT-All outperforms the baseline results in almost every case and consistently provides the best Dice scores for core and enhanced tumor, particularly when the number of tumor cases is extremely low, with 25.9% and 204.09% improvement[4] on core and enhanced tumor over baseline respectively when the number of cases is 20. See Supplementary Materials document for more results. Since lesions are smaller in size when compared to tumors, the results indicate that the network is extracting information from the MS pre-trained network that is relevant to segmenting sub-regions of tumor well, even though lesions present quite differently than brain tumors. As the number of brain tumor samples increase, the gain of FT-All over baseline diminishes. FT-Last Three and FT-Decoder don't perform as well as the baseline. This is likely due to low-level representations not getting updated as per the target task, which in turn fuse with high level representations in the UNet to produce an output. Qualitative segmentation results of the different methods on the local

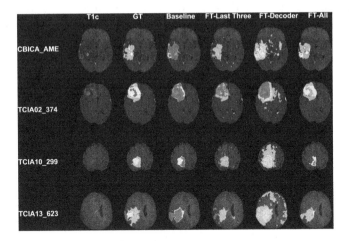

Fig. 3. Examples of visualizations obtained on a local validation set when fine-tuning with 20 BraTS samples for 4 patients (IDs on left). Top two rows and bottom two rows illustrate the segmentation results obtained on HGG and LGG cases respectively. From left to right: T1c MRI (column 1), ground truth segmentation (column 2), results of baseline experiment (column 3), FT-Last Three (column 4), FT-Decoder (column 5) and FT-All (column 6) are shown. Edema, necrotic core and enhancing tumor are shown in green, red and yellow respectively. (Color figure online)

---

[4] The percentage improvement is calculated as the ratio of difference in the baseline and FT-All Dice scores over the baseline.

validation set for the case of 20 target dataset samples are shown in Fig. 3. Note that with just 20 target dataset samples, FT-All is able to capture different substructures of tumor better than the other methods. Performance is better on the HGG over the LGG cases, as more HGG cases are present in the training dataset. More results are presented in the Supplementary Materials document.

4   Conclusions

In this work, we explore different strategies for transfer learning across diseases for the task of focal pathology segmentation. Fine-tuning the entire network trained on a larger MS dataset improves the multi-class brain tumor segmentation results on target MRI datasets, outperforming the baseline method and the other fine-tuning methods, especially when only very small target datasets are available. This outcome indicates that transfer learning methods can have a significant impact, particularly for diseases where there is little access to large scale, annotated datasets needed for training segmentation networks. The public release of more models that have been pre-trained on large proprietary datasets (e.g. where it is not possible to release the images themselves) will permit the community to leverage them for the large set of applications with small datasets.

Acknowledgments. The MS dataset was provided through an award from the International Progressive MS Alliance (PA-1603-08175). The authors would also like to thank Nicholas J. Tustison for his guidance on using ANTs tool.

References

1. Avants, B.B., et al.: A reproducible evaluation of ANTs similarity metric performance in brain image registration. Neuroimage **54**(3), 2033–2044 (2011)
2. Bakas, S., et al.: Advancing the cancer genome atlas glioma MRI collections with expert segmentation labels and radiomic features. Sci. Data **4**, 170117 (2017)
3. Bakas, S., et al.: Segmentation labels and radiomic features for the pre-operative scans of the TCGA-LGG collection. TCIA, vol. 286 (2017)
4. Cheplygina, V., et al.: Not-so-supervised: a survey of semi-supervised, multi-instance, and transfer learning in medical image analysis. MIA **54**, 280–296 (2019)
5. Chu, B., Madhavan, V., Beijbom, O., Hoffman, J., Darrell, T.: Best practices for fine-tuning visual classifiers to new domains. In: Hua, G., Jégou, H. (eds.) ECCV 2016. LNCS, vol. 9915, pp. 435–442. Springer, Cham (2016). https://doi.org/10.1007/978-3-319-49409-8_34
6. Çiçek, Ö., Abdulkadir, A., Lienkamp, S.S., Brox, T., Ronneberger, O.: 3D U-Net: learning dense volumetric segmentation from sparse annotation. In: Ourselin, S., Joskowicz, L., Sabuncu, M.R., Unal, G., Wells, W. (eds.) MICCAI 2016. LNCS, vol. 9901, pp. 424–432. Springer, Cham (2016). https://doi.org/10.1007/978-3-319-46723-8_49
7. Ghafoorian, M., et al.: Transfer learning for domain adaptation in MRI: application in brain lesion segmentation. In: Descoteaux, M., Maier-Hein, L., Franz, A., Jannin, P., Collins, D.L., Duchesne, S. (eds.) MICCAI 2017. LNCS, vol. 10435, pp. 516–524. Springer, Cham (2017). https://doi.org/10.1007/978-3-319-66179-7_59

8. Hussein, S., Cao, K., Song, Q., Bagci, U.: Risk stratification of lung nodules using 3D CNN-based multi-task learning. In: Niethammer, M., et al. (eds.) IPMI 2017. LNCS, vol. 10265, pp. 249–260. Springer, Cham (2017). https://doi.org/10.1007/978-3-319-59050-9_20

9. Huynh, B.Q., et al.: Digital mammographic tumor classification using transfer learning from deep convolutional neural networks. JMI **3**(3), 034501 (2016)

10. Hwang, S., Kim, H.-E.: Self-transfer learning for weakly supervised lesion localization. In: Ourselin, S., Joskowicz, L., Sabuncu, M.R., Unal, G., Wells, W. (eds.) MICCAI 2016. LNCS, vol. 9901, pp. 239–246. Springer, Cham (2016). https://doi.org/10.1007/978-3-319-46723-8_28

11. Ioffe, S., et al.: Batch normalization: accelerating deep network training by reducing internal covariate shift. arXiv preprint arXiv:1502.03167 (2015)

12. Jesson, A., Arbel, T.: Brain tumor segmentation using a 3D FCN with multi-scale loss. In: Crimi, A., Bakas, S., Kuijf, H., Menze, B., Reyes, M. (eds.) BrainLes 2017. LNCS, vol. 10670, pp. 392–402. Springer, Cham (2018). https://doi.org/10.1007/978-3-319-75238-9_34

13. Kamnitsas, K., et al.: Efficient multi-scale 3D CNN with fully connected CRF for accurate brain lesion segmentation. MIA **36**, 61–78 (2017)

14. Mehta, R., Arbel, T.: 3D U-Net for brain tumour segmentation. In: Crimi, A., Bakas, S., Kuijf, H., Keyvan, F., Reyes, M., van Walsum, T. (eds.) BrainLes 2018. LNCS, vol. 11384, pp. 254–266. Springer, Cham (2019). https://doi.org/10.1007/978-3-030-11726-9_23

15. Menegola, A., et al.: Knowledge transfer for melanoma screening with deep learning. ISBI **2017**, 297–300 (2017)

16. Menze, B.H., et al.: The multimodal brain tumor image segmentation benchmark (BraTS). TMI **34**(10), 1993–2024 (2014)

17. Nyúl, L.G., et al.: New variants of a method of MRI scale standardization. TMI **19**(2), 143–150 (2000)

18. Sled, J.G., et al.: A nonparametric method for automatic correction of intensity nonuniformity in MRI data. TMI **17**(1), 87–97 (1998)

19. Smith, S.M.: Fast robust automated brain extraction. HBM **17**(3), 143–155 (2002)

20. Tajbakhsh, N., et al.: Convolutional neural networks for medical image analysis: full training or fine tuning? IEEE TMI **35**(5), 1299–1312 (2016)

21. Yosinski, J., et al.: How transferable are features in deep neural networks? In: Proceeding of NIPS, pp. 3320–3328 (2014)

22. Zhang, D., Shen, D., Alzheimer's Disease Neuroimaging Initiative: Multi-modal multi-task learning for joint prediction of multiple regression and classification variables in Alzheimer's disease. NeuroImage, **59**(2), 895–907 (2012)

Generating Virtual Chromoendoscopic Images and Improving Detectability and Classification Performance of Endoscopic Lesions

Akihiro Fukuda[1(✉)], Tadashi Miyamoto[1], Shunsuke Kamba[2],
and Kazuki Sumiyama[2]

[1] Research and Development Department, LPixel Inc., Tokyo, Japan
fukuda@lpixel.net
[2] Department of Endoscopy, The Jikei University School of Medicine, Tokyo, Japan

Abstract. Endoscopy is a standard method for the diagnosis and detection of colorectal lesions. As a method to enhance the detectability of lesions, the effectiveness of pancolonic chromoendoscopy with indigocarmine has been reported. On the other hand, computer-aided diagnosis (CAD) has attracted attention. However, existing CAD systems are mainly for white light imaging (WLI) endoscopy, and the effect of the combination of CAD and indigocarmine dye spraying is not clear. Besides, it is difficult to gather a lot of indigocarmine dye-sprayed (IC) images for training. Here, we propose image-to-image translation from WLI to virtual indigocarmine dye-sprayed (VIC) images based on unpaired cycle-consistent Generative Adversarial Networks. Using this generator as preprocess part, we constructed detection models to evaluate the effectiveness of VIC translation for localization and classification of lesions. We also compared the localization and classification performance with and without image augmentation by using generated VIC images. Our results show that the model trained on IC and VIC images had the highest performance in both localization and classification. Therefore, VIC images are useful for the augmentation of IC images.

1 Introduction

Medical doctors use endoscopy as the gold standard method to detect digestive lesions. To reduce colorectal cancer deaths, early detection and resection of colorectal adenomas are very important. It has been reported that future colorectal cancer death of the patient would increase significantly if the colonoscopy was performed by an endoscopist with low adenoma detection rate (ADR) [4, 7]. However, it is reported that the adenoma miss rate by conventional colonoscopy

---

A. Fukuda and T. Miyamoto—Contributed equally to this work.

© Springer Nature Switzerland AG 2019
Q. Wang et al. (Eds.): DART 2019/MIL3ID 2019, LNCS 11795, pp. 99–107, 2019.
https://doi.org/10.1007/978-3-030-33391-1_12

is about 20% [2,9]. In addition, previous studies have also found that virtual chromoendoscopy such as Narrow Band Imaging (NBI) and Fujinon Intelligent Chromoendoscopy (FICE) do not improve the adenoma detection rate in comparison with conventional white light imaging (WLI) [1,11,15]. In contrast, pancolonic chromoendoscopy with indigocarmine spraying is reported as effective method increasing the detection rate of colorectal lesions [12].

Computer-aided diagnosis (CAD) is an alternative technology that can be a solution for the low lesion detection rate. A number of studies on automatic polyp detection have been recently reported [8,10,16,17]. However, most published works are trained and evaluated on a small dataset. Moreover, inputs of CAD systems are mostly normal WLI images. One of the reasons is that it is challenging to obtain sufficient dye-sprayed images compared to WLI images. Therefore, it is not clear whether the simultaneous use of dye spraying and CAD system produce the synergistic effect for lesion detection.

In the field of image-to-image translation, Generative Adversarial Networks (GANs) have shown effective results. Recent approaches use Convolutional Neural Networks (CNNs) to learn a parametric translation function. For example, frameworks such as pix2pix require paired images in learning process [6]. On the other hand, frameworks such as DualGAN and CycleGAN can use unpaired images [18,20]. These frameworks translate an image from one domain to another domain and vice versa. As an example of applications to medical image, temp-CycleGAN is reported [5]. It translates a silicone phantom image to real intraoperative image in mitral valve surgery. However, no studies are applying it to endoscopic image enhancement methods such as chromoendoscopy. Also, it is unclear whether this image enhancement technology by using image-to-image translation can be effective preprocess for the colorectal lesions detection model.

In this paper, we propose image-to-image translation from WLI images to virtual indigocarmine dye-sprayed (VIC) images. By using this generator, we constructed detection models of colorectal lesions and validated these CAD systems.

2   Methods

2.1   Image-to-Image Translation

WLI and indigocarmine dye-sprayed (IC) images cannot be taken simultaneously in a clinical setting. Therefore, in this work, the image-to-image translation model was constructed from unpaired images by using CycleGAN [20].

CycleGAN consists of two generators G_1, G_2 and two discriminators D_1, D_2. Generators convert from WLI to IC images and vice versa. The role of each discriminator is to distinguish between real images and converted images.

The loss of CycleGAN consists of the discriminator loss and the cycle consistency loss. In CycleGAN, training process has circular translation flow like the translation from WLI to WLI via IC. The cycle consistency loss expresses differences between an original image and a circularly translated image. This architecture enables CycleGAN to train image-to-image translation by using unpaired images.

2.2   Lesion Detection Model

Any object detection method could be applicable to images generated by Cycle-GAN. However, for real-time lesion detection such as routine endoscopy, high-speed detection is required. In this work, we use YOLOv3 architecture which is a real-time object detector with good precision and speed of detection [13]. Inputs of the neural network are real images or virtual images generated by CycleGAN, and the output is a set of detections (bounding boxes with their respective confidences and class labels).

In addition, we set initial parameters using ImageNet pre-trained model to achieve fast convergence in all cases. For data augmentation, we use random horizontal flips, random resizing, random aspect ratio, random translation, and random erasing [19]. Prediction speed (CycleGAN + YOLOv3) is over 30 fps on TITAN V with the input image size of $512 \times 512 \times 3$.

2.3   Evaluation Metrics

Our detection models localize and classify lesions simultaneously. Thus, we have to evaluate both localization and classification. We then use Average Precision (AP) of localization at intersection-of-union (IoU) threshold of 0.5 (AP_L), AP of the lesion type classification ($AP_{C(A)}, AP_{C(B)}, AP_{C(F)}$), and mean Average Precision of classification (mAP_C). mAP_C is the mean of $AP_{C(A)}, AP_{C(B)}, AP_{C(F)}$, which means the measurement of overall localization performance in three different lesion types (A: cancer, B: adenoma, F: non-tumor).

3   Experiments and Results

3.1   Generating Virtual Indigocarmine Image

We trained CycleGAN by using all WLI and IC images as shown in Table 1. All images were collected in the Jikei university hospital (Tokyo, Japan) from 2017 to 2018. Using these images, we trained the model for 100 epochs. After training, we generated translated IC images from WLI images. We called these translated IC images as virtual indigocarmine (VIC) images in order to differentiate it from original IC images.

To test the VIC image generation, we used paired WLI and IC images of identical lesions taken from similar angles and compared the condition of indigo-carmine dye spraying to the lesions between IC and VIC images. These images are not completely matched because the endoscopy moves during indigocarmine dye spraying.

Compared VIC image with original WLI image, the innominate grooves were dyed blue, and the reddish area of lesions became clearer as shown in Fig. 1. In

Table 1. The number of images for train and test dataset. Each lesion label indicates a type of lesions; A: cancer, B: adenoma, F: non-tumor.

	WLI			IC			VIC		
Label	Train	Test	Total	Train	Test	Total	Train	Test	Total
A	1802	100	1902	918	100	1018	1802	100	1902
B	10377	100	10477	3840	100	3940	10377	100	10477
F	1038	100	1138	451	100	551	1038	100	1138
Total	13317	300	13617	5209	300	5509	13317	300	13617

the case of flat lesions, some grooves were dyed blue, but the lesion was not dyed as shown in Fig. 1(b). This emphasized a boundary between the lesion and normal tissue as the IC image (see Fig. 1(b, d)). However, in VIC images, there was no pooling of indigocarmine unlike real IC images because of no need for spraying indigocarmine (see the white arrow in Fig. 1(f, h)). Therefore, VIC images could provide better visual quality than IC images.

We also tried to generate virtual WLI (VWLI) images from IC images by using trained generator G_2. In translated VWLI image, blue coloration of indigocarmine vanished, and redness in the entire image increased as shown in Fig. 1(c, g).

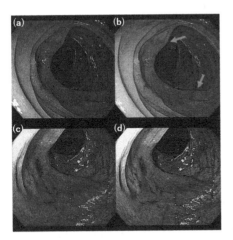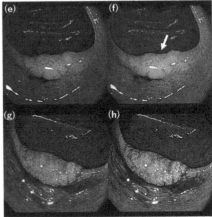

Fig. 1. Visual comparison of (a, e): WLI, (b, f): VIC, (c, g): VWLI, and (d, h): IC. Images (a)–(d) are in the cases of a flat lesion, and Images (e)–(h) are in the cases of a depressed lesion. Yellow arrows in (b) indicate a boundary between the lesion and normal tissue. White arrow in (f) indicates a depression of the lesion. (Color figure online)

3.2 The Effect of VIC Translation in the Lesion Detection

To validate the effectiveness of WLI-to-VIC image translation for localizing and classifying colorectal lesions, we generated VIC images from train dataset of WLI images and trained the model by using it (VIC model). We also constructed a model trained on WLI images (WLI model) to compare the performance of localization and classification with VIC model. Train and test dataset was annotated with bounding box and the class label of three lesion types: cancer, adenoma, and non-tumor. The number of images is as shown in Table 1.

Table 2 shows the evaluation results of the VIC model. Comparing two models, both AP_L and mAP_C of WLI model were higher than that of the VIC model. However, focusing on the performance of classification in each lesion type, only $AP_{C(A)}$ of the VIC model was higher than that of the WLI model. Inversely, $AP_{C(F)}$ of the WLI model was much higher than that of the VIC model, and this difference affected the difference of mAP_C. On the other hand, $AP_{C(B)}$ of both models was low, and there was not much difference.

Table 2. Average precision of lesion localization and classification. AP_L: AP of localization, mAP_C: mean Average Precision of classification, $AP_{C(A)}$: AP of cancer classification, $AP_{C(B)}$: AP of adenoma classification, $AP_{C(F)}$: AP of non-tumor classification.

Train data	WLI	VIC	IC	IC+VIC	IC+WLI
Test data	WLI	VIC		IC	
Localization score: AP_L	0.916	0.876	0.910	0.922	0.897
Classification score of all types: mAP_C	0.635	0.603	0.721	0.733	0.711
Classification score of cancer: $AP_{C(A)}$	0.656	0.720	0.758	0.794	0.776
Classification score of adenoma: $AP_{C(B)}$	0.508	0.486	0.674	0.645	0.601
Classification score of non-tumor: $AP_{C(F)}$	0.743	0.604	0.732	0.760	0.755

Here, we show some results of comparing lesion detection as shown in Fig. 2. In the cases of Fig. 2(a, b), VIC translation deteriorated the detection performance. The redness of the lesion was slightly lighter than that of normal tissue in WLI images. However, the entire image got light in VIC images, which eliminated such slight differences. We could also see blood vessels in WLI images, but it became vague in VIC images. Besides, these VIC images got noisier than WLI images. In contrast, VIC translation improved the detection performance in some cases such as Fig. 2(c, d).

3.3 Augmentation Effect of VIC Images

To verify the usefulness of VIC images for data augmentation, we constructed three models: (i) trained only on IC images; (ii) trained on both IC and VIC images; and (iii) trained on both IC and WLI images. Table 1 shows the number of images for training.

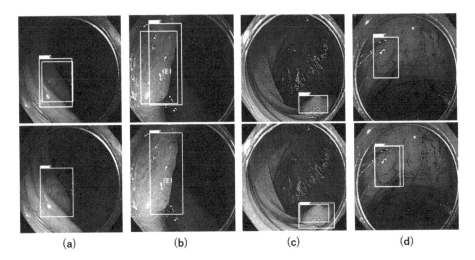

Fig. 2. Detection comparison between WLI and VIC models. Upper row is detection results of WLI model, and lower row is detection results of VIC model. The white and green bounding boxes represent ground truth and detection results, respectively. In the cases of (a) and (b), detection results are deteriorated in VIC model. In contrast, in the cases of (c) and (d), detection results are improved in VIC model. (Color figure online)

Using these trained models, we evaluated the performance of localization and classification against IC images as test data. Table 2 shows the evaluation results. Compared with the IC model, IC+VIC model was high performance in both localization and classification. However, only the performance of adenoma classification ($AP_{C(B)}$) in IC model was higher than that of the VIC model. On the other hand, both AP_L and mAP_C in IC+WLI model were the worst score among three models even though the number of images was much larger than the IC model. Therefore, we found that just adding WLI images was not effective for data augmentation and translating to VIC images were required for performance improvement.

4   Discussion

In this study, we constructed a WLI-to-VIC image generator and vice versa. Generated VIC images were so real that we could not distinguish whether it was fake or not. In comparison between localization and classification results of WLI and VIC models, VIC image translation was not effective. However, it is reported that chromoendoscopy increases the lesion detection rate [3,12,14]. Therefore, this image translation might be useful for medical doctors to detect lesions. For example, by contrast to the background, red lesions get apparent. Also, the excessive accumulation of indigocarmine dye often occurs in reality. VIC images can avoid such a phenomenon and enables medical doctors to observe the depression of lesions which is a critical indicator to evaluate the invasion depth of lesions. Furthermore, VIC images are also effective to recognize the range of lesion compared with WLI images.

We applied our translation models to static images. However, medical doctors use real-time endoscopy in the clinical situation. Hence general input type is not a static image but a video. We consider that we can apply our models to the video input by extracting frames. The translation process is so fast (around 15 msec per image) and a time lag can be negligible. Therefore, medical doctors can always compare WLI image with VIC image during endoscopy by using our translation model, which might increase the medical doctor's detection rate as in the entire colon dye spraying studies [3, 14]. Further studies are needed in order to evaluate the effectiveness of VIC translation for medical doctors in routine endoscopy.

In addition, we can use the VIC generation for secondary interpretation. Our method enables secondary doctors to do virtual indigocarmine dye spraying even if primary doctors did not use indigocarmine dye spraying.

We generated colonoscopic VIC images in this study. However, we consider that image translation is also applicable to other body parts or other endoscopic image enhancing methods. One of the most commonly used image enhancing methods for endoscopy is narrow band imaging (NBI). While NBI requires special hardware, our approach does not require it for generating virtual NBI images.

In our study, the localization and classification performance of the VIC model was not higher than that of the WLI model. In some translation cases, translated images were very noisy or lost the contrast between lesions and normal tissue. These translation behaviors might affect the results of localization and classification in the VIC model. Therefore, we consider that the improvement of VIC generation is required to enhance localization and classification performance.

To improve VIC generation quality, we consider there are two obstacles. First, the dyeing condition varies locationally because Indigocarmine is not necessarily sprayed on the whole image. The unsprayed region in IC images might affect the training of generators and discriminators because we train these models by a single batch. Second, halation in WLI is another obstacle to improving generation quality and remained in VIC image. We regard the halation as a kind of noise, and we need to suppress the degree of halation before translating images.

5   Conclusion

In this paper, we proposed WLI-to-VIC translation and use it as preprocess for lesion detection. Compared with WLI input model, VIC input model did not present the high performance except for the classification of cancer. On the other hand, our results showed that VIC images were useful for data augmentation of IC images because the IC+VIC model had the highest performance in both localization and classification against the IC model. We consider that our study gives clues to apply human-understandable image translation for the performance improvement of CAD.

References

1. Adler, A., Pohl, H., Papanikolaou, I.S., et al: A prospective randomized study on narrow-band imaging versus conventional colonoscopy for adenoma detection: does NBI induce a learning effect? Gut **57** (2008)
2. Ahn, S.B., Han, D.S., Bae, J.H., et al.: The miss rate for colorectal adenoma determined by quality-adjusted, back-to-back colonoscopies. Gut Liver **6**, 64–70 (2012)
3. Brooker, J.C., Saunders, B.P., Shah, S.G., et al.: Total colonic dye-spray increases the detection of diminutive adenomas during routine colonoscopy: a randomized controlled trial. Gastrointest. Endosc. **56**, 333–338 (2002)
4. Corley, D., Jensen, C., Marks, A., et al.: Adenoma detection rate and risk of colorectal cancer and death. N. Engl. J. Med. **370**, 2541 (2014)
5. Engelhardt, S., De Simone, R., Full, P.M., et al.: Improving surgical training phantoms by hyperrealism: deep unpaired image-to-image translation from real surgeries. arXiv pre-prints arXiv:1806.03627 (2018)
6. Isola, P., Zhu, J., Zhou, T., Efros, A.A.: Image-to-image translation with conditional adversarial networks. arXiv preprint arXiv:1611.07004 (2016)
7. Kaminski, M., Regula, J., Kraszewska, E., et al: Quality indicators for colonoscopy and the risk of interval cancer. N. Engl. J. Med. **362** (2010)
8. Ki Min, J., Kwak, M., Myung Cha, J.: Overview of deep learning in gastrointestinal endoscopy. Gut Liver **13**(4), 388–393 (2019)
9. Kumar, S., Thosani, N., Ladabaum, U., et al.: Adenoma miss rates associated with a 3-minute versus 6-minute colonoscopy withdrawal time: a prospective, randomized trial. Gastrointest. Endosc. **85**, 1273–1280 (2017)
10. Mori, Y., Kudo, S.E., Berzin, T.M., et al.: Computer-aided diagnosis for colonoscopy. Endoscopy **49**, 813–819 (2017)
11. Pohl, J., Lotterer, E., Balzer, C., et al.: Computed virtual chromoendoscopy versus standard colonoscopy with targeted indigocarmine chromoscopy: a randomised multicentre trial. Gut **58**, 73–78 (2009)
12. Pohl, J., Schneider, A., Vogell, H., et al.: Pancolonic chromoendoscopy with indigo carmine versus standard colonoscopy for detection of neoplastic lesions: a randomised two-centre trial. Gut **60**, 485–490 (2011)
13. Redmon, J., Farhadi, A.: YoLov3: an incremental improvement. arXiv preprint arXiv:1804.02767 (2018)
14. Repici, A., Wallace, M.B., East, J.E., et al.: Efficacy of per-oral methylene blue formulation for screening colonoscopy[a]. Gastroenterology **S0016−5085**(19), 2198–2207 (2019)
15. Rex, D.K., Helbig, C.C.: High yields of small and flat adenomas with high-definition colonoscopes using either white light or narrow band imaging. Gastroenterology **133**, 42–47 (2007)
16. Urban, G., Tripathi, P., Alkayali, T., et al.: Deep learning localizes and identifies polyps in real time with 96% accuracy in screening colonoscopy. Gastroenterology **155**, 1069–1078 (2018)
17. Wang, P., Xiao, X., Glissen Brown, J.R., et al.: Development and validation of a deep-learning algorithm for the detection of polyps during colonoscopy. Nat. Biomed. Eng. **2**, 741–748 (2018)
18. Yi, Z., Zhang, H., Tan, P., et al.: DualGAN: unsupervised dual learning for image-to-image translation. arXiv preprint arXiv:1704.02510 (2017)

19. Zhong, Z., Zheng, L., Kang, G., et al.: Random erasing data augmentation. arXiv preprint arXiv:1708.04896 (2017)
20. Zhu, J., Park, T., Isola, P., et al.: Unpaired image-to-image translation using cycle-consistent adversarial networks. arXiv preprint arXiv:1703.10593 (2017)

MIL3ID 2019

Self-supervised Learning of Inverse Problem Solvers in Medical Imaging

Ortal Senouf[1], Sanketh Vedula[1(✉)], Tomer Weiss[1], Alex Bronstein[1],
Oleg Michailovich[2], and Michael Zibulevsky[1]

[1] Technion, Haifa, Israel
`sanketh@cs.technion.ac.il`
[2] University of Waterloo, Waterloo, Canada

Abstract. In the past few years, deep learning-based methods have demonstrated enormous success for solving inverse problems in medical imaging. In this work, we address the following question: *Given a set of measurements obtained from real imaging experiments, what is the best way to use a learnable model and the physics of the modality to solve the inverse problem and reconstruct the latent image?* Standard supervised learning based methods approach this problem by collecting data sets of known latent images and their corresponding measurements. However, these methods are often impractical due to the lack of availability of appropriately sized training sets, and, more generally, due to the inherent difficulty in measuring the "groundtruth" latent image. In light of this, we propose a self-supervised approach to training inverse models in medical imaging in the absence of aligned data. Our method only requiring access to the measurements and the forward model at training. We showcase its effectiveness on inverse problems arising in accelerated magnetic resonance imaging (MRI).

Keywords: Deep learning · Inverse problems · Self-supervised learning · Accelerated MRI

1 Introduction

In the past years, there has been an enormous success in deploying deep learning-based methods in imaging, image processing, and computer vision. Most of these tasks, if tackled as a supervised learning problem, require collecting a large dataset of measurements and their corresponding latent variables, which would be referred to as labels in classification and detection tasks, and as ground truth in regression tasks. Whereas the task of labeling images, albeit not simple, can be addressed by using a large number of human annotators, the task of collecting measurements and their corresponding aligned ground-truth images is much

---

O. Senouf and S. Vedula—Contributed equally.

© Springer Nature Switzerland AG 2019
Q. Wang et al. (Eds.): DART 2019/MIL3ID 2019, LNCS 11795, pp. 111–119, 2019.
https://doi.org/10.1007/978-3-030-33391-1_13

harder and often impractical. The acquisition of a groundtruth image typically requires subjecting the same object of interest to a different imaging modality or to the same modality configured to provide more accurate measurements. The need to register such images at the sub-pixel level, coping with the object's natural deformation is often very difficult to surmount.

The limitation of the supervised regime is the main motivation of the present paper. We focus on answering the following question: Given a *single* measurement obtained from a real imaging system, and our knowledge about the forward model embodying the physics of the imaging modality, can we learn an operator solving the inverse problem and reconstructing the latent signal? We henceforth refer to this learning regime as *self-supervised learning* (SSL). It is important to emphasize that the proposed self-supervised learning is cardinally different from *unsupervised learning*, despite the fact that no groundtruth is used in both cases. While the latter relates mostly to generative models which try to estimate the latent data distributions, SSL aims at solving the inverse problem by exploiting internal information within the measurements themselves, and more specifically in our case, trying to explain or dissect the given measurements.

Contributions. We propose an SSL framework, comprising two building blocks: a convolutional neural network (CNN) that serves as the prior, and a forward model, embodying the imaging physics into the pipeline. Several recent studies [5,7] demonstrated that a CNN can serve as a good prior for a wide range of images classes – a line of works that is generally referred to as *deep image prior*. From this perspective, the present solution can be viewed as the embodiment of deep image priors in general inverse problems. We demonstrate and evaluation our method on the case of accelerated magnetic resonance imaging. The forward model in that case is the MR k-space sampling trajectory. By applying SSL to this task, we introduce a significant improvement (around 2–3 dB PSNR) compared to an off-the-shelf total variation-regularized solver, and even some level of proximity to the performance of the fully supervised restoration model.

2   Methods

In this work, we are interested in *inverse problems*, which aim to calculate, from the measurements, the latent signal that produced them. The process of measuring the latent signal is referred to as the *forward model*. We denote the forward model with the operator $\mathcal{F}(\cdot)$ that maps the entities in the domain of latent signals to the measurements. Many types of inverse problems arising in signal and image processing and medical imaging involve a *linear* forward model, which can be straightforwardly expressed as the matrix product

$$\mathbf{y} = \mathbf{F}\mathbf{x} + \eta. \tag{1}$$

Here $\mathbf{x} \in \mathbb{R}^n$ is the latent signal that is measured through the forward model $\mathbf{F} \in \mathbb{R}^{m \times n}$, resulting in the observed measurement $\mathbf{y} \in \mathbb{R}^m$; η denotes additive measurement noise. An inverse problem consists of estimating the latent signal $\mathbf{x}$ from the measurement $\mathbf{y}$.

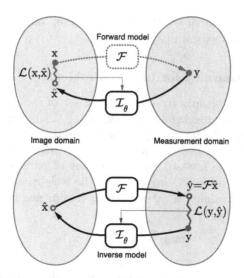

Fig. 1. Comparison of different approaches to learning inverse models. In the standard supervised approach (top), many pairs of latent images **x** and corresponding measurements **y** are available at training, and a loss in the image domain drives the parameters θ of the inverse model such that $\hat{\mathbf{x}} = \mathcal{I}_\theta(\mathbf{y})$ is close to **x**. In the proposed self-supervised approach (bottom) only access to the measurements **y** and the forward model $\mathcal{F}$ is assumed. The loss is formulated in the measurement domain, and the inverse model is trained such that $\mathcal{F}(\mathcal{I}_\theta(\mathbf{y}))$ is close to **y**.

While several important problems (such as denoising, inpainting, compressed sensing, tomography) admit the above structure; linear modeling of $\mathcal{F}$ is not accurate for a range of more exotic problems arising in computational and medical imaging such as multiple-scattering computed tomography, optical diffraction tomography, and wave-propagation inverse problem in ultrasound imaging. The proposed methodology applies to these modalities as well as long as the appropriate forward operator $\mathcal{F}$ is known. Therefore, in order to emphasize the broader applicability of the proposed framework, we will refer to the forward model as $\mathcal{F}$ instead of the matrix **F**.

2.1   Prior-Based Solvers

One of the standard formulations of inverse problems is in the form of maximum *a posteriori* (MAP) estimation the latent signal **x** from the measurements **y**. This formulation allows to introduce information about the latent image through the prior $P_X(\mathbf{x})$, and boils down to the minimization of an objective function comprising the negative log-likelihood and the negative log-prior terms,

$$\hat{\mathbf{x}} = \arg\min_{\mathbf{x}} \ -\log P_{Y|X}(\mathbf{y}|\mathbf{x}) - \log P_X(\mathbf{x}). \tag{2}$$

In the case of additive white Gaussian measurement noise, the first term becomes the Euclidean norm, $\|\mathcal{F}(\mathbf{x}) - \mathbf{y}\|^2$. Famous examples of prior terms include total variation (TV) [4] or sparsity with respect to some dictionary [2], which are regularly employed in medical imaging.

2.2 Supervised Learning for Inverse Problems

As illustrated in Fig. 1 (top), given an aligned set of samples of latent signals and their corresponding measurements $\{(\mathbf{x}_i, \mathbf{y}_i)\}_{i=1}^{N}$, supervised learning methods aim at estimating the inverse operator that maps the measurements to the corresponding latent signals. We denote by $\mathcal{I}_\theta$ the inverse operator that should invert the action of the forward model. The set of parameters θ denotes the trainable degrees of freedom – in our case, the weights of the reconstruction neural network. The training is carried out by minimizing the empirical loss

$$\min_\theta \sum_{i=1}^{N} \mathcal{L}\left(\mathcal{I}_\theta(\mathbf{y}_i), \mathbf{x}_i\right) \tag{3}$$

where $\mathcal{L}$ measures the discrepancy between the estimated latent signal $\mathcal{I}_\theta(\mathbf{y}_i)$ and the groundtruth $\mathbf{x}_i$. Typical choices include the Euclidean and the L_1 distances. In practice, for image restoration tasks, the operator $\mathcal{I}_\theta$ is modeled as a convolutional neural network and the objective (3) is minimized using stochastic gradient-based solvers. Once the optimal set of parameters θ^* has been learned on the training set, the inverse operator $\mathcal{I}_{\theta^*}$ is applied to solve the inverse problem with previously unseen inputs.

2.3 Self-supervised Learning

The focus of this study is the cases where an aligned set of measurements and latent signals is not available or challenging to obtain at the required size (typical supervised training scenarios demand a very large N). In the extreme of such cases, one has access to just one sample of measurements $\mathbf{y}$ and the forward operator $\mathcal{F}$. This exact problem has been traditionally tackled by the prior-based methods that we discussed in the Sect. 2.1. However, a drawback of many prior-based approaches is the need to induce explicit priors on the image instead of learning image- and task-specific priors. On the other hand, in [7] and [5], the authors demonstrated that CNNs by their very own structure can induce a good prior on natural images. The key idea of the proposed self-supervised approach is to find a latent image that is the output of the parametrized inverse operator $\mathcal{I}_\theta$ that best explains the given measurement. Following the ideas in [7] and extending them to a general inverse problem setting, our approach can be formalized as the following optimization problem

$$\min_\theta \mathcal{L}\left(\mathcal{F}(\mathcal{I}_\theta(\mathbf{y})), \mathbf{y}\right). \tag{4}$$

Note that the loss function now operates on the measurement space.

Solving the above optimization problem yields $\hat{\mathbf{x}} = \mathcal{I}_\theta(\mathbf{y})$, i.e., the latent signal at the intermediate stage, as illustrated in Fig. 1 (bottom). Intuitively, we are searching for an image $\hat{\mathbf{x}}$ that is parametrized by $\{\theta, \mathbf{y}\}$ that best explains the measurement $\mathbf{y}$ we have in hand. This approach is referred to as *self-supervised* because the measurements themselves provide the supervision to solve the inverse problem by exploiting the prior induced by the CNN.

3   Problem Setup

We demonstrate the applicability of the above discussed self-supervised solvers on the task of accelerated MRI reconstruction. In accelerated MR imaging, the field-of-view (FOV) is scanned with a reduced number of measurements that can be achieved by acquiring less data in the k-space (Fourier domain) leading to shorter trajectories, which in turn lead to shorter acquisition times. One standard way of designing such acceleration schemes is by acquiring random Cartesian trajectories (that is, directions aligned with the spatial frequency axes) in the k-space.

The forward model of accelerated MRI can be therefore faithfully emulated by sub-sampling the fully sampled k-space, and it is realistic, in this case, to assume that the forward operator is known with high accuracy. Following the terminology described in Sect. 2, we denote the image derived from fully sampled k-space as $\mathbf{x}$ (the latent image), and the image obtained through the sub-sampled k-space is denoted by $\mathbf{y}$ (the measurement). The forward model can therefore be formalized as follows:

$$\mathbf{y} = \mathcal{F}(\mathbf{x}) = \mathbf{\Phi}^{-1}(\mathbf{S} \odot (\mathbf{\Phi}\mathbf{x})) \tag{5}$$

where $\odot$ denotes element-wise (Hadamard) product, and $\mathbf{\Phi}$ and $\mathbf{\Phi}^{-1}$ denote the forward and the inverse Fourier transforms, respectively. The binary matrix $\mathbf{S}$ denotes the sampling operator that embodies the Cartesian trajectories through which the measurements were obtained; we refer to the rate of decimation induced in k-space as the acceleration factor (AF).

We consider the following two inverse problems: (i) *Superresolution (SR)*, consisting of reconstructing a sharp image from measurements containing only the central low frequencies obtained by using the mask $\mathbf{S}$ as in Fig. 2 (a and c); and (ii) *Dealiasing*, in which the obtained mask results in an aliasing artifact due to a coarser sampling in the phase-encoding direction. We use the masks displayed in Fig. 2 (b and d). The inverse problem consists of restoring a finer sampling grid in the phase-encoding direction. Throughout the paper, we denote the experiments specifying the task name (one of the two tasks above) and the acceleration factor.

Loss function. We use the following loss function:

$$\mathcal{L}(\mathbf{y}, \hat{\mathbf{y}}) = \alpha\|\mathbf{y} - \hat{\mathbf{y}}\|_1 + \beta\|\mathbf{\Phi}\mathbf{y} - \mathbf{S} \odot \mathbf{\Phi}(\hat{\mathbf{x}})\|_1 + \gamma\|\mathcal{I}_\theta(\mathbf{y}) - \mathcal{I}_\theta(\hat{\mathbf{y}})\|_1 \tag{6}$$

comprising three terms. The first term essentially treats the task as a *superresolution* problem, enforcing a penalty on the discrepancy between the reconstructed measurement $\hat{\mathbf{y}}$ and the given measurement $\mathbf{y}$. The second term treats the task as an *inpainting* problem in the k-space, penalizing the discrepancy between the masked Fourier transform of the reconstructed latent image and k-space representation of the measurements. The last term enforces cycle consistency on the reconstructed measurement image passing it through the inverse operator $(\mathcal{I}_\theta(\hat{\mathbf{y}}) = \tilde{\mathbf{x}})$ and making it consistent with that of the original measurements $(\mathcal{I}_\theta(\mathbf{y}) = \hat{\mathbf{x}})$. This constraint is similar to the cycle-consistency loss used in [9] for image style transfer. In all the three cases, the L_1 norm measures the discrepancy; the relative importance of each term is governed by the parameters α, β, and γ.

4   Experiments and Discussion

Compared Algorithms. The proposed SSL scheme was compared to the following two baselines: (i) *Total variation*: Similarly to [8], we compare our results to an off-the-shelf accelerated MR reconstruction method with a total variation (TV) regularizer. We used the BART [6] toolkit for calculating the TV-based MR image reconstruction. The regularization weight was set to 0.01, and it was run for 200 iterations per slice. (ii) *Supervised learning*: Since the results of a supervised restoration model would be considered as an upper bound on SSL's performance, we trained a U-Net model [3] on a dataset of aligned reduced measurements and full measurements MRI, and compared our results on samples that were excluded from the training set.

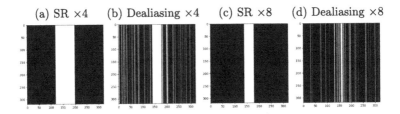

Fig. 2. Visual comparison of the k-space binary masks chosen for different tasks. Tasks ordered from left to right: superresolution $\times 4$, dealiasing $\times 4$, superresolution $\times 8$, and dealiasing $\times 8$

Data. The data used in the preparation of this article were obtained from the NYU fastMRI Initiative database (fastmri.med.nyu.edu) [8]. We have used the fastMRI training set for our experiments and generated two separated sets out of it: one containing 973 volumes (34700 slices) for training and validation, and one containing 8 volumes (48 slices) for testing. Only samples from the test set were used for evaluating all methods: both SSL and the comparison baselines.

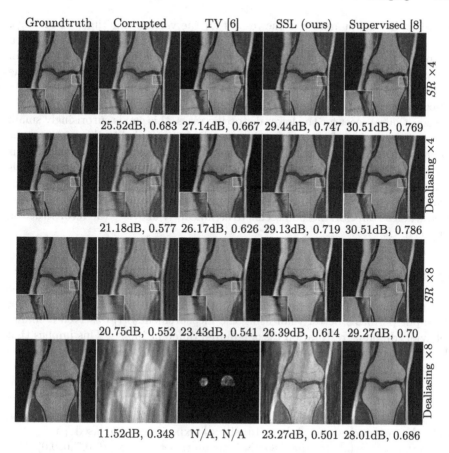

Fig. 3. Comparison of the proposed self-supervised approach (SSL) to ESPIRiT (TV) [6] and supervised trained network [8] on different tasks. From top to bottom the panels depict the tasks: *SR* ×4, dealiasing ×4, *SR* ×8 and dealiasing ×8. From left to right, the columns depict the groundtruth, corrupted (with respective masks), TV-restored [6], SSL-restored(*ours*), and supervised model restored images, along with their corresponding (PSNR, SSIM) metrics mentioned below.

Settings. We performed our experiments with various types of inputs to the inverse operator $\mathcal{I}_\theta$: the measurements themselves $\mathbf{y}$, a gradient-like image which we refer to as "meshgrid" input ($\mathbf{z}$) – similar to what has been used in [7], and a combination of the measurements and the meshgrid input – stacked as two channels, i.e., $[\mathbf{y}\ \mathbf{z}]$. Since cycle-consistency is not valid in the case of a meshgrid (only) input, γ has been set to zero for these experiments. The inverse operator $\mathcal{I}_\theta$ was chosen to be the U-net architecture for all our experiments [3]. We used the Adam optimizer [1] as the update method with learning rate of 10^{-4}.

Results. Table 1 summarizes the results for the various experimental settings, comparing the performance of the above-mentioned benchmarks to ours. When compared to TV [6], our method achieves an improvement of ~2 dB–3 dB in the peak-signal-to-noise ratio (PSNR). Similar results are observed for the structural-similarity measure (SSIM, about 0.05–0.08 points improvement). As expected, the supervised model outperforms the proposed SSL method. However, it seems that at least for the lower distortion rates, this gap is surprisingly small. A visual inspection of the results over one slice is provided in Fig. 3. As can be observed in the zoomed-in region, our method manages to restore finer details better than the TV-based method, and even approaches the restoration levels of the supervised model in the lower distortion rates. As evident both quantitatively and visually, the TV-based method completely fails on the ×8 dealiasing task, whereas our SSL method seems to significantly alleviate the reconstruction artifacts.

Discussion. From the practical perspective, we observed that for lower decimation rates (×4) using the input as the measurements $\mathbf{y}$ (or) [$\mathbf{y}$ $\mathbf{z}$] yielded the best performance. At higher decimation rates (×8), we observed that using $\mathbf{z}$ as the input performs better than using the measurements. [7] observed a similar behavior: different restoration tasks required different inputs. This implies that the input is part of the induced prior, and specifically in our case, the restoration tasks involving higher decimation rates require a smooth input that is distinct from the distorted measurements.

Upon performing a hyper-parameter search for (α, β, γ), we observed that, irrespective of the input, enforcing a higher weight on the k-space loss is crucial relative to the spatial loss. In all ×4 experiments we used $(\alpha, \beta, \gamma) = (1.0, 8.0, 10^{-5})$, while for the ×8 experiments we set them to $(0.0, 7.0, 0.0)$.

Table 1. Quantitative evaluation of the proposed method on 48 slices from 8 volumes. The volumes were chosen randomly from the validation set of the fastMRI dataset [8].

Task	Metrics	Corrupted	TV	SSL (ours)	Supervised
Superresolution ×4	PSNR	25.25	25.61	28.08	28.79
	SSIM	0.683	0.627	0.691	0.701
Dealiasing ×4	PSNR	21.88	25.26	27.56	28.67
	SSIM	0.587	0.579	0.66	0.7056
Superresolution ×8	PSNR	22.16	23.29	25.61	27.25
	SSIM	0.5224	0.5017	0.5541	0.6057
Dealiasing ×8	PSNR	13.74	N/A	22.86	26.72
	SSIM	0.40	N/A	0.47	0.604

5   Conclusion and Future Work

We propose a new learning framework for solving inverse problems in the absence of aligned data. As a proof-of-concept, we demonstrated the applicability of the proposed framework to the use case of accelerated MRI reconstruction, where our approach outperforms standard off-the-shelf solvers by a significant margin. We believe this framework leads to many interesting future directions and can become a tool in solving a new range of inverse problems in the limited/no aligned data regime where the supervised methods are not applicable. One could devise better loss functions that can be imposed in the measurements domain. This framework could be extended to a semi-supervised scenario as well and used for analysing the importance of external (supervised) data.

References

1. Kingma, D.P., et al.: Adam: a method for stochastic optimization. arXiv e-prints arXiv:1412.6980, December 2014
2. Lustig, M., et al.: Sparse MRI: the application of compressed sensing for rapid MR imaging. Magn. Reson. Med. **58**(6), 1182–1195 (2007)
3. Ronneberger, O., Fischer, P., Brox, T.: U-Net: convolutional networks for biomedical image segmentation. In: Navab, N., Hornegger, J., Wells, W.M., Frangi, A.F. (eds.) MICCAI 2015. LNCS, vol. 9351, pp. 234–241. Springer, Cham (2015). https://doi.org/10.1007/978-3-319-24574-4_28
4. Rudin, L.I., et al.: Nonlinear total variation based noise removal algorithms. Physica D **60**(1–4), 259–268 (1992)
5. Shocher, A., et al.: "Zero-Shot" super-resolution using deep internal learning. In: Proceedings CVPR (2018)
6. Uecker, M., et al.: ESPIRiT - an eigenvalue approach to autocalibrating parallel MRI: Where SENSE meets GRAPPA. Magn. Reson. Med. (2014)
7. Ulyanov, D., et al.: Deep image prior. In: Proceedings CVPR (2018)
8. Zbontar, J., et al.: fastMRI: an open dataset and benchmarks for accelerated MRI. arXiv preprint arXiv:1811.08839 (2018)
9. Zhu, J., et al.: Unpaired image-to-image translation using cycle-consistent adversarial networks. In: Proceedings ICCV (2017)

Weakly Supervised Segmentation of Vertebral Bodies with Iterative Slice-Propagation

Shiqi Peng[1], Bolin Lai[1], Guangyu Yao[2], Xiaoyun Zhang[1], Ya Zhang[1(✉)], Yan-Feng Wang[1], and Hui Zhao[2]

[1] Cooperative Medianet Innovation Center, Shanghai Jiao Tong University, Shanghai 200240, People's Republic of China
lai.b.bryan@gmail.com,
{pengshiqi,xiaoyun.zhang,ya_zhang,wangyanfeng}@sjtu.edu.cn
[2] Shanghai Jiao Tong University Affiliated Sixth People's Hospital, Shanghai 200233, People's Republic of China
zhao-hui@sjtu.edu.cn, ygy504187803@126.com

Abstract. Vertebral body (VB) segmentation is an important preliminary step towards medical visual diagnosis for spinal diseases. However, most previous works require pixel/voxel-wise strong supervisions, which is expensive, tedious and time-consuming for experts to annotate. In this paper, we propose a Weakly supervised Iterative Spinal Segmentation (WISS) method leveraging only four corner landmark weak labels on a single sagittal slice to achieve automatic volumetric segmentation from CT images for VBs. WISS first segments VBs on an annotated sagittal slice in an iterative self-training manner. This self-training method alternates between training and refining labels in the training set. Then WISS proceeds to segment the whole VBs slice by slice with a slice-propagation method to obtain volumetric segmentations. We evaluate the performance of WISS on a private spinal metastases CT dataset and the public lumbar CT dataset. On the first dataset, WISS achieves distinct improvements with regard to two different backbones. For the second dataset, WISS achieves dice coefficients of 91.7% and 83.7% for mid-sagittal slices and 3D CT volumes, respectively, saving a lot of labeling costs and only sacrificing a little segmentation performance.

Keywords: Vertebral body segmentation · Weak supervision

1 Introduction

Segmentation of the vertebral bodies (VBs) from CT images is often a prerequisite for many computational spine imaging tasks, such as assessment of spinal deformities, detection of vertebral fractures, and computer-assisted surgical interventions. Previous work of VB segmentation can be generally categorized as model based [12], graph theory based [1] and machine learning based

© Springer Nature Switzerland AG 2019
Q. Wang et al. (Eds.): DART 2019/MIL3ID 2019, LNCS 11795, pp. 120–128, 2019.
https://doi.org/10.1007/978-3-030-33391-1_14

methods [3]. Most recently, convolutional neural networks (CNNs) achieve better performances and thus have been widely used. U-Net incorporated with VB location prior knowledge for automatic vertebrae segmentation is explored in an iterative fashion [9]. Nevertheless, all these methods have a same drawback that they require pixel/voxel-wise labeled CT/MR scans to train models. It is desired to leverage less fine-grained labels for segmentation so as to save the labeling cost.

In this paper, we explore a Weakly supervised Iterative Spinal Segmentation (WISS) method for VB segmentation. Considering that the normal VBs without fractures are roughly quadrilateral from the sagittal view, we thus propose to annotate the position of a VB with four corner landmarks in the mid-sagittal slice and utilize them as weak labels for segmentation.

From any input CT volume with an annotated slice, we first segment the VBs on the annotated slices in a self-training manner [8]. The segmentation model is improved iteratively by confident prediction selection and densely connected CRF [7]. After the segmentation model converges on the mid-sagittal slices, we then adopt a slice-wise propagation method [2] to generalize this process to other successive slices to obtain the full volumetric segmentation. We apply the segmentation model to adjacent slices and create initial masks for them as extra training data, ultimately producing the final segmentations when the model converges. As this process iterates, segmentation results of all CT slices can be obtained and thus 3D VB segmentation is achieved.

The proposed WISS method for 2D slices is evaluated on a private spinal metastases CT dataset, and the 3D volumetric segmentation is evaluated on the public lumbar spine CT dataset [6]. On the first dataset, WISS achieves an improvement in dice coefficient of $+2.1\%$ and $+3.7\%$ with regard to two different segmentation backbones, respectively. Furthermore, experimental results on random noise disturbed dataset show that WISS is robust to weak and noisy supervision, which is very essential for medical diagnosis. For the second dataset, WISS achieves dice coefficients of 91.7% and 83.7% on the mid-sagittal slices and 3D CT volumes, respectively. Compared with state-of-the-art strongly supervised VB segmentation methods [9], WISS saves huge costs of labeling and sacrifices a little segmentation performance, which is very worthwhile in the practical applications.

2 Method

In the spinal metastases dataset, each CT volume contains a mid-sagittal slice with four corner landmark annotations. We aim to leverage such weak supervisions on a single slice to achieve the volumetric segmentation.

2.1 Sagittal Slice Segmentation via Self-training

We first connect four corner landmarks to construct the coarse quadrilateral training labels for the mid-sagittal slices. Then a base segmentation model is trained using these coarse labels. Such labels are refined by selecting the most confident predictions and recovering the boundaries by fully connected conditional random field (CRF) [7], thus additional supervisions are obtained. By repeating training and refining procedures, we can achieve better segmentation results and get a better segmentation model.

Segmentation Backbone: In our method, Mask R-CNN [5] is selected as the segmentation backbone for its quite good performances on object detection task and instance segmentation task. The probability map prediction from Mask R-CNN is utilized for the confidence computation.

Mask R-CNN is a two stage network: the first stage scans image and generates region of interest (ROI) proposals, and the second classifies the proposals and generates bounding boxes and masks. Formally, during training, a multi-task loss is defined on each sampled ROI as

$$\mathcal{L} = \mathcal{L}_{cls} + \mathcal{L}_{box} + \mathcal{L}_{mask} + \alpha \mathcal{L}_{edge}. \tag{1}$$

The classification loss $\mathcal{L}_{cls}$, bounding-box regression loss $\mathcal{L}_{box}$, and mask loss $\mathcal{L}_{mask}$ are defined in [5]. Besides, to preserve the object boundaries, we compared the magnitude and orientation of the edges of the predicted mask with the ground truth. Thus an edge loss [11] is added to the loss function as

$$L_{edge} = \sqrt{(M_x - G_x)^2 + (M_y - G_y)^2}, \tag{2}$$

where M is a generated mask and G is the corresponding ground truth. (M_x, M_y) and (G_x, G_y) are the first derivatives of M and G, respectively in x and y directions. α is a weighted coefficient. Although the edges of the annotations might not be accurate at the beginning, $\mathcal{L}_{edge}$ can be considered as an attention of the possible edge areas. As the iteration proceeds, the annotations will be more and more accurate, thus edge loss will help model converge to the optimal solution.

Confident Prediction Selection: We propose a confident prediction selection method to avoid passing errors to the next iteration. During inference, Mask R-CNN generates three outputs for each predicted ROI: the probability $\mathcal{P}$ to contain a VB, bounding box coordinates $\mathcal{C}$ and a probability map $\mathcal{M}$ of each pixel. First, we select the most confident ROIs where the object probability $\mathcal{P}$ exceeds a threshold $\mathcal{T}_1$. For each ROI, we select the confident pixels as mask where the probability map $\mathcal{M}$ exceeds another threshold $\mathcal{T}_2$. Considering the prior knowledge that VBs are generally arranged in a column, we then fit a curve based on the center points of the confident ROIs. ROIs close to this curve are selected as final predictions, and ROIs away from this curve are rejected. As shown in Fig. 1, the colored regions are the predicted ROIs and the red line is the fitted curve. The leftmost green region is a false positive prediction and thus it is discarded.

Error Alleviation by CRF: Since the initial coarse quadrilateral labels are imperfect, the output probability maps are not tend to converge to the optimal

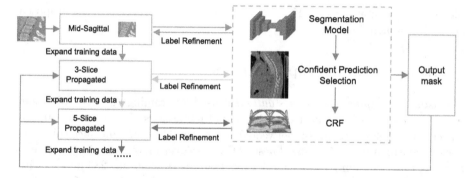

Fig. 1. Overview of the proposed method. We use segmentation output mask incorporating with confident prediction selection and CRF refinements to gradually generate extra training data for VB segmentation. Arrows colored in orange, green and purple represent slice-propagated training at its 1st, 2nd and 3rd iterations, respectively. For each iteration, training and refining procedures are repeated in a self-training manner until the model converges. Best viewed in color. (Color figure online)

solution. We thus adopt the densely connected conditional random fields (CRF) to overcome such a problem. The CRF model establishes pairwise potentials, which take both pixel positions and intensities into account, on all pairs of pixels in the image. Therefore low-level appearances, such as VB boundaries, are incorporated into the refined predictions. CRF recovers the object boundaries by correcting the oversegmentation regions and undersegmentation regions, thus providing extra training information and alleviating the impact of error amplification.

2.2 Slice-Propagated Segmentation

In order to generate VB segmentations for all sagittal CT slices, we train the segmentation model in a slice-propagated manner. Formally, we denote X_i, Y_i and $\hat{Y}_i$ as the ith sagittal slices, corresponding labels and the model outputs for all the CT volumes in the training set, respectively. m is the mid-sagittal index. The segmentation model first learns VB appearances based on the mid-sagittal slices $[X_m]$ via the self-training method introduced above. After the model converges, we then apply this model to $[X_{m-1}, X_{m+1}]$ from the entire training set to compute initial predicted probability maps $[\hat{Y}_{m-1}, \hat{Y}_{m+1}]$. Given these probability maps, refined VB segmentations $[Y_{m-1}, Y_{m+1}]$ are created using the confident prediction selection and densely connected CRF explained above. These segmentations are employed as training labels for the segmentation model on the $[X_{m-1}, X_{m+1}]$ slices, ultimately producing the updated segmentations $[\hat{Y}_{m-1}, \hat{Y}_{m+1}]$ once the model converges. As this procedure proceeds iteratively, we can gradually obtain the converged VB segmentation results across all CT slices, and then a volumetric segmentation can be produced by stacking the slice-wise segmentations $[\ldots, \hat{Y}_{m-1}, \hat{Y}_m, \hat{Y}_{m+1}, \ldots]$. The overview of the proposed method is depicted in Fig. 1.

3   Experimental Setup and Results

Datasets. *The spinal metastases dataset* is used for training and 2D evaluation. All CT scans come from patients with spinal metastases. The scans are reconstructed to in-plane resolution between 0.234 mm and 2.0 mm, and slice thickness between 0.314 mm and 5.0 mm. These CT scans cover all of the spine, including cervical, thoracic, lumbar and sacral VBs. Training set contains 284 images with 3400 VBs, and testing set contains 95 images with 1109 VBs. The four points annotations and reference segmentations are annotated by three radiologists.

The lumbar spine dataset consists of 10 scans of healthy subjects of the lumbar vertebraes. The scans are reconstructed to in-plane resolutions of 0.282 mm to 0.791 mm and slice thickness of 0.725 mm to 1.530 mm. We manually edit the reference segmentation to keep only VBs. The segmentation models are trained on the spinal metastases dataset and directly evaluated on the lumbar dataset.

Table 1. Performances evaluated on the spinal metastases CT dataset with two segmentation backbones. *M* denotes Mask R-CNN backbone. *E* means using the edge loss (Eq. 1). *R* means using confident prediction selection and fully connected CRF refinements. *ST* stands for self-training. For the last four rows, prefix *n-* represents for experiments on the noisy dataset where the four corner landmark labels are randomly shifted by 0 to 1 mm.

Methods	DIC	ACC	SEN	SPE
UNet [10]	86.5	95.1	79.3	**98.8**
UNet-ST	**88.6**	**95.5**	**86.8**	97.5
M [5]	87.6	97.8	81.2	**99.6**
M-E	87.8	97.8	82.3	99.4
M-E-R	89.6	98.0	**89.8**	98.8
M-E-R-ST	**90.1**	**98.1**	88.8	99.1
n-M	85.6	97.4	79.6	99.3
n-M-E	86.2	97.6	79.4	**99.5**
n-M-E-R	86.2	97.6	79.5	**99.5**
***n*-M-E-R-ST**	**89.3**	**97.9**	**90.6**	98.6

Evaluation Metrics. For the spinal metastases dataset, we use Dice coefficient (DIC), Accuracy (ACC), Sensitivity (SEN), and Specificity (SPE) metrics to evaluate the segmentation performances [4]. Larger values mean better segmentation accuracy. DIC is the most important criterion.

For the lumbar spine dataset, the segmentation performance is evaluated with Dice similarity coefficient (DIC), average symmetric surface distance (ASD), and Hausdorff distance (HSD). All metrics are calculated for individual vertebrae and then averaged over all scans.

Implementation. The proposed method is implemented using the TensorFlow library[1]. Stochastic gradient descent optimizer is used to optimize parameters with a learning rate and momentum of 0.001 and 0.9, respectively. Transfer learning technique is applied since the model is quite large but the training set is relatively small. We adopt weights pre-trained on MSCOCO dataset and only trained the head network, which help the model converge faster and achieve better results. Training for 50 epochs on an NVIDIA TITAN X GPU with 12 GB memory takes approximately 2 h, and testing takes about 0.5 s per image. As for self-training, the number of iterations is set to be 2. Confident thresholds T_1 and T_2 are set to be 0.9 and 0.5 respectively. Edge loss coefficient α is set to be 0.1.

Mid-sagittal Slices Segmentation via Self-training. Quantitative results on the spinal metastases CT dataset are shown in Table 1. We compare the performances of U-Net [10] and Mask R-CNN [5] as segmentation backbones. As for U-Net backbone, we adopt the same quadrilateral coarse labels, but don't use the confident prediction selection and CRF techniques. The results demonstrate that our proposed method improves the performances effectively. For U-Net backbone, DIC is improved by 2.1%. And for Mask R-CNN backbone, our method outperforms backbone 2.5% in DIC.

In practice, errors are inevitable in the manual annotations. A generic segmentation method should be robust enough against these labeling noises. To prove such robustness of our method, we build a noisy dataset by randomly shifting the four corner landmarks by 0 to 1 mm and conduct experiments again on this noisy dataset. The experimental results show that though the overall performance is decreased, self-training is still effective. The performance of Mask R-CNN is improved by +2.8% in DIC. The results on this noisy dataset are reported in Table 1 with prefix n-.

Figure 2 shows segmentation results of four typical kinds of images of the spinal metastases dataset. The four examples are cervical, sacral, thoracic and lumbar VBs. Although the appearances of cervical VBs and sacral VBs are quite different from thoracic VBs and lumbar VBs, especially for C1 and C2, our model is robust enough to successfully detect and segment these two difficult cases as demonstrated in Fig. 2(a). In Fig. 2(b), two lumbar VBs and five sacral VBs are segmented, but segmentation for S3 is not accurate enough due to its irregular shape. Besides, in Fig. 2(d), a lumbar VB (the yellow one) suffers metastatic tumor and is therefore collapsed. Its original texture and shape have been destroyed. Even so, our model detects this collapsed VB and segments it successfully, indicating that our model is highly tolerant and robust.

Weakly Supervised Slice-Propagated Segmentation. We conduct the proposed slice-propagated training on the spinal metastases dataset. Then we

---

[1] https://www.tensorflow.org/.

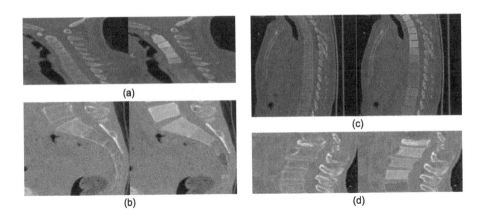

Fig. 2. Qualitative results for the spinal metastases dataset. For each case, *left* is the input image and *right* is the segmentation result. *(a) Cervical VBs; (b) Sacral VBs; (c) Thoracic VBs; (d) Lumbar VBs with collapse.* Best viewed in color. (Color figure online)

directly evaluate the 3D segmentation performance on the lumbar spine CT dataset. We report the results with propagating 5 sagittal slices. The dice score for 2D mid-sagittal slices on the lumbar dataset is $91.7 \pm 2.3\%$, and the volumetric segmentation results are tabulated in Table 2. We achieve a dice score of $83.71 \pm 1.50\%$, which is a little lower than the 2D segmentation because the marginal slices is quite difficult than mid-sagittal slices. State-of-the-art 3D VB segmentation on the lumbar dataset is reported in [9] with 96.5% dice score and 0.2 mm ASD. It should be noted that our method only bases on four corner landmark weak labels but [9] requires strong voxel-wise annotations. We save huge labeling costs and achieve volumetric VB segmentation at the cost of a little decrease in performance, which is very worthwhile.

Table 2. Volumetric segmentation results for 10 subjects of the lumbar spine CT dataset.

Metrics	#1	#2	#3	#4	#5	#6	#7	#8	#9	#10	MEAN ± STD
DIC (%)	83.21	83.26	82.25	83.72	82.78	84.95	85.48	83.09	86.77	81.59	**83.71 ± 1.50**
ASD (mm)	0.50	0.50	0.51	0.48	0.49	0.43	0.52	0.50	0.46	0.88	**0.53 ± 0.12**
HSD (mm)	4.54	5.30	4.30	3.89	4.50	4.49	5.77	4.63	4.17	4.76	**4.64 ± 0.52**

In addition, we display qualitative segmentation results of mid-sagittal slices for a good case and a bad case in Fig. 3. For the good case, all five lumbar VBs are properly detected and the edges are accurately segmented. However, regarding to the bad case, VBs are successfully detected as well, but some edge regions are missing due to the low image contrast, resulting in a relatively low value of the dice coefficient.

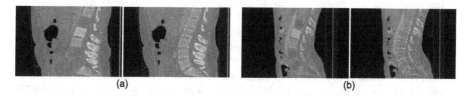

(a)   (b)

Fig. 3. Qualitative results for the lumbar spine CT dataset. (a) *A good case (#4)*; (b) *A bad case (#10)*. For each case, left is the segmentation result as color overlay with different colors for different instances, and right is the segmentation results as difference maps with oversegmentation errors marked in red and undersegmentation errors in yellow. Best viewed in color. (Color figure online)

4 Conclusion

In this paper, we proposed a Weakly supervised Iterative Spinal Segmentation (WISS) method leveraging only four corner landmark weak labels on a single sagittal slice to achieve volumetric segmentation from CT images of VBs. WISS first segments the VBs on the annotated mid-sagittal slices in a self-training manner. Then a slice-wise propagation method is adopted to generalize this process to other successive slices to obtain the full volumetric segmentation. The experiments have demonstrated that WISS is effective and robust to weak and noisy supervision. Furthermore, WISS saves huge labeling costs and only sacrifices a little segmentation performance, which is very valuable in practical applications. In future works, the proposed WISS method will be applied to other medical applications to prove its versatility.

References

1. Ali, A.M., Aslan, M.S., Farag, A.A.: Vertebral body segmentation with prior shape constraints for accurate BMD measurements. Comput. Med. Imaging Graph. **38**(7), 586–595 (2014)
2. Cai, J., et al.: Accurate weakly-supervised deep lesion segmentation using large-scale clinical annotations: slice-propagated 3D mask generation from 2D RECIST. In: Frangi, A.F., Schnabel, J.A., Davatzikos, C., Alberola-López, C., Fichtinger, G. (eds.) MICCAI 2018. LNCS, vol. 11073, pp. 396–404. Springer, Cham (2018). https://doi.org/10.1007/978-3-030-00937-3_46
3. Chu, C., Belavỳ, D.L., Armbrecht, G., Bansmann, M., Felsenberg, D., Zheng, G.: Fully automatic localization and segmentation of 3d vertebral bodies from CT/MR images via a learning-based method. PLoS ONE **10**(11), e0143327 (2015)
4. Gutman, D., et al.: Skin lesion analysis toward melanoma detection: A challenge at the international symposium on biomedical imaging (ISBI) 2016, hosted by the international skin imaging collaboration (ISIC). arXiv preprint arXiv:1605.01397 (2016)

5. He, K., Gkioxari, G., Dollár, P., Girshick, R.: Mask R-CNN. In: Proceedings of the IEEE International Conference on Computer Vision, pp. 2961–2969 (2017)
6. Ibragimov, B., Likar, B., Pernuš, F., Vrtovec, T.: Shape representation for efficient landmark-based segmentation in 3-D. IEEE Trans. Med. Imaging **33**(4), 861–874 (2014)
7. Krähenbühl, P., Koltun, V.: Efficient inference in fully connected CRFs with Gaussian edge potentials. In: Advances in Neural Information Processing Systems, pp. 109–117 (2011)
8. Lee, H.W., Kim, N.R., Lee, J.H.: Deep neural network self-training based on unsupervised learning and dropout. Int. J. Fuzzy Logic Intell. Syst. **17**(1), 1–9 (2017)
9. Lessmann, N., van Ginneken, B., de Jong, P.A., Išgum, I.: Iterative fully convolutional neural networks for automatic vertebra segmentation. arXiv preprint arXiv:1804.04383 (2018)
10. Ronneberger, O., Fischer, P., Brox, T.: U-net: convolutional networks for biomedical image segmentation. In: Navab, N., Hornegger, J., Wells, W.M., Frangi, A.F. (eds.) MICCAI 2015. LNCS, vol. 9351, pp. 234–241. Springer, Cham (2015). https://doi.org/10.1007/978-3-319-24574-4_28
11. Sarker, M.M.K., et al.: SLSDeep: skin lesion segmentation based on dilated residual and pyramid pooling networks. In: Frangi, A.F., Schnabel, J.A., Davatzikos, C., Alberola-López, C., Fichtinger, G. (eds.) MICCAI 2018. LNCS, vol. 11071, pp. 21–29. Springer, Cham (2018). https://doi.org/10.1007/978-3-030-00934-2_3
12. Štern, D., Likar, B., Pernuš, F., Vrtovec, T.: Parametric modelling and segmentation of vertebral bodies in 3D CT and MR spine images. Phys. Med. Biol. **56**(23), 7505 (2011)

A Cascade Attention Network for Liver Lesion Classification in Weakly-Labeled Multi-phase CT Images

Xiao Chen[1,3], Lanfen Lin[1(✉)], Hongjie Hu[2(✉)], Qiaowei Zhang[2], Yutaro Iwamoto[3], Xianhua Han[3], Yen-Wei Chen[1,3,4(✉)], Ruofeng Tong[1], and Jian Wu[1]

[1] College of Computer Science and Technology, Zhejiang University, Hangzhou, China
llf@zju.edu.cn, chen@is.ritsumei.ac.jp
[2] Department of Radiology, Sir Run Run Shaw Hospital, Hangzhou, China
hongjiehu@zju.edu.cn
[3] College of Information Science and Engineering, Ritsumeikan University, Kyoto, Japan
[4] Zhejiang Lab, Hangzhou, China

Abstract. Focal liver lesion classification is important to the diagnostics of liver disease. In clinics, lesion type is usually determined by multi-phase contrast-enhanced CT images. Previous methods of automatic liver lesion classification are conducted on lesion-level, which rely heavily on lesion-level annotations. In order to reduce the burden of annotation, in this paper, we explore automatic liver lesion classification with weakly-labeled CT images (i.e. with only image-level labels). The major challenge is how to localize the region of interests (ROIs) accurately by using only coarse image-level annotations and accordingly make the right lesion classification decision. We propose a cascade attention network to address the challenge by two stages: Firstly, a dual-attention dilated residual network (DADRN) is proposed to generate a class-specific lesion localization map, which incorporates spatial attention and channel attention blocks for capturing the high-level feature map's long-range dependencies and helps to synthesize a more semantic-consistent feature map, and thereby boosting weakly-supervised lesion localization and classification performance; Secondly, a multi-channel dilated residual network (MCDRN) embedded with a convolutional long short-term memory (CLSTM) block is proposed to extract temporal enhancement information and make the final classification decision. The experiment results show that our method could achieve a mean classification accuracy of 89.68%, which significantly mitigates the performance gap between weakly-supervised approaches and fully supervised counterparts.

Keywords: Liver lesion classification · Channel attention · Spatial attention · Weakly-labeled · Multi-phase CT images · CLSTM

© Springer Nature Switzerland AG 2019
Q. Wang et al. (Eds.): DART 2019/MIL3ID 2019, LNCS 11795, pp. 129–138, 2019.
https://doi.org/10.1007/978-3-030-33391-1_15

1 Introduction

Globally, liver cancer ranks the sixth in cancer incidence and the second in tumor-related mortality. Multi-phase computed tomography (CT)images containing the enhancement pattern of focal liver lesions usually provide guidance for early liver cancer diagnosis. The main phases include the non-contrast (NC) phase, arterial (ART) phase, portal venous (PV) phase and delayed (DL) phase. Typically, to reduce the radiation dose, the DL phase is not required in clinical diagnosis.

Several previous studies have investigated liver lesion classification performance using multi-phase CT images with full annotations (lesion-level annotations). Most studies first selected or detected ROIs and then extracted low-level features [1, 2] or mid-level features [3–5] from ROIs. Some recent studies have explored the diagnostic performance of deep convolutional neural networks (DCNN) for liver lesion classification in multi-phase CT images. Yasaka et al. [6] proposed a multi-channel CNN for liver lesion classification on multi-phase CT images. Frid-Arar et al. [7] proposed a multi-class patch-based CNN for liver lesion detection. Liang et al. [8] proposed a residual network integrated with bi-directional LSTM model to learn the enhancement pattern of different kinds of lesions. Nevertheless, all of these methods must first identify or localize a lesion ROI on a CT image and then build classifiers based on the extracted ROIs. The first step is finished either by an expert radiologist's manual effort or an automatic lesion detection or segmentation algorithm [9]. However, lesion-level annotations are both labor-intensive and time-consuming, which pose obstacles for preparing large training datasets. In this paper, we explore address liver lesion classification using merely image-level label (with only the lesion class label, but without the lesion localization or boundary information), which is called as weakly-labeled annotations. Note that the annotation with both the lesion class label and lesion localization or boundary information is called as fully-labeled annotation or lesion-level annotation.

Given only the weakly-labeled multi-phase CT images, the major challenge of building a robust and well-performing lesion classification model is how to focus on the lesion area and then make classifications by the temporal enhancement pattern. In this paper, we propose a cascade attention classification framework. A dual-attention dilated residual network (DADRN) is proposed to automatically enhance the important region (lesion region). Then, another multi-channel dilated residual network (MCDRN) embedded with convolutional long short-term memory (CLSTM) block is used to extract spatiotemporal features of the guided attention region (lesion region) and produce the final liver lesion classification decision. Here, to provide a more semantic-accurate localization map, spatial attention and channel attention blocks are incorporated into DADRN. In many studies, attention mechanism has demonstrated its ability to focus on the most discriminative area and improve the feature representation of ROIs. Hu et al. [10] proposed a light-weight squeeze-and-excitation block that enhances channel-wise dependencies of high-level features, considering that each channel map can be regarded as a class-specific response. Woo et al. [11] proposed a convolutional block attention module that emphasizes meaningful features in both spatial and cross-channel axes. Their proposed module achieved the best classification accuracy on ImageNet-1K when integrated with a state-of-the-art CNN network. Our primary contributions can be summarized as follows.

A Cascade Attention Classification Framework: We propose a cascade attention classification method for focal liver lesion classification with weakly-labeled multiphase CT images, which consists of following two networks: (1) a *dual-attention dilated residual network (DADRN)*for localize the most class-specific discriminative region (lesion region) and improve the feature representation for classification; (2) a *multi-channel dilated residual network (MCDRN)* embedded with convolutional long short-term memory (CLSTM) block for fine classification that extract spatiotemporal features of the guided attention region (lesion region) for further improvement of feature representation.

Novel Attention Network (DADRN): We propose a novel dual-attention dilated residual network (DADRN) for multi-phase CT images analysis, which incorporates spatial attention and channel attention blocks for modeling the spatial and channel interdependencies of the high-level feature map and selectively aggregate similar semantic features.

State-of-the-Art Classification Accuracy: The proposed cascade attention classification framework achieved a mean lesion classification accuracy 89.68%, which is state-of-the-art performance in weakly-supervised approaches and is comparable to the performance obtained by fully-supervised lesion classification methods.

2 Methodology

As shown in Fig. 1, given multi-phase CT images without any lesion location information, firstly, the DADRN is trained (Sect. 2.1) with the concatenation of multi-phase images and its image-level annotation as a multi-class classification task. The well-trained DADRN can not only predict the lesion type of the RGB-like multi-phase input, but also can generate the class-specific localization map (Sect. 2.1.3). The generated localization map can be used as a guided attention mask of the multi-channel input of MCDRN (Sect. 2.2). The backbone of DADRN and MCDRN are based on DRN-d-50 [12], the average pooling layer and fully-connected layers are removed from the original architecture so as to obtain high-resolution global feature maps, which is four times larger than non-dilated residual network and thus facilitate consideration of small lesions at the course of its prediction.

2.1 Dual-Attention Dilated Residual Network (DADRN)

DADRN (upper part of Fig. 1) [15], is used for lesion classification and weakly-supervised localization. It includes two attention blocks, i.e., the channel attention block (CAB) and the spatial attention block (SAB) (Fig. 2). The attention blocks take the global feature map $A \in \mathbb{R}^{512 \times 28 \times 28}$ produced by DRN backbone as input. The output feature maps of two attention blocks are concatenated in channel dimension as

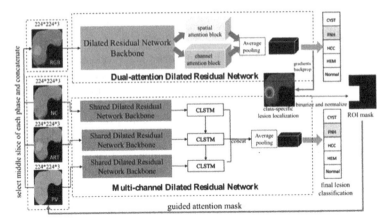

Fig. 1. Overview of the cascade attention classification network

$x \in \mathbb{R}^{(512\times2)\times28\times28}$, which serves as the global feature representation of input image and is used for lesion classification and localization in the first stage.

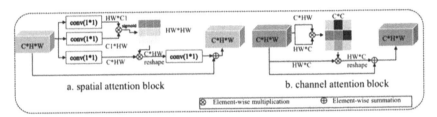

Fig. 2. Illustration of spatial and channel attention blocks

2.1.1 Channel Attention Block (CAB)

Since each channel map in the global feature can be considered as a class-specific response, the CAB aims to emphasize the similarity between channel maps. We first reshape $A \in \mathbb{R}^{C\times H\times W}$ into $A' \in \mathbb{R}^{C\times(H\times W)}$, and perform a matrix multiplication to calculate channel similarity map $\alpha_{ij} \in \mathbb{R}^{C\times C}$ as,

$$\alpha_{ji} = \frac{1}{1+e^{-S_{ij}}}, \text{ where } S_{ij} = A'A'^{T} \tag{1}$$

where α_{ij} indicates the cosine similarity of the ith and j^{th} channel map. Here, we adopt the sigmoid function to normalize the similarity map because noise is present in the target medical images. The sigmoid function can avoid oversensitivity to local intensity changes and can disseminate more information than that of softmax function. Subsequently, the feature attention map is obtained by a matrix multiplication of A and α, where A_j represents the jth channel map of the input feature A. We then multiply the feature attention map by a scale parameter η, and perform an element-wise sum operation with the original input A as,

$$y_j = \eta \sum_{i=1}^{c} (\alpha_{ji} A_i) + A_j \qquad (2)$$

The parameter η is first initialized as 0 and was gradually assigned more weight in the training phase via back-propagation. The final output of CAB is $y \in \mathbb{R}^{C \times H \times W}$.

2.1.2 Spatial Attention Block (SAB)

The SAB is designed to model long-range dependencies in the spatial dimension. Here, spatial regions with the same pattern are benefited from each other via the spatial attention mechanism. Given the global feature map A, it is fed into 1×1 conv layer and transformed into two feature spaces $B_1, B_2 \in \mathbb{R}^{C1 \times H \times W}$, which are then flattened in the spatial dimension $B_1', B_2' \in \mathbb{R}^{C1 \times (H \times W)}$ and calculate the spatial similarity map as,

$$\beta_{ji} = \frac{1}{1 + e^{-S_{ij}}}, \; where \; S_{ij} = B_1'^T B_2' \qquad (3)$$

where $\beta_{ji} \in \mathbb{R}^{N \times N}$ and $N = H \times W$. Meanwhile, A was also transformed into feature map $C \in \mathbb{R}^{C \times H \times W}$ Then, a matrix multiplication is performed between β and the concatenated feature maps C to generate a new feature attention map z_j as,

$$z_j = \gamma \sum_{i=1}^{N} \beta_{ji} B_i + B_j \qquad (4)$$

Note that all other spatial positions are included when synthesizing the jth position feature vector in z_j. Here, more similar positions have higher attention weights. The final output of the spatial attention module $z \in \mathbb{R}^{C \times H \times W}$ is the element-wise sum result between the feature attention and original feature maps. The adaptive scale parameter γ is first initialized as 0.

2.1.3 Class-Specific Lesion Localization

The well-trained classification network can be used for weakly-supervised localization. Grad-CAM [13] is generally used to localize the attended regions in the global feature map, which uses gradients of the prediction score for a specific class and the global feature map to calculate the importance of spatial locations in the convolutional layers.

The process of weakly-supervised lesion localization is (Fig. 3): First, DADRN predicts the type of the concatenated multi-phase image and produce a class-specific Grad-CAM heatmap; Then, the heatmap is normalized and binarized with a threshold of 0.25, considering cover possible lesion area as much as possible; After that, the heatmap is resized to 224×224 and a bounding box is generated that covers all positive pixels in the binarized heatmap. Finally, the guided attention mask that covers the bounding box is generated as $M' \in \mathbb{R}^{1 \times 224 \times 224} \left(where \; M'_{ijk} \in \{0, 1\} \right)$.

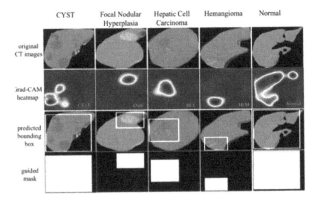

Fig. 3. Illustration of class-specific lesion localization process

2.2   Multi-channel Dilated Residual Network (MCDRN)

The architecture of MCDRN is shown in the lower part of Fig. 1. MCDRN has three channels corresponding to three phases. Each phase's liver slice image $T \in \mathbb{R}^{3 \times 224 \times 224}$ is multiplied by the guided attention mask $M' \in \mathbb{R}^{1 \times 224 \times 224}$ and the result is fed into a shared-weight DRN for extraction of high-level feature map. Each CLSTM cell in MCDRN takes each phase's global feature map $F^n \in \mathbb{R}^{512 \times 28 \times 28}$ as input. The output of CLSTM cells are concatenated as $F \in \mathbb{R}^{1536 \times 28 \times 28}$ and is fed into a 1×1 conv layer to extract the spatiotemporal features of the guided attention region (lesion region) and facilitate improve liver lesion classification performance in the second stage.

Training Process. In the training phase, DADRN is trained with weakly-labeled multi-phase CT images (RGB format). Weighted cross entropy loss is adopted as the objective function for this multi-class classification task. After DADRN is well trained, the network parameters of DADRN are fixed. Secondly, MCDRN is trained with guidance from DADRN. The final lesion classification result is determined by MCDRN, but the performance would be influenced by the classification and weakly-supervised localization performance of DADRN.

3   Experimental Results

3.1   Materials

The multi-phase CT images used in this study were collected from 156 patients. The CT scans were acquired with a slice collimation of 5–7 mm, a matrix of 512×512 pixels, and an in-plane resolution of 0.57–0.89 mm. There were a total of 1091 CT liver slice images corresponding to each phase, which consisted of five types, namely Normal, CYST, Focal Nodular Hyperplasia (FNH), Hepatic Cell Carcinoma (HCC), and Hemangioma (HEM)). Notice that, each liver slice image only contains one type of liver lesions or neither. We first conducted liver registration on multi-phase CT images with a non-rigid registration algorithm. Then, an iterative probabilistic atlas model [14] is applied to automatically segment liver tissue from the original CT volume data. Details of the dataset considered in this study are shown in Table 1.

Table 1. Details of multi-phase CT images dataset, slices number (CT volumes) in each phase.

Type	Train		Validation		Test		Total
	Set1	Set2	Set1	Set2	Set1	Set2	
Normal	135(58)	126(51)	41(16)	57(22)	51(19)	44(20)	227(93)
CYST	168(64)	166(61)	56(25)	59(26)	69(25)	68(27)	293(114)
FNH	75 (43)	75(35)	29(10)	27(18)	26(14)	28(14)	130(67)
HCC	149(57)	143(65)	52(23)	57(18)	50(21)	51(18)	251(101)
HEM	112(53)	114(62)	38(20)	37(16)	40(20)	39(15)	190(93)

3.2 Performance Analysis of the Proposed Method

3.2.1 Comparison Between DADRN and Other Attention-Based Models

In the proposed cascade network, the localization (loc) and classification (cls) accuracy of DADRN is essential for the final fine classification performance. To evaluate the effectiveness of the attention blocks in DADRN, we compared it with other attention blocks in Table 2. We chose pure DRN-d-50 (DRN) as the baseline and DRN-d-50 embedded with two state-of-the art attention blocks for comparison, i.e., SEDRN (DRN+Squeeze Excitation (SE) block [10]), CBAMDRN (DRN+convolutional block attention block [11]).

In Table 2, the localization accuracy of each class is calculated as Eq. (5). Since the resized localization map is often larger than ground-truth bounding box (bbox). We chose intersection over the detected bounding box area ratio (IoBB) as the evaluation metrics. A predicted bbox is considered accurate when its IoBB is greater than 0.3. If there are multiple ROIs in a liver slice image, it will be viewed as correct localized if the number of correct predicted lesions is more than 1. The best macro localization and classification accuracy is achieved by the proposed DADRN.

$$loc\ accuracy_{class\,c} = \frac{total\ num\ of\ correct\ localized\ slices\ for\ class\,c}{total\ num\ of\ slices\ for\ class\,c} \quad (5)$$

Table 2. The class-wise loc accuracy, macro average loc and cls accuracy of DADRN (%)

Method	CYST	FNH	HCC	HEM	Loc accuracy	cls accuracy
DRN [12]	88.40	96.30	92.00	64.86	85.39	84.21
SEDRN [10]	82.61	96.30	94.00	72.97	86.47	86.95
CBAMDRN [11]	85.51	92.59	**94.00**	75.68	86.94	85.49
DADRN	**94.20**	**96.30**	90.00	**86.49**	**92.11**	**87.64**

3.2.2 Ablation Study of the Proposed Cascade Attention Network

Table 3 presents the cls accuracy comparison results. Compared to single MCDRN with no guided attention mask, the proposed cascade network obtains marginally better cls accuracy (macro average 4.8%). Compared to single DADRN, the proposed method also showed better performance in most classes (average 2.04%). Compared to the cascade network without CLSTM block, the proposed method achieved better cls performance in all categories (average 2.5%).

Table 3. class-wise and macro average cls accuracy of each network (%) (weakly labeled data)

Method	CYST	FNH	HCC	HEM	Normal	Accuracy
DADRN	93.86	85.45	78.29	**85.16**	95.45	87.64
MCDRN (w/o guidance)	95.45	85.45	77.29	68.57	97.62	84.88
DADRN+MCDRN (w/o CLSTM)	95.65	81.81	82.25	79.53	96.64	87.18
DADRN+MCDRN	**96.31**	**89.09**	**84.29**	80.92	**97.83**	**89.68**

3.2.3 Comparison with State-of-the-Art Lesion Classification Models

In Table 4, we also compared the proposed method based on weak labels to state-of-the-art lesion classification methods based on full labels including both deep learning-based methods [6–8] and non-deep learning-based methods [1, 4, 5]. The ROIs of lesions were first extracted from the whole liver slice images in our dataset by doctors. Then we performed ROI-level classifications by using the state-of-the-art methods. As shown in Table 4, the macro lesion accuracy of our method using only weak labels is close to that of the traditional methods using full-labels, which motivates us to explore the potential of using liver slice images directly for the liver lesion classification task.

Table 4. The class-wise and macro average classification accuracy (%) compared to state-of-the-art methods with fully labeled multi-phase CT images.

		Method	CYST	FNH	HCC	HEM	Accuracy
Weak annotations		DADRN +MCDRN	96.31	89.09	84.29	80.92	87.65
Full annotations	Non-deep learning methods	Roy et al. [1]	95.71	70.84	58.44	56.45	70.36
		Diamant et al. [4]	82.41	68.20	78.84	76.90	76.59
		Xu et al. [5]	92.15	69.08	85.04	84.31	82.65
	Deep learning methods	Yasaka et al. [6]	96.96	83.66	86.82	84.16	87.90
		Frid-Adar et al. [7]	97.75	76.39	84.37	40.67	74.80
		Liang et al. [8]	98.02	86.74	88.82	87.75	90.33

4 Conclusions

In this paper, we proposed a cascade attention network to address focal liver lesion classification in weakly-labeled multi-phase CT images. The attention-based DADRN learns what and where to emphasize or suppress in a global feature map and enhances the lesion area. The MCDRN strengthens the focal lesion's contrast-enhanced pattern. In future, we will extend the proposed method to multi-label classification task.

Acknowledgements. This work was supported in part by Major Scientific Research Project of Zhejiang Lab under the Grant No. 2018DG0ZX01, in part by the Science and Technology Support Program of Hangzhou under the Grant No. 20172011A038, and in part by the Grant-in Aid for Scientific Research from the Japanese Ministry for Education, Science, Culture and Sports (MEXT) under the Grant No. 18H03267.

References

1. Roy, S., et al.: Three-dimensional spatiotemporal features for fast content-based retrieval of focal liver lesions. IEEE Trans. Biomed. Eng. **61**(11), 2768–2778 (2014)
2. Xu, Y., et al.: Combined density, texture and shape features of multi-phase contrast-enhanced CT images for CBIR of focal liver lesions: a preliminary study. Innov. Med. Healthc. **2015**, 215–224 (2015)
3. Yang, W., et al.: Content-based retrieval of focal liver lesions using bag-of-visual-words representations of single-and multiphase contrast-enhanced CT images. J. Digit. Imaging **25** (6), 708–719 (2012)
4. Diamant, I., et al.: Improved patch-based automated liver lesion classification by separate analysis of the interior and boundary regions. IEEE J. Biomed. Health Inf. **20**(6), 1585–1594 (2016)
5. Xu, Y., et al.: Texture-specific bag of visual words model and spatial cone matching-based method for the retrieval of focal liver lesions using multiphase contrast-enhanced CT images. Int. J. Comput. Assist. Radiol. Surg. **13**(1), 151–164 (2018)
6. Yasaka, K., et al.: Deep learning with convolutional neural network for differentiation of liver masses at dynamic contrast-enhanced CT: a preliminary study. Radiology **286**(3), 887–896 (2017)
7. Frid-Adar, M., Diamant, I., Klang, E., Amitai, M., Goldberger, J., Greenspan, H.: Modeling the intra-class variability for liver lesion detection using a multi-class patch-based CNN. In: Wu, G., Munsell, B.C., Zhan, Y., Bai, W., Sanroma, G., Coupé, P. (eds.) Patch-MI 2017. LNCS, vol. 10530, pp. 129–137. Springer, Cham (2017). https://doi.org/10.1007/978-3-319-67434-6_15
8. Liang, D., et al.: Combining convolutional and recurrent neural networks for classification of focal liver lesions in multi-phase CT images. In: Frangi, A.F., Schnabel, J.A., Davatzikos, C., Alberola-López, C., Fichtinger, G. (eds.) MICCAI 2018. LNCS, vol. 11071, pp. 666–675. Springer, Cham (2018). https://doi.org/10.1007/978-3-030-00934-2_74
9. Li, X., et al.: H-DenseUNet: hybrid densely connected UNet for liver and tumor segmentation from CT volumes. IEEE Trans. Med. Imaging **37**(12), 2663–2674 (2018)
10. Hu, J., Shen, L., Sun, G.: Squeeze-and-Excitation networks. In: IEEE Conference on Computer Vision and Pattern Recognition (CVPR), pp. 7132–7141 (2017)

11. Woo, S., Park, J., Lee, J.-Y., Kweon, I.S.: CBAM: convolutional block attention module. In: Ferrari, V., Hebert, M., Sminchisescu, C., Weiss, Y. (eds.) ECCV 2018. LNCS, vol. 11211, pp. 3–19. Springer, Cham (2018). https://doi.org/10.1007/978-3-030-01234-2_1
12. Yu, F., Koltun, V., Funkhouser, T.A.: Dilated residual networks. In: IEEE Conference on Computer Vision and Pattern Recognition (CVPR), pp. 472–480 (2017)
13. Selvaraju, R., Cogswell, M., Das, A., et al.: Grad-CAM: visual explanations from deep networks via gradient-based localization. In: Proceedings of ICCV 2017, pp. 618–626 (2017)
14. Dong, C., Chen, Y., Lin, L., et al.: Segmentation of liver and spleen based on computational anatomy models. Comput. Biol. Med. **67**, 146–160 (2015)
15. Chen, X., et al.: A dual-attention dilated residual network for liver lesion classification and localization on CT images. In: Proceedings of IEEE ICIP 2019 (2019, in press)

CT Data Curation for Liver Patients: Phase Recognition in Dynamic Contrast-Enhanced CT

Bo Zhou[1,2], Adam P. Harrison[2(✉)], Jiawen Yao[2], Chi-Tung Cheng[4],
Jing Xiao[3], Chien-Hung Liao[4], and Le Lu[2]

[1] Biomedical Engineering, Yale University, New Haven, CT, USA
[2] PAII Inc., Bethesda, MD, USA
`adam.p.harrison@gmail.com`
[3] PingAn Technology, Shenzhen, China
[4] Chang Gung Memorial Hospital, Linkou, Taiwan, ROC

Abstract. As the demand for more descriptive machine learning models grows within medical imaging, bottlenecks due to data paucity will exacerbate. Thus, collecting enough large-scale data will require automated tools to harvest data/label pairs from messy and real-world datasets, such as hospital picture archiving and communication systems (PACSs). This is the focus of our work, where we present a principled data curation tool to extract multi-phase computed tomography (CT) liver studies and identify each scan's phase from a real-world and heterogenous hospital PACS dataset. Emulating a typical deployment scenario, we first obtain a set of noisy labels from our institutional partners that are text mined using simple rules from DICOM tags. We train a deep learning system, using a customized and streamlined 3D squeeze and excitation (SE) architecture, to identify non-contrast, arterial, venous, and delay phase dynamic CT liver scans, filtering out anything else, including other types of liver contrast studies. To exploit as much training data as possible, we also introduce an aggregated cross entropy loss that can learn from scans only identified as "contrast". Extensive experiments on a dataset of 43K scans of 7680 patient imaging studies demonstrate that our 3DSE architecture, armed with our aggregated loss, can achieve a mean F1 of 0.977 and can correctly harvest up to 92.7% of studies, which significantly outperforms the text-mined and standard-loss approach, and also outperforms other, and more complex, model architectures.

Keywords: Data curation · PACS · Dynamic CT · Phase recognition

Electronic supplementary material The online version of this chapter (https://doi.org/10.1007/978-3-030-33391-1_16) contains supplementary material, which is available to authorized users.

Q. Wang et al. (Eds.): DART 2019/MIL3ID 2019, LNCS 11795, pp. 139–147, 2019.
https://doi.org/10.1007/978-3-030-33391-1_16

1 Introduction

Over the last decade, deep learning techniques have seen success in automatically interpreting biomedical and diagnostic imaging data [1,2]. However, robust performance often requires training from large-scale data. Unlike computer vision datasets, which can rely on crowd-sourcing [3], the collection of large-scale medical imaging datasets must typically involve physician labor. Thus, there exists a tension between modeling power and data requirements that only promises to increase [4]. An enticing prospect is mining physician expertise by collecting retrospective data from picture archiving and communication systems (PACSs), but the current generation of PACSs do not properly address the curation of large-scale data for machine learning. In PACSs, DICOM tags regarding scan descriptions are typically hand inputted, non-standardized, and often incomplete, which leads to the need for extensive data curation [5]. These limitations frequently produce high mislabeling rates, *e.g.*, the 15% rate reported by Gueld *et al.*, meaning that simply selecting the scans of interest (SOIs) from a large set of studies can be prohibitively laborious. This has spurred efforts to automatically text mine image/label pairs from PACSs [6–8], but these efforts rely on complicated and customized natural language processing (NLP) technology to extract labels. Apart from the barriers put forth by this complexity, these solutions address contexts where it is possible to extract the information of interest from accompanying text. This is not always possible, as NLP parsers [8,9] cannot always straightforwardly correct errors in the original reports or fill in missing information. As such, collecting large-scale data will also require developing automated, but robust, tools that go beyond mining from DICOM tags and/or reports.

This is the topic of our work, where we articulate a robust approach to large-scale data curation based on visual information. In our case, we focus on a hospital PACS dataset we collected that consists of 43 010 computed tomography (CT) scans of 7 680 imaging studies from 4 666 unique patients with liver lesions, along with pathological diagnoses. Its makeup is highly heterogeneous, comprising studies of multiple organs, protocols, and reconstruction types. Very simple and accessible text matching rules applied to the DICOM tags can accurately extract scan descriptions; however omissions and errors in the text mean these labels are noisy and unreliable. Without loss of generality, we focus on extracting a large-scale and well curated dataset of dynamic liver CT studies from our PACS data. Dynamic CT is the most common protocol to categorize and assess liver lesions [10], and we expect a large-scale dataset to prove highly valuable for the development of computer-aided diagnosis systems, *provided it is well curated*. Thus, the goal is to use the noisy labels to train a visual recognition system that can much more robustly identify dynamic liver CT studies, extract the corresponding axial-reconstructed scans, and identify the phase of each as being non-contrast (NC), arterial (A), venous (V), or delay (D). Figure 1 shows examples of each phase and discriminating features of each.

Unlike prior work, we focus on extracting multi-phase volumetric SOIs of a certain type, rather than on extracting disease tags or labels. This places a

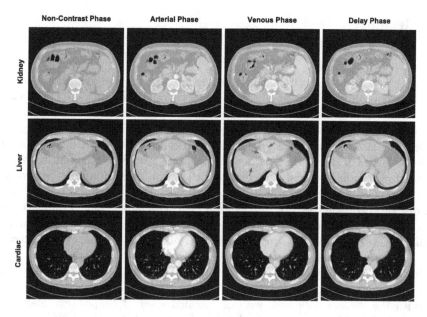

Fig. 1. Non-contrast (NC), arterial (A), venous (V), and delay (D) phases are the SOIs in dynamic CT. Radiologists use contrast information in several organs to determine the phase, such as contrast in the heart/aorta (red arrows), portal veins (green arrows), and kidneys (yellow arrows). (Color figure online)

high expectation on performance, *i.e.*, F1 scores of 0.95, or higher. To tackle this problem, we develop a principled phase recognition system whose contributions are threefold. First, we collect the aforementioned large-scale dataset from a hospital PACS, that includes more than 43 010 scans. Second, we introduce a customized phase-recognition deep-learning model, comprised of a streamlined version of C3D [11] with squeeze and excitation (SE) layers. We show that this simple, yet effective model, can outperform much more complicated models. Third, we address a common issue facing data curation systems, where many text mined labels are too general. In our case, these are labels that indicate only "contrast" rather than the more specific NC, A, V, or D SOIs. So that we can still use these images for training, along with their weak supervisory signals, we design an aggregated cross entropy (ACE) loss that incorporates the hierarchical relationship within annotations. Our experimental results demonstrate that our 3DSE model, in combination with our ACE loss, can achieve significantly better phase recognition performance than the text-mined method and other deep-learning based approaches. To the best of our knowledge, this is the first work investigating visual-information based data curation methods in PACS, and we expect that our data curation system would also prove a useful curation approach in domains other than liver dynamic CT.

2   Methods

2.1   Dataset

Our goal is to reliably curate as large as possible a dataset of liver dynamic CT scans, with minimal labor. To do this, we first extracted a dataset of CT studies from the PACS of *Anomymized*, corresponding to patients who had pathological diagnoses of liver lesions, with the hope that such a dataset would be of great interest for later downstream analysis. This resulted in 7 680 studies of 4 666 patients. For each study, the number of scans range from 4 to 30 and there are one to three studies per patient. The resulting dataset is highly heterogenous, containing several types of reconstructions, projections, anatomical regions, and contrast protocols that we not interested in, *e.g.*, computed tomography arterial portography. Studies containing dynamic CT scans may have anywhere from one or all of NC, A, V, and D contrast phase SOIs. Our aim is to identify and extract the axial-reconstructed versions of these scans from each study, should they exist. As such, this task exemplifies many of the general demands and challenges of data curation across medical domains.

With the dataset collected, we next applied a set of simple text matching rules to the DICOM tags to noisily label each scan as being either NC, A, V, D or other (O). The full set of rules are tabulated in our supplemental materials. The text-matching rules are more than sufficient to reliably extract labels *based on text alone*, due to the extremely simple structure and vocabulary of DICOM tags. However, because the source DICOM tags are themselves error-prone and unreliable [12], these labels suffer from inaccuracies, which we demonstrate later in our results. Finally, we filter out any scans that have less than 10 slices, with a spatial resolution coarser than 5mm, or were taken after or during a biopsy or transplant procedure. As a result, we found 1728, 1703, 1504 and 1736 A, V, D and NC scans, respectively, with 326 scans labeled as 'contrast'. We then manually annotated a validation set and a test set, comprising 801 and 1262 scans; 150 and 231 studies; and 101 and 196 patients, respectively. This left a training set of 29 891 scans from 5 164 studies of 3 267 patients with noisy text-mined annotations.

2.2   3DSE Network

As Fig. 1 illustrates, visual cues indicating the phase can be located in different anatomical areas. Given this, we opt for a 3D classification network. State of the art 3D classification networks, such as 3D-Resnet [13] and C3D [11], are often quite large, adding to the training time and increasing overfitting tendencies.

Instead, we use a streamlined but effective architecture we call 3DSE, which is illustrated in Fig. 2. To begin, we first downsample all volumes to $128 \times 128 \times 32$. From these, image features are extracted using two convolutional layers, each followed by a rectified linear unit and max pooling layers. With such a streamlined feature extracter, activation maps are highly local [14]. Thus, we add squeeze and excitation (SE) [14] layers. These scale each feature channel with multiplicative

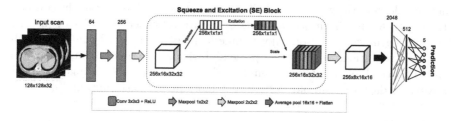

Fig. 2. Our 3DSE network is designed to have a relatively small amount of parameters and consists of three parts, including two 3D convolution layers, one SE layer, and two fully connected layers.

factors computed using global pooling, providing an efficient means to increase descriptive capacity and inject global information. Subsequent pooling layers and a two fully connected layers provide the five output phase predictions. The total parameter size 19.22 MB which is significantly smaller than 3D-Resnet [13] and C3D [11].

2.3 Aggregated Cross Entropy

Frequently, text-mined labels are only able to provide a more general label of "contrast" for a scan, indicating that it could be any of A, V, or D SOIs. Since our goal is to determine the exact phase, the easiest way to handle such scans is to simply remove them from training, at the cost of using less data. Yet, such weakly supervised data still provides useful information, which should ideally be exploited to use as much training data as possible. To do this, we formulate a simple aggregated cross entropy (ACE) loss that can execute a cross entropy (CE) loss, but these weakly supervised instances. We formulate the probability of "contrast" as equalling the sum of the probabilities of all contrast phases:

$$p_C = p_A + p_V + p_D, \tag{1}$$

$$= \frac{\exp(\mathbf{w}_A) + \exp(\mathbf{w}_V) + \exp(\mathbf{w}_D)}{\sum_i \exp(\mathbf{w}_i)}, \tag{2}$$

where (2) assumes a pseudo-probability calculated using softmax, $\mathbf{w}_{(.)}$ denotes the logit outputs, and i indexes all five outputs.

The p_C can be naively used in a CE loss, but that would preclude using a numerically stable "softmax with CE" formulation. Instead, for scans that can only be labelled as "contrast", the CE loss can be written as:

$$\ell_{CE} = -y_{NC} \log(p_{NC}) - y_O \log(p_O) - y_C \log(p_C), \tag{3}$$

$$= -\log\left(\frac{\exp(\mathbf{w}_A) + \exp(\mathbf{w}_V) + \exp(\mathbf{w}_D)}{\sum_i \exp(\mathbf{w}_i)}\right), \tag{4}$$

$$= \text{logsumexp}(\{\mathbf{w}_i\}) - \text{logsumexp}(\{\mathbf{w}_A, \mathbf{w}_V, \mathbf{w}_D\}), \tag{5}$$

where $y_{(.)}$ denotes the ground truth. The elimination of all terms but the contrast term in (4), follows from y_C equalling one, with all other $y_{(.)}$ values equalling zero. The logsumexp function enjoys numerically stable forward- and backward-pass implementations. Thus, when presented with a "contrast" scan, our model uses (5) for the loss, providing a simple and numerically stable means to exploit all available data to train our desired, but more fine-grained, outputs.

3   Results

We tested our 3DSE network, with and without the ACE loss, on our dataset, and compared it to both the noisy text-mined labels and also 3D-Resnet-101 [13] and C3D [11]. For all models we perform a sweep of learning rates and report results corresponding to the best setting and stopping point based on the validation set.

Focusing first on scan-level comparisons, Table 1 presents F1 scores across the different phase types. As can be observed from the text-mined results, many scans are misclassified as O and many D scans are missed, demonstrating the shortfalls of relying on labels based on DICOM tags. In contrast, the vision-based 3DSE significantly reduces classification errors, improving the mean F1 score from 0.938 (via text mining) to 0.967. In particular, V's F1 score is improved from 0.868 to 0.956. Performance is increased even further when we use the ACE loss to include the "contrast" scans in training, boosting the mean F1 score to 0.977. While tests show a degradation of performance for the D phase, these differences do not meet statistical significance, unlike the statistically significant improvements seen in the NC, V, and O phases. Thus, these results validate the use of our ACE formulation to exploit as much training data as possible.

Table 1. Quantitative comparison of scan-level performance. Best results are marked in bold. For the 3DSE + ACE F1 phase-level scores, we use ∗and † to indicate if differences were statistically significant ($\alpha < 0.05$) compared to the text-mining and 3DSE model, respectively. Significance was calculated using randomized tests [15] and adjusted using the multiple comparison correction of Holm-Bonferroni [16].

	Text mining			3DSE			3DSE + ACE		
	Precision	Recall	F1 score	Precision	Recall	F1 score	Precision	Recall	F1 score
NC	0.977	0.895	0.934	0.965	0.965	0.964	0.993	0.986	**0.988**∗†
A	0.966	0.983	0.974	0.974	0.966	0.970	0.991	0.991	**0.992**
V	0.975	0.782	0.868	0.965	0.946	0.956	0.930	0.993	**0.963**∗
D	0.964	0.956	0.960	0.964	0.956	**0.960**	0.972	0.930	0.951
O	0.926	0.986	0.955	0.981	0.989	0.985	0.997	0.990	**0.993**∗†
Mean	0.962	0.920	0.938	0.970	0.964	0.967	0.977	0.978	**0.977**

Shifting focus to across-model comparisons, Table 2 compares our 3DSE model, with and without SE, against other state-of-the-art 3D deep models [11,13]. As can be seen, 3D-Resnet is nearly 17 times larger than 3DSE and performs poorly, which we observed was due to overfitting. Moving down in model

Table 2. Across-model quantitative evaluation using the F1 score. Best and second-best results are marked in bold and italic, respectively.

	NC	A	V	D	O	Mean	Model size (MB)
3DResnet [13]	0.560	0.866	0.259	0.052	0.929	0.533	325.22
C3D [11]	0.972	0.965	0.920	0.895	0.989	0.948	33.56
3DSE-SE	0.954	0.953	0.924	0.914	0.985	0.946	11.44
3DSE	0.964	0.970	0.956	0.960	0.985	*0.967*	19.22
3DSE+ACE	0.988	0.992	0.963	0.951	0.993	**0.977**	19.22

size, C3D [11] performs better than 3D-Resnet, but is still unable to match 3DSE. If we remove the SE layer from our 3DSE model, performance considerably suffers, which demonstrates that the SE layer is important in achieving high performance. Despite this, performance still matches C3D even though a significantly smaller number of parameters are used. Finally, the last rows show 3DSE with and without the ACE loss, with latter achieving the highest performance at a model size much smaller than competitors. Finally, as Fig. 3 illustrates, the 3DSE model focuses on anatomical regions that are consistent with clinical practice. More visualizations can be found in our supplementary material.

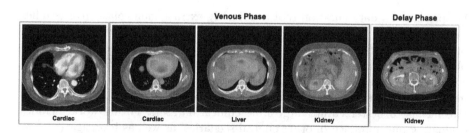

Fig. 3. Respond-CAM [17] visualizations of 3DSE from three different dynamic CT scans. (A) the 3DSE focuses on contrast accumulation in the cardiac region; (V): 3DSE focuses on contrast remnants in the cardiac blood pool, liver portal veins, and kidney veins; (D): 3DSE focuses on contrast accumulation in the ureters of the kidney.

These boosts in scan-level performance are important, but arguably the study-level performance is even more important, as the ultimate goal is to identify and extract as many dynamic liver CT studies as possible for downstream analysis. Thus, we also evaluate how many studies are correctly extracted, meaning all of their corresponding SOIs are correctly classified. As Table 3 demonstrates, 90.5% of studies have all of their scans correctly classified by our 3DSE model. Including the wealky supervised data using the ACE loss, we can further improve this to 92.7%. If we extrapolate these results to entire dataset of 7 680 studies, this means that the 3DSE model, armed with the ACE loss, can

Table 3. Study-level performance of text mining and 3DSE. Each row groups studies based on the number of dynamic CT scans of interest (SOIs) they possess. Each column counts the number of studies based on how many scans were misclassified, if any. Best results for each SOI number are marked in bold.

	Text mining			3DSE			3DSE + ACE		
	0 Errs.	1 Err.	≥2 Errs.	0 Errs.	1 Err.	≥2 Errs.	0 Errs.	1 Err.	≥2 Errs.
0 SOIs	35	8	10	47	4	2	**48**	5	0
1 SOI	36	13	1	47	1	2	**49**	1	0
2 SOIs	0	1	0	1	0	0	**1**	0	0
3 SOIs	15	3	1	19	0	0	**19**	0	0
4 SOIs	**101**	6	1	95	12	1	97	10	1
Total	186	32	13	209	16	6	**214**	16	1
Accuracy	80.9%	–	–	90.5%	–	–	92.7%	–	–

correctly identify and extract 609 more studies than the text mining approach. This is a significant boost of study numbers for any subsequent analyses.

4   Conclusion

We presented a data curation tool to robustly extract multi-phase liver studies from a real-world and heterogenous hospital PACS. This includes a streamlined, but powerful, 3DSE model and a principled ACE loss designed to handle incompletely labelled data. Experiments demonstrated that our 3DSE model, along with the ACE loss, can outperform both text mining and also more complex deep models. These results indicate that our vision-based approach can be an effective means to better curate large-scale clinical datasets. Future work includes evaluating our approach in other clinical scenarios, as well as investigating how to harmonize text-mined features with our visual-based system.

References

1. Litjens, G.J.S., et al.: A survey on deep learning in medical image analysis. Med. Image Anal. **42**, 60–88 (2017)
2. Zhou, B., Lin, X., Eck, B., Hou, J., Wilson, D.: Generation of virtual dual energy images from standard single-shot radiographs using multi-scale and conditional adversarial network. In: Jawahar, C.V., Li, H., Mori, G., Schindler, K. (eds.) ACCV 2018. LNCS, vol. 11361, pp. 298–313. Springer, Cham (2019). https://doi.org/10.1007/978-3-030-20887-5_19
3. Deng, J., Dong, W., Socher, R., Li, L.J., Li, K., Fei-Fei, L.: Imagenet: a large-scale hierarchical image database. In: IEEE CVPR, pp. 248–255 (2009)
4. Kohli, M.D., Summers, R.M., Geis, J.R.: Medical image data and datasets in the era of machine learning: Whitepaper from the 2016 C-MIMI meeting dataset session. J. Digital Imaging **30**(4), 392–399 (2017)

5. Harvey, H., Glocker, B.: A standardised approach for preparing imaging data for machine learning tasks in radiology. In: Ranschaert, E.R., Morozov, S., Algra, P.R. (eds.) Artificial Intelligence in Medical Imaging, pp. 61–72. Springer, Cham (2019). https://doi.org/10.1007/978-3-319-94878-2_6
6. Yan, K., Wang, X., Lu, L., Summers, R.M.: Deeplesion: automated mining of large-scale lesion annotations and universal lesion detection with deep learning. J. Med. Imaging **5**(3), 036501 (2018)
7. Zhou, B., Chen, A., Crawford, R., Dogdas, B., Goldmarcher, G.: A progressively-trained scale-invariant and boundary-aware deep neural network for the automatic 3D segmentation of lung lesions. In: 2019 IEEE Winter Conference on Applications of Computer Vision (WACV), pp. 1–10. IEEE (2019)
8. Irvin, J., Rajpurkar, P., et al.: Chexpert: a large chest radiograph dataset with uncertainty labels and expert comparison. In: AAAI (2019)
9. Peng, Y., Wang, X., Lu, L., Bagheri, M., Summers, R., Lu, Z.: NegBio: a high-performance tool for negation and uncertainty detection in radiology reports. AMIA Jt Summits Transl. Sci. Proc. **2018**, 188–196 (2018)
10. Burrowes, D.P., Medellin, A., Harris, A.C., Milot, L., Wilson, S.R.: Contrast-enhanced us approach to the diagnosis of focal liver masses. RadioGraphics **37**(5), 1388–1400 (2017)
11. Tran, D., Bourdev, L., Fergus, R., Torresani, L., Paluri, M.: Learning spatiotemporal features with 3D convolutional networks. In: IEEE International Conference on Computer Vision, pp. 4489–4497 (2015)
12. Gueld, M.O., et al.: Quality of DICOM header information for image categorization. In: Proceedings of SPIE Medical Imaging (2002)
13. Hara, K., Kataoka, H., Satoh, Y.: Learning spatio-temporal features with 3D residual networks for action recognition. In: IEEE CVPR, pp. 3154–3160 (2017)
14. Hu, J., Shen, L., Sun, G.: Squeeze-and-excitation networks. In: IEEE Conference on Computer Vision and Pattern Recognition, pp. 7132–7141 (2018)
15. Yeh, A.: More accurate tests for the statistical significance of result differences. In: Proceedings of the 18th Conference on Computational Linguistics - Volume 2. COLING 2000, Stroudsburg, PA, USA, pp. 947–953 (2000)
16. Holm, S.: A simple sequentially rejective multiple test procedure. Scand. J. Stat. **6**, 65–70 (1979)
17. Zhao, G., Zhou, B., Wang, K., Jiang, R., Xu, M.: Respond-CAM: analyzing deep models for 3D imaging data by visualizations. In: Frangi, A.F., Schnabel, J.A., Davatzikos, C., Alberola-López, C., Fichtinger, G. (eds.) MICCAI 2018. LNCS, vol. 11070, pp. 485–492. Springer, Cham (2018). https://doi.org/10.1007/978-3-030-00928-1_55

Active Learning Technique for Multimodal Brain Tumor Segmentation Using Limited Labeled Images

Dhruv Sharma[1,2], Zahil Shanis[1], Chandan K. Reddy[2], Samuel Gerber[1], and Andinet Enquobahrie[1(✉)]

[1] Kitware, Inc., Carrboro, NC 27510, USA
andinet.enqu@kitware.com
[2] Virginia Polytechnic Institute and State University, Blacksburg, VA 24060, USA

Abstract. Image segmentation is an essential step in biomedical image analysis. In recent years, deep learning models have achieved significant success in segmentation. However, deep learning requires the availability of large annotated data to train these models, which can be challenging in biomedical imaging domain. In this paper, we aim to accomplish biomedical image segmentation with limited labeled data using active learning. We present a deep active learning framework that selects additional data points to be annotated by combining U-Net with an efficient and effective query strategy to capture the most uncertain and representative points. This algorithm decouples the representative part by first finding the core points in the unlabeled pool and then selecting the most uncertain points from the reduced pool, which are different from the labeled pool. In our experiment, only 13% of the dataset was required with active learning to outperform the model trained on the entire 2018 MICCAI Brain Tumor Segmentation (BraTS) dataset. Thus, active learning reduced the amount of labeled data required for image segmentation without a significant loss in the accuracy.

Keywords: Deep learning · Active learning · Segmentation

1 Introduction

Image segmentation is a critical task in computer vision as it helps us understand the image at a semantic level. While there have been various algorithms devised to carry out semantic segmentation [1], deep learning models have become the main choice because of their supreme performance and generalization [2,3]. The recent advances in deep learning have motivated some encouraging works for medical image segmentation [4–6] as well. But the deep learning models require large volumes of training data, which can be difficult to collect. The problem becomes more challenging for medical image segmentation as the data needs to be labelled at a pixel level. Annotating the data can be tedious for the human

© Springer Nature Switzerland AG 2019
Q. Wang et al. (Eds.): DART 2019/MIL3ID 2019, LNCS 11795, pp. 148–156, 2019.
https://doi.org/10.1007/978-3-030-33391-1_17

expert, thus, affecting the labeling accuracy. The limited number of domain experts in medical imaging adds more challenge to the process of collecting labelled data.

In biomedical imaging, domain expertise is required for labeling the data. Thus, it is very important to get only those data points labeled which contribute the most in the learning of the model. Active learning [7] is a paradigm that helps in querying the labels of only the most informative data points. Two factors - uncertainty and representativeness, define the informativeness of a data point. When working with deep neural networks, a single query point is not enough to fine-tune the weights of the model. Thus, pool-based strategies such as ranked batch-mode sampling, exploration-exploitation [8] are commonly used with the deep learning models. In past couple of years, there have been several efforts in applying active learning for medical image segmentation. Suggestive Annotation [9] is one of the initial frameworks for biomedical image segmentation using deep active learning for the MICCAI 2015 gland challenge. It uses the Fully Convolutional Network (FCN) and formulates the representativeness as the maximum set-cover problem. In a similar way, Representative Annotation [10] reduces the computational complexity of finding the most representative points by first using agglomerative clustering and then applying the maximum set-cover over each cluster. Both of these works require 50% of the labeled data. In this work, we show that the amount of labelled data can be reduced further.

In our work, we focus on applying active learning for brain tumor lesion segmentation from MR images by using a very limited amount of labeled data and computation time. We hypothesize that the data required to train a machine learning model can be reduced by selecting the training points intelligently, at a cost of a reduced accuracy within a certain limit. To test this hypothesis, we used the 2018 Brain Tumor Segmentation (BraTS) MICCAI challenge [11] dataset. We also devised our own query strategy: A Coreset based Ranked Batch Mode Sampling algorithm to reduce the computational cost of selecting the query points, yet selecting the best ones. We used U-Net as the base deep learning model to perform the lesion segmentation task. Figure 1 summarizes the entire proposed deep active learning framework.

2   Methodology

The two major components of our framework are the deep learning model and the query strategy. In this section, we will discuss them in detail.

2.1   Model Architecture

U-Net [6] is one of the first successful models used for medical image segmentation. It is a classic encoder-decoder model, where the encoder captures the spatial information into a reduced form using Convolutional Neural Network (CNN). This is similar to any CNN model being used for classification, which first encodes the important features and then uses them for classification.

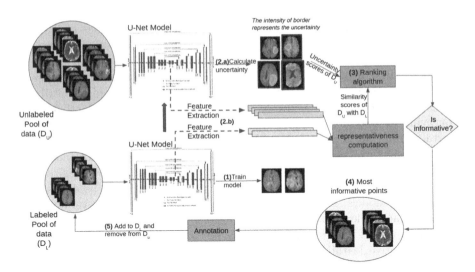

Fig. 1. Our active learning framework for MRI image segmentation. (1) The model is trained on the labeled pool. (2) Find the (a) uncertainty and (b) representative scores for the unlabeled pool using the trained model weights. (3) The query strategy combines these scores (4) and yields the query points, (5) which are the annotated and included in labeled pool. This process is repeated until required.

But U-Net uses these encoded spatial features to reconstruct an output of same size as of input. This captures the semantic information by combining the high-level features from the encoder feature maps with the decoder using skip connections. We used a modified version of U-Net as explained in [12]. This model uses a dice loss function. The dice loss function directly aims at maximizing the dice coefficient metric, thus performing better for data with class imbalance.

2.2 Query Strategies

Query strategy is an essential part of active learning and is used to find the most informative data points in the unlabeled pool. The two major factors that determine the informativeness of a data point are *uncertainty* - the confidence of the model in predicting the correct output of the unlabeled data point, and *representativeness* - there should be minimal similarity between the query pool and the labeled pool, as well as diversity within the query pool. There have been various approaches used to estimate the uncertainty of the model, like classification uncertainty and entropy based uncertainty. Exploration-exploitation [13], batch-mode sampling [14] are some query strategies that also capture the representativeness. We used uncertainty sampling, ranked batch mode sampling, and proposed coreset based ranked batch mode sampling, as described below.

Uncertainty Sampling. Uncertainty sampling [15] is the most common and one of the first query strategies. It is a classic stream-based selective sampling strategy that selects one query point at a time. Hence, it is more famous with traditional ML models that can be fine-tuned by a single data point. But we need a batch of data points with deep learning models. For this, all the points in unlabeled pool are ranked according to their uncertainty and top n data points with the highest uncertainty are sampled.

This algorithm uses the prediction of the model to capture the uncertainty. There are three ways of doing this - least confidence, margin sampling, and entropy. We used the least confidence approach for the experiments as it is computationally cheap and yields good results empirically.

Ranked Batch-Mode Sampling (RBM). Uncertainty sampling is not the best strategy to mine the most informative query points as it fails to capture the representativeness. Batch Mode Active Learning (BMAL) [14] is a query strategy that incorporates reprsentativeness into its selection strategy. BMAL has its own drawbacks as discussed in [16]. Ranked batch-mode sampling algorithm describes a novel way of sampling points, keeping the major factors of uncertainty and representativeness in mind. It calculates the scores of the two factors and take the weighted mean by maintaining a running ratio. The points in the unlabeled pool are ranked based on this combined score. To increase the diversity in the labeled pool, it selects those points from the unlabeled pool which don't have a high similarity with the labeled pool and the query pool, thus capturing the intra- and the inter-diversity of the unlabeled pool as explained in Fig. 2. Initially, the algorithm gives higher preference to the diversity factor, but as the sampling continues, the weighting scheme (α) shifts to the uncertainty scores.

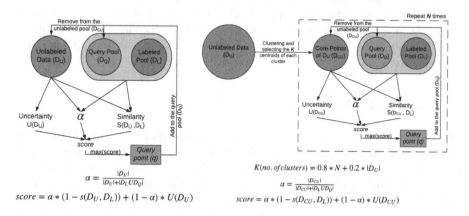

Fig. 2. (left) Ranked batch-mode sampling algorithm and (right) coreset based ranked batch-mode sampling algorithm

Coreset Based Ranked Batch-Mode Sampling. The ranked batch-mode algorithm [16] performs well because it captures both, uncertainty and representativeness. But because of the exhaustive similarity computation between the two pools, labeled and unlabeled, for selecting each query point, it slows down the process and also requires a large amount of memory. We propose a refined version of the ranked batch-mode algorithm by decoupling the step of finding the representative points to capture intra-pool diversity and inter-pool diversity. First, K-means is used to reduce the size of the unlabeled pool and keep the most diverse points. The K is decided by using the following formula - $K = 0.8N_q + 0.2N_u$, where N_q is the number of data points in the query pool and N_u is the number of data points in the unlabeled pool. Then, we choose the data points closest to the centroid of each cluster. The reduced pool is then used to select the data points most dissimilar to the labeled pool and capture the inter-diversity as shown in Fig. 2.

2.3   Training Process

We divided the available annotated data into two pools - labeled data and unlabeled data to emulate the active learning process. The entire process was then run as explained in Fig. 1. The model was trained on the labeled pool of data. Predictions from the trained model are then used to determine the uncertainty scores of the of the data points in the unlabeled pool. For the representativeness computation, the encoder output of the same trained model was used to extract the features of the data points of the two pools. The uncertainty scores and the representativeness scores were then fed into the query strategy to find the most informative points. The model was trained from scratch after including annotated query points to the labeled pool. Also, the number of training epochs were increased by 2 after each query to compensate for the increased training dataset size. The batch-mode sampling techniques used Euclidean distance to determine representativeness.

3   Data and Experiments

We used the 2018 Brain Tumor Segmentation (BraTS) MICCAI challenge dataset to train and evaluate our algorithm. It consists of 210 cases of High Grade Gliomas (HGG) and 75 cases of Low Grade Gliomas (LGG) along with the ground-truth markings for the tumor. Each slice has been manually annotated into 4 categories - enhancing tumor, tumor core, whole tumor, and the background and normal brain pixels. Each case has 4 modalities - T1, T1 contrast enhanced (T1ce), T2 and FLAIR. The dataset is skull-stripped, interpolated to the same resolution of $1 \, mm^3$, and registered to the same dimension of $240 \times 240 \times 155$.

The data is randomly split into the train-validation-test parts in the ratio of 80:10:10 on case level. The training data has 166 HGG and 62 LGG cases, validation data with 22 HGG and 6 LGG cases, and testing data with 22 HGG and 7 LGG cases after the split. Each slice of the four modalities for every case is normalized to have zero mean and unit variance. The tumor is present only in a small part of the brain. The healthy voxels comprise 98% of total voxels,0.18% belongs to necrosis, 1.1% to edema and non-enhanced, and 0.38% to enhanced tumor. Patches of size $128 * 128 * 4$ are randomly sampled from each slice after eliminating the zero-intensity pixels to tackle this class-imbalance problem. This populates the **training data** with **99,864 patches, validation data** with **12,264 patches**, and **testing data** with **12,702 patches**.

Table 1. Experiments conducted and the hyperparameters setting for each experiment

Exp. no	Model	Training data used	Hyperparameters
1	Vanilla U-Net	99k + patches	Epochs = 40
2	U-Net with uncertainty sampling	7k patches (~7% data)	Initial Epochs = 10 Initial pool size = 2k patches Number of queries = 10 Patches labeled/query = 500
3	U-Net with RBM sampling	15k patches (~15% data)	Initial Epochs = 10 Initial pool size = 9k patches **Number of queries = 10** Patches labeled/query = 600
4	U-Net with coreset based RBM sampling	13k patches (~13% data)	Initial Epochs = 10 Initial pool size = 10k patches **Number of queries = 5** Patches labeled/query = 600

We conducted four experiments as in Table 1. First, we used the entire data for training and trained the model for 40 epochs. In the second experiment, we used uncertainty sampling as the query strategy, 7% of the training data, and conducted 10 queries. In third experiment, ranked batch-mode sampling was used as the query strategy using 15% of the data and required 10 queries. Finally, we used the coreset based ranked batch mode sampling which used only 13% of the entire data and only 5 queries.

4   Results and Discussion

Table 2 presents the results for the experiments conducted. The Coreset based Ranked Batch Mode sampling outperformed all the other methods with the dice coefficient scores of 0.844 for whole tumor, 0.83 for tumor core, and 0.799 for enhancing tumor with a reduced average query time of just 43 min. The Ranked Batch Mode sampling gives somewhat closer results, but at a cost of greater computation time and memory.

Table 2. The dice coefficients for the three tumors for each experiment

Exp. no	Model	Whole tumor dice coefficient	Tumor core dice coefficient	Enhancing tumor dice coefficient	Avg query time
1	Vanilla U-Net	0.815	0.689	0.608	–
2	U-Net with uncertainty sampling	0.802	0.724	0.727	–
3	U-Net with RBM sampling	0.829	0.812	0.788	1 hr 50 mins
4	U-Net with coreset based RBM sampling	**0.844**	**0.83**	**0.799**	**43 mins**

With our coreset based ranked batch-mode algorithm, we were able to achieve better results with the limited labeled data (only ~13%) and query computation time. We have also tackled the much prevalent issue of class imbalance using active learning: Our algorithm selects the under-represented data points to be included in the labeled pool, thus reducing the imbalance as much as possible. This is evident from the comparable dice coefficient scores of the three tumors for our algorithm, versus the large difference in them when no active learning is used. Also, the increased scores of the coreset based approach empirically validates the fact that the points being selected are more informative as compared to using the previous strategies. Furthermore, decoupling the selection steps of the intra-pool and inter-pool diverse points yields a faster convergence as we require only 5 queries to reach the final accuracy scores, with average query time also reduced by one hour.

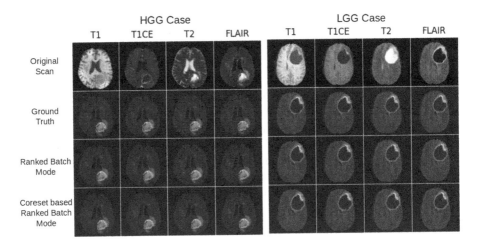

Fig. 3. The test results for HGG (left) and LGG (right) cases.

5   Conclusion and Future Work

In this paper, we presented a deep active learning based solution for MRI brain tumor image segmentation. Our contributions are (1) a more efficient and effective query strategy, and (2) method to tackle the class-imbalance problem using active learning. This improved the results as shown in Fig. 3 and Table 2 as our algorithm is able to capture even the minute details of the enhancing tumor. In future work, we will evaluate our framework with other datasets and explore bayesian networks [17] which can provide a better estimate of uncertainty of the unlabeled data points.

References

1. Zaitoun, N., et al.: Survey on image segmentation techniques. Procedia Comput. Sci. **65**, 797–806 (2015)
2. Long, J., et al.: Fully convolutional networks for semantic segmentation. In: The IEEE Conference on Computer Vision and Pattern Recognition (CVPR) (2015)
3. Girshick, R.B. et al.: Rich feature hierarchies for accurate object detection and semantic segmentation. CoRR. abs/1311.2524 (2013)
4. Chen, H., Qi, X., Cheng, J.Z., Heng, P.A.: Deep contextual networks for neuronal structure segmentation. In: AAAI, pp. 1167–1173 (2016)
5. Chen, H., Qi, X., Yu, L., Heng, P.A.: DCAN: deep contour-aware networks for accurate gland segmentation. In: CVPR, pp. 2487–2496 (2016)
6. Ronneberger, O., Fischer, P., Brox, T.: U-Net: convolutional networks for biomedical image segmentation. In: Navab, N., Hornegger, J., Wells, W.M., Frangi, A.F. (eds.) MICCAI 2015. LNCS, vol. 9351, pp. 234–241. Springer, Cham (2015). https://doi.org/10.1007/978-3-319-24574-4_28
7. Settles, B.: Active Learning Literature Survey. University of Wisconsin-Madison (2009)
8. Yin, C., et al.: Deep similarity-based batch mode active learning with exploration-exploitation. In: Raghavan, V. et al. (ed.) ICDM, pp. 575–584. IEEE Computer Society (2017)
9. Yang, L., et al.: Suggestive Annotation: A Deep Active Learning Framework for Biomedical Image Segmentation. CoRR. abs/1706.04737 (2017)
10. Zheng, H., et al.: Biomedical Image Segmentation via Representative Annotation (2019)
11. Multimodal Brain Tumor Segmentation Challenge (2018). https://www.med.upenn.edu/sbia/brats2018/data.html
12. Isensee, F., Kickingereder, P., Wick, W., Bendszus, M., Maier-Hein, K.H.: Brain tumor segmentation and radiomics survival prediction: contribution to the BRATS 2017 challenge. In: Crimi, A., Bakas, S., Kuijf, H., Menze, B., Reyes, M. (eds.) BrainLes 2017. LNCS, vol. 10670, pp. 287–297. Springer, Cham (2018). https://doi.org/10.1007/978-3-319-75238-9_25
13. Loy, C.C., et al.: Stream-based joint exploration-exploitation active learning. In: CVPR, pp. 1560–1567. IEEE Computer Society (2012)
14. Guo, Y., Schuurmans, D.: Discriminative batch mode active learning. In: Platt, J.C. et al. (ed.) NIPS, pp. 593–600. Curran Associates, Inc. (2007)

15. Xu, H., Wang, X., Liao, Y., Zheng, C.: An uncertainty sampling-based active learning approach for support vector machines. In: International Conference on Artificial Intelligence and Computational Intelligence, Shanghai 2009, pp. 208–213 (2009)
16. Cardoso, T.N.C., et al.: Ranked batch-mode active learning. Inf. Sci. **379**, 313–337 (2017)
17. Gal, Y. et al.: Deep Bayesian Active Learning with Image Data. CoRR. abs/1703.02910 (2017)

Semi-supervised Learning of Fetal Anatomy from Ultrasound

Jeremy Tan[✉], Anselm Au, Qingjie Meng, and Bernhard Kainz

Imperial College London, London SW7 2AZ, UK
j.tan17@imperial.ac.uk

Abstract. Semi-supervised learning methods have achieved excellent performance on standard benchmark datasets using very few labelled images. Anatomy classification in fetal 2D ultrasound is an ideal problem setting to test whether these results translate to *non*-ideal data. Our results indicate that inclusion of a challenging background class can be detrimental and that semi-supervised learning mostly benefits classes that are already distinct, sometimes at the expense of more similar classes.

Keywords: Semi-supervised learning · Fetal ultrasound

1 Introduction

Fetal ultrasound is the most widespread screening tool for congenital abnormalities and is a key recommendation in the World Health Organization's guidelines for antenatal care [13]. Classification of standardized tomographic 2D planes is a key step in nearly all screening exams. However, low image quality and shortage of experts can compromise screening efficacy or in the least make quality heterogeneous across sites. To democratize care, several efforts have been made to automate standard plane detection using deep learning [2–4,8]. However, many of these methods still rely on large amounts of labelled data.

Because labelling is expensive, semi-supervised learning (SSL) methods have become an active area of research, particularly for image data [9,14] and in the medical domain [5]. Recent methods have achieved remarkable performance by learning from unlabelled data. This added information can help to push decision boundaries into lower density regions, resulting in better generalization. Amidst this progress, Oliver et al. call for more "realistic evaluation" [10]. One key concern is that benchmark datasets (e.g. CIFAR10, SVHN) do not reflect realistic scenarios.

We study the use of SSL for standard plane classification in fetal ultrasound [2]. This task includes a challenging background class, class imbalance, and different levels of inter-class similarity. In accordance with Oliver et al. we demonstrate that supervised baselines can cope with surprisingly few labelled images; that a background class can cause SSL to become detrimental; and that SSL is effective for distinct classes, but can weaken performance on classes which are prone to confusion.

Q. Wang et al. (Eds.): DART 2019/MIL3ID 2019, LNCS 11795, pp. 157–164, 2019.
https://doi.org/10.1007/978-3-030-33391-1_18

2   Related Work

Automatic anatomy detection from ultrasound videos is a popular topic with many successful approaches using convolutional neural networks [2]. Further advancements have added multi-task learning to predict sonographer gaze [3] or multi-scale networks to exploit lower and higher level features [8]. Some methods have also studied the challenge of limited labelled data by pretraining on natural images [4]. However there has been little investigation into the use of SSL. Exploring this avenue can reveal what benefits SSL can bring, and conversely, what challenges remain for SSL in non-ideal data scenarios.

Recently, SSL methods have gained momentum. Underlying many of these methods is a consistency loss which minimizes sensitivity to perturbations (in input/weight space). Examples of perturbations include image augmentations, gaussian noise, weight dropout [9], targeted augmentations [14], and mixup augmentations (interpolation between images) [12]. Input perturbations have been shown to minimize the input-output Jacobian (linked to better generalization) [1]. Despite these advances, Oliver et al. point out that real unlabelled data is likely to be more irregular than the perfectly balanced benchmark datasets. It may also include out-of-distribution or confounding data that could hurt SSL [11]. We aim to study the ways in which SSL might help in a real problem which stands to benefit from SSL.

3   Methods

The architecture used in this study, Sononet [2], is a convolutional neural network (similar to VGG) that has been tailored for the task of anatomical standard plane detection in fetal ultrasound. It contains 15 convolutional layers, 4 max-pooling layers, and ends with global average pooling. This acts as a strong fully supervised baseline. Supervised methods are trained using Adam with a learning rate of 1E-3. All models are trained for 50 epochs with a batch size of 32.

For the SSL method, we use the consistency loss employed in both the Π model [9] and the unsupervised data augmentation (UDA) method [14] which are among the state of the art for standard benchmark datasets. This consistency loss uses the softmax predictions for unlabelled data, $\mathcal{D}_U$, as labels for the same images under augmentations. This consistency loss can be formalized as

$$\mathcal{L}_{\mathrm{KL}}(x_u, w) = KL(f(x_u; w) \| f(x'_u; w)). \tag{1}$$

This is added to the typical supervised (cross-entropy) loss with some proportion λ (in all our experiments $\lambda = 0.5$). Note that the weights w are the same for inference on both the original image x_u (drawn from $\mathcal{D}_U$) and the corresponding augmented image x'_u. In this case the augmentations include random combinations of the following operations:

– Horizontal flipping
– Random contrast adjustment by a factor within [0.7, 1.3]

- Random rotation by an angle within $[-\frac{\pi}{4}, \frac{\pi}{4}]$
- Random cropping ranging from 1% to 20%

The same augmentation is applied to all methods, including supervised baselines. These augmentations are not specially tailored to the data as is the case in UDA. For the best performance, UDA uses AutoAugment [6], a reinforcement learning method that finds the optimal augmentation policies. This would likely improve both SSL and fully supervised regimes. However, as shown in the results, the scores of the supervised baselines are already very high with surprisingly few labelled images; applying AutoAugment to both SSL and fully supervised methods may truncate the margin for potential improvement that we wish to study. We include (a) training signal annealing (TSA), (b) confidence-based masking (CBM), (c) entropy minimization, and (d) softmax temperature controlling [14]. Since these are proposed in [14], we refer to the combination of (i) the consistency loss with (ii) these additional techniques, as UDA for simplicity and to acknowledge their contributions.

TSA [14] uses a threshold, η_{tsa}, to mask the contribution of a given labelled image, x_l (drawn from $\mathcal{D}_L$), to the supervised gradient. Specifically, an example only contributes to the gradient if the softmax probability in the ground truth class is greater than the threshold, $p(y^*|x_l) > \eta_{tsa}$. The threshold η_{tsa} starts at $\frac{1}{\#of classes}$ and is increased to 1 following a linear, log, or exponential schedule across the total number of epochs.

CBM [14] uses a confidence threshold on unlabelled images. An unlabelled image only contributes to the consistency gradient if, $\max(p(y|x_u)) > \eta_{cbm}$. A η_{cbm} of 0.75 is used for all SSL experiments.

Entropy minimization [7] is applied to $p(y|x'_u)$, the prediction for an augmented unlabelled image. Also the prediction for original unlabelled image is sharpened by using a softmax temperature of 0.8.

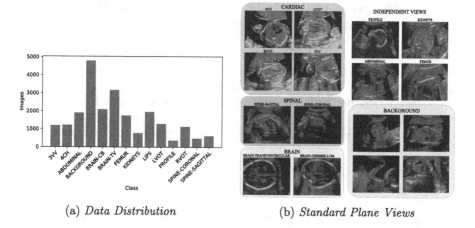

(a) *Data Distribution*   (b) *Standard Plane Views*

Fig. 1. Distribution of the training data (a) and examples of standard views (b).

3.1   Dataset

Our dataset contains 13 anatomical classes plus 1 background class. The entire training dataset consists of 22757 images (class distribution shown in Fig. 1a). For SSL, 100 images are extracted from each class to make up the labelled data $\mathcal{D}_L$. The remaining images are treated as unlabelled data $\mathcal{D}_U$. Experiments are performed using subsets of $\mathcal{D}_L$, specifically using 1, 5, 20, 50, and 100 images per class. The test set follows the same distribution, but totals to 5737 images. Each image is 224 × 288 pixels. These image frames are derived from a dataset containing 2438 videos from over 2000 volunteers.

Examples of some of the classes are displayed in Fig. 1b. The cardiac classes are among the most difficult to distinguish. While the spine and brain also span multiple classes, these images are generally more clear and can have significant pose differences (spine). The background class contains a diverse range of images sampled from the videos (excluding frames of standard planes). All extracted samples satisfy a minimum image-space distance between neighbouring frames. This means that most background frames are extracted during rapid probe movement and not when the sonographer slows down to home in on the standard planes. However, some images that resemble standard planes still make it through this naïve filtering approach. Also, the background class is larger than any anatomical class (Fig. 1a). In short, the background class introduces class imbalance; is not easily characterized by a single common feature; and contains examples which resemble other classes.

3.2   Evaluation

Fully supervised methods are evaluated with 1, 5, 20, 50, and 100 labelled images per class. Another experiment is performed using the entire labelled training set (total 22757 images). The SSL framework is applied to the cases of 5, 20, and 50 labelled images per class, where there is a large margin for potential improvement. These cases represent a very feasible labelling task compared to labelling all 22757 images.

Each evaluation is done with and without the background class. To measure the impact of the background class on anatomical classes, accuracy is reported only for the anatomical classes (not background). Accuracy is also reported with a single merged cardiac class. In this case, any cardiac view that is classified as any of the four cardiac views is considered correct. Comparing the overall and grouped cardiac accuracies gives an indication of whether improvements extend to the cardiac classes.

4   Results

Accuracy for fully supervised baseline methods is shown in Fig. 2. With only 20 labelled examples per class, overall accuracy is near 70% and grouped cardiac accuracy is over 80%. All baselines are trained for 50 epochs and did not grossly overfit (except for 1 image per class which was trained for 5 epochs).

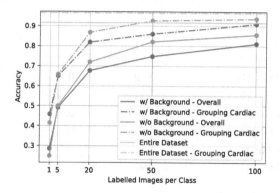

Fig. 2. Supervised baselines with varying number of labelled images per class. Inclusion of the background class increases the difficulty of the classification task. Accuracy is reported as either overall or grouping all cardiac classes into a single class.

When applying the SSL consistency loss, we find the performance is sensitive to the consistency loss masking threshold, η_{cbm}. This is particularly true for the cardiac classes. Table 1 compares the performance of different thresholds for the cardiac classes. The threshold for all other classes remains constant at 0.75. A cardiac threshold of 0.25 gives best performance and is used for all further experiments.

Table 1. Confidence mask threshold values for cardiac classes. These experiments use 20 labelled images per class and exclude the background class.

Method	Cardiac confidence mask threshold	Grouping cardiac	Overall
Supervised	N/A	**0.868**	**0.720**
Basic UDA	η_{cbm}	0.849	0.665
	$\frac{1}{2} \cdot \eta_{cbm}$	0.840	0.661
	$\frac{1}{3} \cdot \eta_{cbm}$	**0.905**	**0.728**
	$\frac{1}{4} \cdot \eta_{cbm}$	0.831	0.664
	>1 (disabled)	0.631	0.631
UDA best configuration	η_{cbm}	0.915	0.720
	$\frac{1}{3} \cdot \eta_{cbm}$	**0.936**	**0.754**

Further experiments are performed with different UDA settings to find the optimal configuration (Table 2). We find that a log TSA schedule gives the best performance. Log schedules are suggested for cases when the network is less likely to quickly overfit [14].

Table 2. Different configurations for the case of 20 labelled images per class without the background class.

Method	Optimizer	TSA schedule	Grouping cardiac	Overall
Supervised	Adam: 1E-3	N/A	**0.868**	**0.720**
UDA	Adam: 1E-3	Linear	0.905	0.728
	Momentum: 1E-3	Linear	0.891	0.692
	SGD cyclic: [7E-3, 5E-2]	Linear	0.921	0.735
	Adam: 1E-3	Log	**0.936**	**0.754**
	SGD cyclic: [7E-3, 5E-2]	Log	0.935	0.744

The best found configuration is then used with 5, 20, and 50 labelled images per class, with and without the background class. Accuracies are reported in Fig. 3.

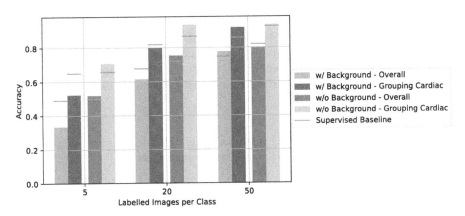

Fig. 3. Overall and grouped cardiac accuracies with and without the background class for 5, 20, and 50 labelled images per class. Red bars indicate supervised baseline performance. Without the background class (green bars), SSL accuracy is almost always above supervised baslines (red). Inclusion of the background class can cause SSL performance to drop below supervised baselines. (Color figure online)

Confusion matrices are displayed in Fig. 4. SSL improves accuracy for distinct classes such as brain, femur, kidney, and lips from mid 0.80 (a - supervised) to mid 0.90 (b - UDA), which approaches the fully supervised performance shown in (c). However, for cardiac classes, confusion is increased when using SSL.

5   Discussion

Similarly to Oliver et al. [10], we show that supervised baselines are surprisingly accurate (Fig. 2). There is also a clear diminishing return of increasing the number of labelled images, which starts as early as 20 examples per class. Inclusion

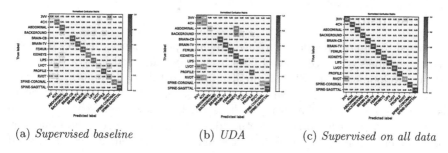

    (a) *Supervised baseline*   (b) *UDA*   (c) *Supervised on all data*

Fig. 4. Confusion matrices for the case of 20 labelled images per class without background. The supervised baseline (a) performs surprisingly well given the limited data. SSL (b) is able to make considerable improvement for distinct classes, but can increase confusion of cardiac classes. Even when trained on the entire labelled dataset (c), some cardiac classes are prone to confusion.

of the background class decreases accuracy in almost all cases. This indicates that the background class adds difficulty even in the fully supervised case.

Investigating sensitivity to confidence thresholds (Table 1), we see that $\frac{1}{3}$ · η_{cbm} (0.25) is the only setting that improves both grouped cardiac and overall accuracy for the basic UDA implementation. A value near 0.25 is reasonable given that the network must divide its confidence over 4 very similar cardiac classes. Even for the best UDA configuration, a threshold of 0.25 for the cardiac classes makes a considerable difference; without it, overall accuracy does not improve from the supervised baseline.

Figure 3 displays that without the background class (green bars), the SSL regime can almost always improve upon the fully supervised baseline. The only exception being the overall accuracy for 50 labelled examples. In this case the supervised baseline is already quite high and any further improvement would likely depend on the cardiac classes which the SSL method struggles with. In contrast, the inclusion of the background class (blue bars), not only reduces the accuracy of the fully supervised baselines, but tends to be harmful to the SSL method. For most of the blue bars, the SSL method fails to match, let alone surpass, the baseline accuracy. This illustrates the negative impact of including confounding images in the unlabelled data. Again, the case with 50 labelled examples is the exception. Perhaps 50 labelled examples is sufficient to capture the majority of the variation in the background class, preventing it from having a negative impact on the SSL loss.

While the SSL has been shown to increase both grouped cardiac and overall accuracies, the confusion matrices in Fig. 4 clearly show that these improvements are often at the expense of the cardiac classes. It seems unlabelled data can help the network to learn when the classes are inherently more distinct, but can cause harm when classes are inherently similar.

6   Conclusion

Supervised baselines provide surprisingly reliable performance even in extremely low data regimes (e.g. accuracy of 50% from only 5 labelled images per class). Recent developments in SSL can further improve this performance. However, having irregular data can cause SSL to be detrimental rather than beneficial. Also, classes with high similarity, such as cardiac views, can see an increase in confusion. For such classes, injecting domain knowledge (e.g. lowering cardiac confidence thresholds) may be necessary to supplement a lack of labelled examples.

Acknowledgments. Support from Wellcome Trust IEH Award iFind project [102431]. JT is supported by the ICL President's Scholarship.

References

1. Athiwaratkun, B., Finzi, M., Izmailov, P., Wilson, A.G.: There are many consistent explanations of unlabeled data: why you should average. In: ICLR (2019)
2. Baumgartner, C.F., et al.: SonoNet: real-time detection and localisation of fetal standard scan planes in freehand ultrasound. IEEE Trans. Med. Imaging **36**(11), 2204–2215 (2017)
3. Cai, Y., Sharma, H., Chatelain, P., Noble, J.A.: Multi-task SonoEyeNet: detection of fetal standardized planes assisted by generated sonographer attention maps. In: International Conference on Medical Image Computing and Computer-Assisted Intervention, pp. 871–879 (2018)
4. Chen, H., et al.: Standard plane localization in fetal ultrasound via domain transferred deep neural networks. IEEE J. Biomed. Health Inform. **19**, 1627–1636 (2015)
5. Cheplygina, V., de Bruijne, M., Pluim, J.P.: Not-so-supervised: a survey of semi-supervised, multi-instance, and transfer learning in medical image analysis. Med. Image Anal. **54**, 280–296 (2019)
6. Cubuk, E.D., Zoph, B., Mane, D., Vasudevan, V., Le, Q.V.: AutoAugment: learning augmentation policies from data. In: CVPR (2019)
7. Grandvalet, Y., Bengio, Y.: Semi-supervised learning by entropy minimization. In: NeurIPS (2005)
8. Kong, P., Ni, D., Chen, S., Li, S., Wang, T., Lei, B.: Automatic and efficient standard plane recognition in fetal ultrasound images via multi-scale dense networks. In: Melbourne, A., et al. (eds.) PIPPI/DATRA -2018. LNCS, vol. 11076, pp. 160–168. Springer, Cham (2018). https://doi.org/10.1007/978-3-030-00807-9_16
9. Laine, S., Aila, T.: Temporal ensembling for semi-supervised learning. In: ICLR (2017)
10. Oliver, A., Odena, A., Raffel, C., Cubuk, E.D., Goodfellow, I.J.: Realistic evaluation of deep semi-supervised learning algorithms. In: NeurIPS (2018)
11. Singh, A., Nowak, R., Zhu, J.: Unlabeled data: now it helps, now it doesn't. In: NeurIPS (2008)
12. Verma, V., Lamb, A., Kannala, J., Bengio, Y.: Interpolation consistency training for semi-supervised learning. In: IJCAI (2019)
13. World Health Organization, et al.: WHO recommendations on antenatal care for a positive pregnancy experience. World Health Organization (2016)
14. Xie, Q., Dai, Z., Hovy, E., Luong, M.T., Le, Q.V.: Unsupervised data augmentation for consistency training. arXiv preprint arXiv:1904.12848 (2019)

Multi-modal Segmentation with Missing MR Sequences Using Pre-trained Fusion Networks

Karin van Garderen[1,3(✉)], Marion Smits[1], and Stefan Klein[1,2]

[1] Department of Radiology and Nuclear Medicine, Erasmus MC,
Rotterdam, The Netherlands
k.vangarderen@erasmusmc.nl
[2] Department of Medical Informatics, Erasmus MC, Rotterdam, The Netherlands
[3] Medical Delta, Delft, The Netherlands

Abstract. Missing data is a common problem in machine learning and in retrospective imaging research it is often encountered in the form of missing imaging modalities. We propose to take into account missing modalities in the design and training of neural networks, to ensure that they are capable of providing the best possible prediction even when multiple images are not available. The proposed network combines three modifications to the standard 3D UNet architecture: a training scheme with dropout of modalities, a multi-pathway architecture with fusion layer in the final stage, and the separate pre-training of these pathways. These modifications are evaluated incrementally in terms of performance on full and missing data, using the BraTS multi-modal segmentation challenge. The final model shows significant improvement with respect to the state of the art on missing data and requires less memory during training.

Keywords: Convolutional neural network · Glioma segmentation · Missing data

1 Introduction

Tumor segmentation is a key task in brain imaging research, as it is a prerequisite for obtaining quantitative features of the tumor. Since manual segmentation by radiologists is time-consuming and prone to inter-observer variation, there is a clear need for effective automatic segmentation methods. Research into these methods for glioma has been accelerated by the recurring BraTS multi-modal segmentation challenge on low-grade glioma (LGG) and glioblastoma (GBM) [8]. The best performing methods in recent editions were all based on 3D convolutional neural networks (CNNs) with the encoder-decoder shape of the UNet.

While the BraTS challenge focuses on improving performance, there are practical problems to overcome before automatic segmentation can be applied in

© Springer Nature Switzerland AG 2019
Q. Wang et al. (Eds.): DART 2019/MIL3ID 2019, LNCS 11795, pp. 165–172, 2019.
https://doi.org/10.1007/978-3-030-33391-1_19

practice. One of these challenges is dealing with missing data. The BraTS benchmark contains four MR modalities: a T1-weighted image (T1W), a T1-weighted image with contrast agent (T1WC), a T2-weighted image (T2W) and a T2-weighted FLAIR image (FLAIR), which are co-registered so that corresponding voxels in the image are aligned and a CNN can learn to segment a tumor from the specific combination of modalities. Although these images are complementary, a radiologist is still able to perform a partial segmentation if one of these modalities is missing, while for a CNN this is not guaranteed. Especially in retrospective and multi-center studies it is not unlikely that images are either missing or have quality issues.

There are two ways in general to deal with the problem of missing data. The most common way is to impute the missing values by an estimate, which can be as simple as the mean value. More advanced techniques for missing image imputation is to generate a new image from remaining modalities, which can be achieved through neural networks [5,10].

However, it is also possible to train a CNN to be inherently robust to missing data. The HeMis model [3] is an example of this, where the modalities are each passed through a separate pathway before being merged in a so-called abstraction layer which extracts the mean and variance of the resulting features. This network architecture enforces a shared feature representation of the modalities, though it may be of additional value to include a similarity term in the loss function to enforce a true shared representation [9].

1.1   Contribution

Building on the existing work on shared representations, we provide a careful experimental evaluation of different aspects that make the network robust to missing images. We evaluate four modifications to a state-of-the-art UNet architecture and evaluate their effect incrementally. A first adaptation is to train with missing data in a curriculum learning approach. Secondly, a multi-path architecture is evaluated where the information of different modalities is fused in a later stage. Thirdly, within this architecture, a shared representation layer is compared to a concatenation of feature maps. Finally, we propose a training procedure where each pathway is trained separately before combining them and training the final classification layer. This approach enforces each path to form an informative feature represenation. The separate training also reduces the demand on GPU memory, which is the main bottleneck in state-of-the-art segmentation networks. The modified architectures are compared to the baseline architecture, in a situation where it is trained with the entire dataset but also when it is specifically trained for each combination of modalities.

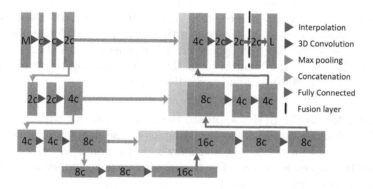

Fig. 1. Illustration of the UNet architecture. The number of feature maps, as a function of the parameter c, is indicated for each step. The fusion and shared representation networks contain one UNet per modality, which are fused at the indicated location. M indicates the number of input modalities and L the number of output labels. In this study $M = 4$ and $L = 4$.

2   Methodology

2.1   Network Architecture

The 3D UNet architecture [2] is a well-established segmentation network and still was one of the best performing architectures at the most recent 2018 BraTS challenge [4]. Therefore the UNet forms the baseline for our research. One UNet is trained on all modalities and evaluated with missing data, but also a dedicated UNet is trained and evaluated for each specific combination of modalities. The number of trainable parameters in the model depends on the number of feature maps in each convolution, which we chose to parameterize by a single variable c. The first convolution has c kernels, and as the size of the feature maps decreases the number of kernels is increased. Figure 1 shows the UNet architecture with the number of feature maps per convolution layer expressed as a multiple of c.

In the reference UNet architecture each 3D convolution block contains a batch normalization, a 3D unpadded convolution layer with kernels of size 3^3, and Leaky ReLu activation. The last fully connected layers are implemented as a 3D convolution with kernels of size 1^3. The downsampling step is a max-pooling layer of stride 2 and size 2^3 and the upsampling is a tri-linear interpolation. For this UNet architecture each target voxel has a receptive field of 88^3 voxels.

Modality Dropout. To make a network robust to missing data it needs to train with missing data. To this end, a specific modality dropout scheme was implemented which removes entire input channels (MR sequences) with a probability p. The features from missing sequences are removed by setting the input to zero and scaling the other inputs by m_o/M, where m_o is the number of original input images and M is the number of remaining inputs. A curriculum learning approach is used to aid convergence: starting from $p = 0.125$ the probability of dropout is doubled every 50 epochs until it reaches $p = 0.5$. This method is applied to directly to the input layer in the Dropout network, but also to the fusion layers in the Multipath and SharedRep networks.

Multipath Network. In this approach the network has one pathway for each of the $M = 4$ modalities and the feature maps of the final convolutional layer are concatenated to an output of $8c$ channels in a fusion layer, which is where the modality dropout is applied. The final prediction is performed again by a 1^3 convolution layer with $4c$ channels.

For a fair comparison it is important to consider the number of trainable parameters, which scales quadratically with the number of channels per layer. To create a multi-path network of the same size as a single reference network, the UNets that form the pathways have half the number of channels per layer. As the UNet was implemented with $c = 32$, the separate pathways are a quarter of the size with $c = 16$. Note that whereas parameter size scales quadratically, the memory usage scales approximately linear with the number of feature maps. The multi-pathway networks (with $M = 4$) therefore require approximately twice the amount of GPU memory during training compared to the single UNet.

Shared Representation. The Shared Representation (SharedRep) network is a multi-path network with a specific fusion layer, based on the HeMIS model [3]. Instead of concatenating, the fusion layer takes the mean and variance of each feature map and therefore encourages a common feature represenation between the modalities. To enable fair comparison to the fusion network, the last layer of each pathway has double the amount of feature maps ($4c$), leading to $8c$ features in the fusion layer. The network is trained with modality dropout of the pathways and the variance is set to zero if only a single pathway is available.

Pre-trained Paths. Pre-training the paths means that a UNet is trained for each individual MR modality and the separate prediction layers are replaced by one fusion layer. These are trained with modality dropout ($p = 0.5$), while freezing the parameters of the single pathways. When fusing the pathways with a shared representation layer, the final convolutional layers of the networks are also replaced and trained in order to learn a new shared feature representation. Using the pre-training scheme greatly reduces the demand on GPU memory, as the pathways require a quarter of the memory of the whole network and half that of the full UNet with $c = 32$. The combined training scheme took approximately 50% longer than without pre-training, though with parallel training of the paths on separate devices it was even faster than the baseline.

2.2   Data and Preprocessing

The networks were trained and evaluated on the training set of the BraTS challenge 2018 [1], which is a benchmark dataset of pre-operative scans of 278 patients with low-grade glioma (LGG, 75) or glioblastoma (GBM, 203). The images in this benchmark are skull-stripped, co-registered and resampled to a size of 240 by 240 by 155 voxels. The target areas for evaluation are the whole tumor, tumor core and enhancing core. The non-background voxels of each separate image were normalized to zero mean and unit standard deviation. Random patches of 108^3 voxels were extracted, which correspond to 20^3 target voxels. With a probability of 50% a patch was selected from a tumor area, meaning that the center voxel was part of the tumor, and with 50% probability the center voxel was located outside of the tumor but inside the brain.

2.3   Training and Evaluation

The networks were optimized with the Adam optimizer [6] and the cross-entropy loss function. An epoch is defined as an iteration over 100 batches with 4 random patches, and the models were trained for 150 epochs. For pre-trained pathways, the separate pathways and the final combination layer were trained for 100 epochs each. The dataset was divided into five cross-validation folds, so that 20% of the subjects were always selected for testing and never used during training. The folds are random, but the same for each experiment. Evaluation took place on the whole image, although it was classified by the network in patches to limit memory usage. To assess whether the models are indeed more robust to missing data, we evaluated the same models in a situation where any combination of sequences is removed.

2.4   Visualizing Shared Representations

To validate the concept of a shared representation layer in the context of missing data, we would like to know whether the feature representation of such a layer is indeed robust to missing data. We evaluated this in a qualitative way by looking at the t-SNE [7] maps of the activations of the final fully connected layer. Feature maps from the final fully connected layer were extracted for 40,000 random voxels originating from 16 random patches. A t-SNE map was computed to map the 64-dimensional feature vectors to a 2D representation. These maps can be interpreted as a representation of the distances between voxels in the specific feature representation of each model. The same set of voxels was used for both maps.

3   Results

Six networks were trained and evaluated in five-fold cross-validation and, as an additional reference, a dedicated UNet was trained for each combination of sequences. The results are summarized in Table 1. On the full dataset, the simple UNet without dropout performs best, and every modification to the network comes with a decreased performance in this case. For missing data scenarios, the regular UNet suffers while the other networks are able to maintain a better performance. None of the networks is able to outperform a dedicated UNet trained for each specific combination of sequences.

There is no architecture that consistently outperforms the others, though the pre-trained multipath networks seem to perform best overall and especially on cases with few available modalities. However, when considering performance on the full dataset, the UNet baseline still performs best and the SharedRep model without pretraining performs better than pretrained paths on the tumor core. Training only with modality dropout greatly decreases performance on the full dataset while only providing minor improvement on missing data.

Table 1. Numeric results in terms of mean Dice percentage on the three different regions of interest. Color scales (see online) are adapted to each region, defined by the best and worst results on that region.

	All	All but T1W	All but T1WC	All but T2W	All but FLAIR	T2W, FLAIR	T1WC, FLAIR	T1WC, T2W	T1W, FLAIR	T1W, T2W	T1W, T1WC	FLAIR	T2W	T1WC	T1W
Whole tumor															
UNet	83	65	78	74	43	65	43	46	63	23	18	37	30	14	4
Dropout	77	76	81	76	59	73	62	59	77	61	33	51	60	21	8
Multipath	82	81	82	77	70	80	74	69	77	70	42	69	63	32	25
SharedRep	83	82	82	79	72	81	74	71	76	71	48	72	69	36	29
Multipath + Pretraining	84	83	83	82	75	82	78	74	78	73	56	72	70	49	44
SharedRep + Pretraining	83	83	82	81	74	81	77	72	79	73	58	75	69	52	44
Dedicated	83	81	81	79	73	79	77	74	76	72	59	73	71	49	48
Tumor core															
UNet	71	47	43	59	46	43	26	36	35	23	26	28	27	9	2
Dropout	57	59	33	56	50	36	42	43	20	39	42	28	40	13	9
Multipath	69	67	44	64	61	44	58	57	40	33	46	36	34	31	25
SharedRep	70	69	43	66	64	41	60	59	38	37	50	30	31	38	20
Multipath + Pretraining	66	65	42	64	64	42	61	61	40	37	53	34	36	43	29
SharedRep + Pretraining	67	66	42	64	63	43	59	60	37	37	53	34	29	49	23
Dedicated	71	64	46	64	63	45	61	63	42	43	56	37	43	43	25
Enhancing core															
UNet	63	40	6	55	43	2	21	36	6	4	25	7	6	6	3
Dropout	57	56	7	58	55	5	39	46	9	8	44	4	6	13	9
Multipath	61	61	7	58	56	5	55	54	7	8	44	9	6	33	9
SharedRep	62	61	8	60	58	7	54	55	10	7	48	5	5	39	6
Multipath + Pretraining	62	62	12	60	60	12	57	58	16	6	50	17	1	39	9
SharedRep + Pretraining	60	60	10	58	59	12	54	57	9	8	50	9	8	48	9
Dedicated	63	60	17	63	59	18	60	58	17	14	56	10	16	45	9

3.1   t-SNE Visualizations

The resulting t-SNE representations are shown in Fig. 2 for the pretrained Multipath and SharedRep model. The predicted and true labels are highlighted in red, showing that the mapped representation is meaningful to the network prediction and ground truth. Also, the feature maps generated with missing data are highlighted to see whether they lead to distinct feature representations. Whereas the multipath fusion model maps the different missing data scenarios to specific parts of the feature space, the shared representation model seems to have less distinction between complete and incomplete data. This visualization supports the notion that the shared representation layer does indeed lead to a feature representation that is consistent, even when images are removed.

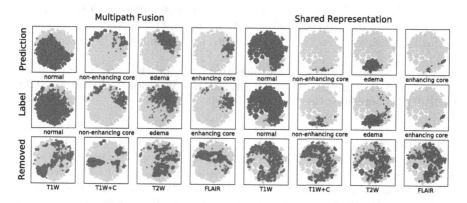

Fig. 2. t-SNE results for pretrained network with fusion by concatenation (left) and shared representation (right). Specific subsets of the voxels are indicated in red. (Color figure online)

4   Discussion and Conclusion

We have carefully evaluated different approaches for training a CNN to be robust to missing imaging modalities, in the context of the BraTs multi-modal segmentation challenge with four MR sequences. Applying modality dropout on the input channels is a simple way to achieve some robustness, but it has a significant impact on performance with full data. More advanced multimodal architectures, with a separate pathway for each modality, give a better balance between performance and robustness.

The pathways can be fused either through a simple concatenation or using their statistical moments (mean and variance), thereby enforcing a shared feature representation. Although qualitative visual results show that the shared representation layer forces the feature maps of different combinations of modalities toward a common space, the performance results give no conclusive evidence that it should be preferred over a simple concatenation. The pretraining of the separate paths with a single modality seems to increase the performance mostly in the more difficult cases with fewer modalities. It is also in these cases that a dedicated UNet trained for the specific combination of modalities performs best in comparison, showing that there is still room for improvement.

However, it must be noted that the performance achieved by multipath models do not match the best performance on the most recent BraTS training set, as measured on the full dataset. Further improvements on the UNet core are expected to increase the performance further, on both full and partial datasets. The evaluation in this paper has focussed on a systematic comparison of model architectures with the same hyperparameters and size. However, the demand on GPU memory is different between networks. The pre-training of paths in the multipath networks drastically reduces the required memory, so they could be trained with more channels per layer, a larger batch size, a larger patch size or simply a less expensive GPU. It should be preferred for this reason and for its consistent good performance with any combination of modalities.

Acknowledgements. This work was supported by the Dutch Cancer Society (project number 11026, GLASS-NL), the Dutch Organization for Scientific Research (NWO) and NVIDIA Corporation (by donating a GPU).

References

1. Bakas, S., et al.: Advancing the cancer genome atlas glioma MRI collections with expert segmentation labels and radiomic features. Sci. Data **4**, 170117 (2017)
2. Çiçek, Ö., Abdulkadir, A., Lienkamp, S.S., Brox, T., Ronneberger, O.: 3D U-Net: learning dense volumetric segmentation from sparse annotation. In: Ourselin, S., Joskowicz, L., Sabuncu, M.R., Unal, G., Wells, W. (eds.) MICCAI 2016. LNCS, vol. 9901, pp. 424–432. Springer, Cham (2016). https://doi.org/10.1007/978-3-319-46723-8_49
3. Havaei, M., Guizard, N., Chapados, N., Bengio, Y.: HeMIS: hetero-modal image segmentation. In: Ourselin, S., Joskowicz, L., Sabuncu, M.R., Unal, G., Wells, W. (eds.) MICCAI 2016. LNCS, vol. 9901, pp. 469–477. Springer, Cham (2016). https://doi.org/10.1007/978-3-319-46723-8_54
4. Isensee, F., Kickingereder, P., Wick, W., Bendszus, M., Maier-Hein, K.H.: No New-Net. ArXiv e-prints, September 2018
5. Jerez, J., et al.: Missing data imputation using statistical and machine learning methods in a real breast cancer problem. Artif. Intell. Med. **50**(2), 105–115 (2010)
6. Kingma, D., Ba, J.: Adam: a method for stochastic optimization. In: International Conference on Learning Representations (2014)
7. Maaten, L.V.D., Hinton, G., Visualizing data using t-SNE: Visualizing data using t-SNE. J. Mach. Learn. Res. **9**, 2579–2605 (2008)
8. Menze, B.H., Jakab, A., Bauer, S., et al.: The multimodal brain tumor image segmentation benchmark (BRATS). IEEE Trans. Med. Imaging **34**(10), 1993–2024 (2015)
9. van Tulder, G., de Bruijne, M.: Representation learning for cross-modality classification. In: Muller, H., et al. (eds.) Medical Computer Vision and Bayesian and Graphical Models for Biomedical Imaging, pp. 126–136. Springer, Cham (2017). https://doi.org/10.1007/978-3-319-61188-4_12
10. Van Nguyen, H., Zhou, K., Vemulapalli, R.: Cross-domain synthesis of medical images using efficient location-sensitive deep network. In: Navab, N., Hornegger, J., Wells, W.M., Frangi, A.F. (eds.) MICCAI 2015. LNCS, vol. 9349, pp. 677–684. Springer, Cham (2015). https://doi.org/10.1007/978-3-319-24553-9_83

More Unlabelled Data or Label More Data? A Study on Semi-supervised Laparoscopic Image Segmentation

Yunguan Fu[1,2](✉), Maria R. Robu[1], Bongjin Koo[1], Crispin Schneider[3],
Stijn van Laarhoven[3], Danail Stoyanov[1], Brian Davidson[3],
Matthew J. Clarkson[1], and Yipeng Hu[1]

[1] Wellcome/EPSRC Centre for Interventional and Surgical Sciences,
Centre for Medical Image Computing, University College London, London, UK
`yunguan.fu.18@ucl.ac.uk`
[2] InstaDeep, London, UK
[3] Division of Surgery and Interventional Science, University College London,
London, UK

Abstract. Improving a semi-supervised image segmentation task has
the option of adding more unlabelled images, labelling the unlabelled
images or combining both, as neither image acquisition nor expert
labelling can be considered trivial in most clinical applications. With
a laparoscopic liver image segmentation application, we investigate the
performance impact by altering the quantities of labelled and unlabelled
training data, using a semi-supervised segmentation algorithm based on
the mean teacher learning paradigm. We first report a significantly higher
segmentation accuracy, compared with supervised learning. Interestingly,
this comparison reveals that the training strategy adopted in the semi-
supervised algorithm is also responsible for this observed improvement,
in addition to the added unlabelled data. We then compare different
combinations of labelled and unlabelled data set sizes for training semi-
supervised segmentation networks, to provide a quantitative example of
the practically useful trade-off between the two data planning strategies
in this surgical guidance application.

Keywords: Semi-supervised · Laparoscopic video · Image
segmentation

1 Introduction

Deep convolutional neural networks have been proposed to segment livers from
surgical video images [6], a significant step towards fully-automated computer-
assisted guidance for liver resection procedures. The automatically segmented
liver surfaces can be used to reconstruct anatomical structures for assisting real-
time navigation and for registering with preoperative 3D medical images, such as

Q. Wang et al. (Eds.): DART 2019/MIL3ID 2019, LNCS 11795, pp. 173–180, 2019.
https://doi.org/10.1007/978-3-030-33391-1_20

diagnostic CT or MR, to locate the target of operative interest. Precise image-guidance has the potential to increase the number of patients that can be offered laparoscopic liver resection over open surgery, thereby significantly reducing the surgery-related stress and risk.

Further improving the segmentation accuracy may resort to more labelled data or unlabelled data with semi-supervised learning. Like many other medical image segmentation tasks, deep-learning-based approaches often require a substantial amount of labelled data for training, which rely on human experts with specialised clinical knowledge and multidisciplinary experience. On the other hand, acquiring more unlabelled image data from more patients or prolonging procedures may have a significant impact on workflow and patient safety. Therefore the data planning decision in relation to performance improvement needs to be carefully considered.

Semi-supervised approaches have been successfully applied in medical image segmentation [2,3,8]. However, comparing semi-supervised methods directly with the supervised counterparts has to consider multiple factors, such as added unlabelled data and a different network with its training strategy that is often more complex and specific to application. We postulate that this could lead to inconclusive correlation between confounding factors and the observed performance improvement. Based on the 'mean teacher' method [11], which has been adapted into several medical imaging applications [5,8], we decomposed the effects into those caused by the change of network (training and architectures) and those by adding unlabelled data. The mean teacher approach averages model weights to produce perturbed predictions as pseudo labels for regularising the training [7], a strategy that can be applied with or without ground-truth labels. In this work, we use the aforementioned surgical application as a real-world example to provide a quantitative analysis of the performance impact on the quantities of labelled and unlabelled training data.

Using real patient data from liver surgery cases, we summaries the contributions in this study as follows: (a) A statistically significant higher segmentation accuracy is reported in terms of Dice score and Hausdorff distance, compared with a previously proposed supervised method [6]; (b) We demonstrate the possibility that the change of training strategy specific to semi-supervised learning could result in significantly better segmentation results without adding any labelled or unlabelled data; (c) We show that adding more unlabelled data potentially can reach the improvement made with more labels, providing a practically important quantitative basis for data planning decisions.

2   Method

2.1   Supervised Segmentation Network Architecture

To analyse the effect with different training data set sizes in this work, we consistently use an exemplar neural network throughout our experiment, which is adapted from a U-Net variant [1]. Like the original U-Net [9], it consists of a

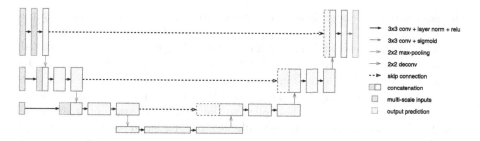

Fig. 1. U-Net architecture with multi-scale inputs (depth = 3).

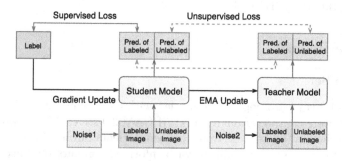

Fig. 2. Mean teacher structure

downsampling path (encoder) and an upsampling path (decoder), with skip connections added between the two paths. In addition, a multi-scale input image pyramid is added at each encoder layer except for the bottom one. For the decoder, the attention gate and deep supervision are omitted in this network for faster training. The details of the network architecture are illustrated in Fig. 1. The two-class Dice [10] with L_2 regularization is adopted for classifying the foreground pixels representing liver from the background pixels.

2.2 Semi-supervised Mean Teacher Training

Denote the labelled input as x_l, with its label as y_l, and the unlabelled input as x_u. Let $x_m = [x_l; x_u]$ be the mixed input. Two identical segmentation networks, the student network $f(x_m, \eta_m^1; \theta_s)$ and the teacher network $f(x_m, \eta_m^2; \theta_t)$ are illustrated in Fig. 2, with different input noise η and network weights θ.

During the training, the student network's weights θ_s are optimized using back-propagated gradients with respect to a regularised segmentation loss:

$$L_s = L_l(f(x_l, \eta_l^1; \theta_s), y_l) + \lambda \ L_u(f(x_m, \eta_m^1; \theta_s), f(x_m, \eta_m^2; \theta_t)),$$

where λ is a hyper-parameter balancing the contributions of a supervised loss L_l and an unsupervised loss L_u, both based on the two-class soft Dice loss [10]. L_l measures the overlap between the prediction and the ground-truth label, while L_u measures the discrepancy between student and teacher's predictions.

The teacher network is updated using exponential moving average (EMA): after each training step, $\theta_t = \alpha\theta_t + (1-\alpha)\theta_s$, where α controls the smoothing.

One important mechanism of this method is adding noise η_l^i and η_u^i to labelled and unlabelled image input, respectively, and $\eta_m^i = [\eta_l^i; \eta_u^i]$ for $i \in \{1,2\}$. In this work, we propose to use random affine transformation as the noise in the spatial domain. We apply two independently-drawn affine transformations to the input data as follows: one is applied to the student network input, with the same transformation applied to the available labels for supervised loss; while the second is composed with the first and applied to the teacher network input. The second transformation is then applied to the student network's prediction for computing the unsupervised loss.

3   Experiment

3.1   Data Set

A total of 41,994 laparoscopic video frames, with a sampling rate of four frames-per-second, were captured from a Storz TIPCAM 3D stereo laparoscope camera in our experiment. These were from thirteen patients during six liver resection and seven liver staging procedures, with informed consents obtained from all patients, and the data collection was approved by our institutional research ethics board. In addition, 2,209 images were selected on which, the regions of liver were manually contoured by an expert clinical research fellow in General Surgery to provide ground-truth segmentation labels. The annotation was performed in NiftyIGI [4], resulting in 67, 156, 148, 168, 246, 180, 140, 260, 198, 178, 166, 144, 158 labelled frames for each patient respectively. The original size of frame images were 1920×540 pixels in RGB channels with black borders on both sides. For computational and memory efficiency, all images were linearly re-sampled to 128×384 for each channel after cropping out the border to 1660×540 pixels.

3.2   Network Implementation and Training

The depth of network was 4 and each network was trained for $10,000$ iterations with a mini-batch size of 32, using the Adam optimizer with an initial learning rate at 10^{-4}. The weight of L_2 loss was fixed to 10^{-5} throughout the experiments. The network output has the same size as the re-sampled input image, larger than 81×21 used in previous work [6]. In the loss used in the mean teacher training, $\lambda = 0.1\beta$ with β increasing progressively, i.e. $\beta = \exp(-5(\max(1-\frac{S}{L}, 0))^2)$, where S is the current training step and $L = 1000$ is the ramp-up length. The EMA decay α was fixed to 0.99 during the initial ramp-up phase and 0.999 afterwards. All networks were implemented in TensorFlow and trained using Nvidia Tesla V100 general-purpose graphics process units on a DGX-1 workstation. To avoid over-fitting the entire data set, all the reported hyper-parameter values were configured empirically without extensive tuning.

3.3   Evaluation

All experiment results reported in this paper were based on 13-fold leave-one-patient-out cross-validations: for each fold, data from one patient was used for evaluation and the network was trained on the remaining data. The predicted binary masks representing segmentation were first re-sampled to 1660 × 540 and then processed by filling the holes before evaluation. Commonly-adopted data augmentation strategies for surgical video applications, including contrast and brightness adjustment and standardization, were also used before feeding the input data. The segmentation performance was measured by the Dice score and the 95th-percentile Hausdorff distance. The reported Hausdorff distance is in pixels and 100 pixels correspond approximately 1.5 mm to 6.0 mm, depending on the typical object-to-camera distance range in this application.

To test different data set sizes, 2%, 10%, 25%, 50% and 100% of the labelled data set were randomly sampled from each patients for semi-supervised networks, while 0%, 6.25%, 25% and 100% of the unlabelled data set were sampled with 0% indicating the mean teacher models trained without unlabelled data, which are fully supervised. A single network without the mean teacher model (hereafter referred to as the *baseline supervised network*) was also tested. In practice, however, the availability of the labelled and unlabelled image data would be influenced by other practical factors, such as cost and patient cohort sampling, and is highly application-dependent. This controlled experiment was designed with a simplified condition that excludes potential anatomical-variation-introduced difference between patients and should be considered as the first step towards a more comprehensive experiment design considering both inter- and intra-patient variation. We also report the statistical significance using non-parametric Wilcoxon signed-rank tests at a significance level of 0.05.

4   Result

Baseline Supervised Network (SL). The median Dice scores on 13 folds from the baseline supervised network trained using all labelled images ranged from 0.85 to 0.98 with a median of 0.95, compared with 0.78, 0.98 and 0.97 from the previous study [6], respectively. The difference was probably due to the change of loss function and the adoption of the U-net variant. When varying the quantity of the training (labelled) data from 2% to 100%, the segmentation performance was improved, from 0.9250 to 0.9594 and from 137.00 to 91.61, for Dice score and Hausdorff distance, respectively.

Mean Teacher (MT). The results for SL and MT with 100% unlabelled data are given in Table 1. Both the medians of Dice score and Hausdorff distance from MT were significantly better (both p-values < 0.001). The median Dice scores on 13 folds ranged from 0.87 to 0.98, with a median of 0.97, therefore surpassed the previous study [6] (p-value = 0.008). Examples are shown in Fig. 3.

Table 1. Supervised model (SL) and mean teacher (MT) with all data.

Metric	Method	Median	Mean	Std	Wilcoxon
Dice score	SL	0.9594	0.8792	0.1819	9.27e−28
	MT	**0.9646**	**0.9032**	0.1483	
Hausdorff distance	SL	91.61	148.23	166.86	4.40e−07
	MT	**81.49**	**137.57**	163.16	

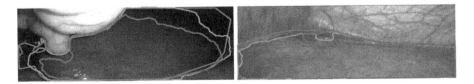

Fig. 3. Two examples with ground truth (green) and the predictions of the supervised model (blue) and mean teacher trained with all labelled and unlabelled data (orange). (Color figure online)

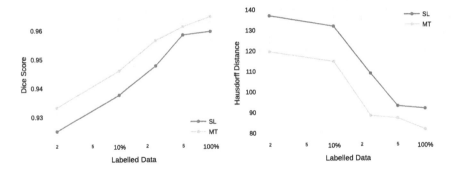

Fig. 4. Supervised model and mean teacher with different quantities of labels.

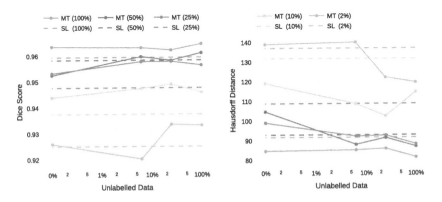

Fig. 5. Supervised model (SL) and mean teacher (MT) with different quantities of unlabelled data. The quantity of labelled data used is indicated in brackets.

Mean Teacher with Different Labelled Data Set Sizes. The median Dice scores for the MT models, trained with all available unlabelled data and different quantities of labelled data, varied from 0.9332 to 0.9646. It consistently outperformed SL with the same labelled data set sizes sampled, as shown in Fig. 4. The Hausdorff distance results also showed a consistent difference. In addition, a clear overall trend for both segmentation metrics can be observed: the performance improves as the number of labelled data increases.

Mean Teacher with Different Unlabelled Data Set Sizes. Median Dice scores are plotted in Fig. 5 with the quantity of labelled data indicated in the brackets. Without using any unlabelled data, MT generally outperformed SL; with more unlabelled data, MT produced better segmentation in general, but it was not monotonic. For instance, using 6.25% of unlabelled data improves MT (10%) from 0.9438 to 0.9473 in terms of Dice score, but for MT (2%) the score decreases from 0.9259 to 0.9202. This may be caused by (a) high correlation between unlabelled data due to the nature of the procedure and the omitted inter-patient variation (also discussed in Sect. 3.3); (b) the lack of optimised semi-supervised training and hyper-parameter tuning, which was not pursued further for the purpose of this work. Practically important, perhaps more interesting, results can be found to quantify the trade-off between the labelled and unlabelled data. For example, using 100% unlabelled data, MT (50%) reached a Dice score of 0.9611 which was higher than SL (100%), 0.9594, depicting a scenario in which more unlabelled data achieve a comparable performance as adding labels would.

5   Conclusion

The quantified differences showed in this work, such as the improvement due to more labelled and/or unlabelled data, are useful in developing machine learning applications that in turn assist clinical procedures. To summarise, we have shown a statistically significant improvement in segmenting liver from laparoscopic video images using a semi-supervised mean teacher method. Whilst adding more labelled data generally improves the segmentation, it is possible to use more unlabelled data, instead of labelling more data, to achieve comparable level of segmentation accuracy. To the best of our knowledge, it is the first time these conclusions are presented with quantitative evidence based on real patient data.

These results, however, should be interpreted with the limitations of the experiment design due to practical constraints. We suspect that non-optimised semi-supervised training and sampling intra-patient variation, also discussed in Sects. 3.2 and 3.3, respectively, are possible reasons for the perturbing segmentation performance as unlabelled data increase, which limited potentially larger improvement. Nevertheless, the reported high segmentation accuracy warrants a high applicability of these presented models for clinical use. Thus, the statistical significance found in the performance changes, measured on independent test data, suggest potential clinical value in planning data for training these semi-supervised models. These experiments produced a set of quantitative results, on which future work can be built to answer further multidisciplinary questions.

Acknowledgement. This work is supported by the Wellcome/EPSRC Centre for Interventional and Surgical Sciences (WEISS) (203145Z/16/Z). DS receives funding from EPSRC [EP/P012841/1]. MC receives funding from EPSRC [EP/P034454/1]. BD was supported by the NIHR Biomedical Research Centre at University College London Hospitals NHS Foundations Trust and University College London. The imaging data used for this work were obtained with funding from the Health Innovation Challenge Fund [HICF-T4-317], a parallel funding partnership between the Wellcome Trust and the Department of Health.

References

1. Abraham, N., Khan, N.M.: A novel focal tversky loss function with improved attention u-net for lesion segmentation. arXiv preprint arXiv:1810.07842 (2018)
2. Bai, W., et al.: Semi-supervised learning for network-based cardiac MR image segmentation. In: Descoteaux, M., Maier-Hein, L., Franz, A., Jannin, P., Collins, D.L., Duchesne, S. (eds.) MICCAI 2017. LNCS, vol. 10434, pp. 253–260. Springer, Cham (2017). https://doi.org/10.1007/978-3-319-66185-8_29
3. Cheplygina, V., de Bruijne, M., Pluim, J.P.: Not-so-supervised: a survey of semi-supervised, multi-instance, and transfer learning in medical image analysis. Med. Image Anal. **54**, 280–296 (2019)
4. Clarkson, M.J., et al.: The NifTK software platform for image-guided interventions: platform overview and NiftyLink messaging. Int. J. Comput. Assist. Radiol. Surg. **10**(3), 301–316 (2015)
5. Cui, W., et al.: Semi-supervised brain lesion segmentation with an adapted mean teacher model. arXiv preprint arXiv:1903.01248 (2019)
6. Gibson, E., et al.: Deep residual networks for automatic segmentation of laparoscopic videos of the liver. In: Medical Imaging 2017: Image-Guided Procedures, Robotic Interventions, and Modeling, vol. 10135, p. 101351M. International Society for Optics and Photonics (2017)
7. Lee, D.H.: Pseudo-label: the simple and efficient semi-supervised learning method for deep neural networks. In: Workshop on Challenges in Representation Learning, ICML, vol. 3, p. 2 (2013)
8. Perone, C.S., Cohen-Adad, J.: Deep semi-supervised segmentation with weight-averaged consistency targets. In: Stoyanov, D., et al. (eds.) DLMIA/ML-CDS-2018. LNCS, vol. 11045, pp. 12–19. Springer, Cham (2018). https://doi.org/10.1007/978-3-030-00889-5_2
9. Ronneberger, O., Fischer, P., Brox, T.: U-Net: convolutional networks for biomedical image segmentation. In: Navab, N., Hornegger, J., Wells, W.M., Frangi, A.F. (eds.) MICCAI 2015. LNCS, vol. 9351, pp. 234–241. Springer, Cham (2015). https://doi.org/10.1007/978-3-319-24574-4_28
10. Sudre, C.H., Li, W., Vercauteren, T., Ourselin, S., Jorge Cardoso, M.: Generalised dice overlap as a deep learning loss function for highly unbalanced segmentations. In: Cardoso, M.J., et al. (eds.) DLMIA/ML-CDS -2017. LNCS, vol. 10553, pp. 240–248. Springer, Cham (2017). https://doi.org/10.1007/978-3-319-67558-9_28
11. Tarvainen, A., Valpola, H.: Mean teachers are better role models: weight-averaged consistency targets improve semi-supervised deep learning results. In: Advances in Neural Information Processing Systems, pp. 1195–1204 (2017)

Few-Shot Learning with Deep Triplet Networks for Brain Imaging Modality Recognition

Santi Puch$^{(\boxtimes)}$, Irina Sánchez, and Matt Rowe

QMENTA, Boston, MA, USA
{santi,irina,matt}@qmenta.com

Abstract. Image modality recognition is essential for efficient imaging workflows in current clinical environments, where multiple imaging modalities are used to better comprehend complex diseases. Emerging biomarkers from novel, rare modalities are being developed to aid in such understanding, however the availability of these images is often limited. This scenario raises the necessity of recognising new imaging modalities without them being collected and annotated in large amounts. In this work, we present a few-shot learning model for limited training examples based on Deep Triplet Networks. We show that the proposed model is more accurate in distinguishing different modalities than a traditional Convolutional Neural Network classifier when limited samples are available. Furthermore, we evaluate the performance of both classifiers when presented with noisy samples and provide an initial inspection of how the proposed model can incorporate measures of uncertainty to be more robust against out-of-sample examples.

Keywords: Brain imaging · Modality recognition · Few-shot learning · Triplet loss · Uncertainty · Noise

1 Introduction

In recent decades, many useful imaging biomarkers have emerged from multiple imaging modalities such as CT, PET, SPECT and MRI (and its many sub-modalities) to assist with differential diagnosis, disease monitoring and measuring the efficacy of pharmaceutical treatments. Diagnostic workflows and clinical trials have therefore become dependent on the simultaneous use of multiple modalities to augment the clinical understanding of complex diseases. This diversity of imaging modalities creates complexity for image archival systems such as PACS, VNAs and cloud-based solutions, and the institutions or businesses that use them.

Classification of modalities and sub-modalities is important for efficient imaging workflows, a particularly difficult problem in MRI as the many distinct sub-modalities are not differentiated in a simple and consistent manner by image

© Springer Nature Switzerland AG 2019
Q. Wang et al. (Eds.): DART 2019/MIL3ID 2019, LNCS 11795, pp. 181–189, 2019.
https://doi.org/10.1007/978-3-030-33391-1_21

header information. For example, the use of contrast enhancing agents is a field often accidentally omitted or improperly populated in DICOM headers, meaning the use of a contrast enhancing agent can only be determined from the features of the image itself. In molecular imaging, an increasing variety of radioligands are being developed for monitoring different disease processes with each having distinct patterns of uptake or deposition. A human expert can easily distinguish them by their distinct visual features, however, scanner, vendor and center-specific idiosyncrasies in sequence implementation result in inconsistencies in DICOM header information that make automatic classification from DICOM headers alone highly challenging.

Due to the importance of the visual features of the images to classify, the problem lends itself to Convolutional Neural Networks (CNNs), which have proved to be highly successful at achieving near human-level performance at classifying images based on visual features [2]. A challenge to using CNNs for this kind of application is that they require large volumes of annotated data, which can be difficult to obtain for novel imaging biomarkers or rare modalities. For example, in a clinical trial utilising a novel imaging biomarker, it might be difficult to collect more than a handful of examples of the associated imaging sequence at startup. However, during the course of the trial, thousands of images may be acquired, requiring specific expertise to properly classify each sequence. Few-shot learning techniques offer a solution to creating robust classifiers from a limited amount of training data.

In this paper, we propose a few-shot learning model based on Deep Triplet Networks, capable of capturing the most relevant imaging features that enable the differentiation between modalities even if the amount of training examples is limited.

2   Methods

2.1   Data

We collect a brain imaging dataset that consists of 7 MRI sequences (T1, T2, post-contrast T1, T2-FLAIR, PD, PASL and MRA), CT and FDG-PET imaging, sourced from several public datasets that include brain scans from healthy and diseased individuals. We consider two categories for these modalities: base modalities, that includes T1, T2, CT and FDG-PET, and are the most abundant and have the most distinctive imaging traits; and few-shot modalities, which includes T1-post, T2-FLAIR, PD, PASL and MRA modalities.

To train and evaluate the models, we extract 2D slices by sampling a normal distribution centered around the middle slice of the brain along the sagittal, coronal and axial axes. We sample 30874 slices of T1, 231759 of T2, 18541 of CT, 15432 of FDG-PET, 8017 of T1-post, 9828 of T2-FLAIR, 8370 of PD, 5321 of PASL and 8462 of MRA images. We used 70% for training, 10% for evaluation and 20% for test.

2.2   Deep Triplet Networks

We approach the few-shot learning problem with Triplet Networks [4]. A Triplet Network is a type of metric learning algorithm designed to learn a metric embedding $\phi(x)$ and a corresponding distance function $d(x, x')$ induced by a normed metric, so that given a triplet of samples (x, x^+, x^-) and a similarity measure $r(x, x')$ that satisfies $r(x, x^+) > r(x, x^-)$, the learned distance function satisfies $d(x, x^+) < d(x, x^-)$. In essence, Triplet Networks learn to project samples in a embedding space in which similar samples are closer and dissimilar samples are farther apart with respect to a normed metric.

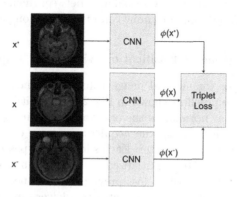

Fig. 1. A Deep Triplet Network takes an *anchor*, a *positive* and a *negative* sample, computes their embeddings with a deep CNN and then learns a distance function that satisfies the similarities between the samples of the triplet.

In our experimental setting, which corresponds to a multi-class image classification problem, the similarity measure $r(x, x')$ is defined by the labeling of our samples, that is, $r(x, x') = 1$ if x and x' belong to the same class and $r(x, x') = 0$ if x and x' belong to different classes. We define our distance function using the L_1 normed metric as follows:

$$d(x, x') = ||\phi(x) - \phi(x')||_1 \tag{1}$$

where $\phi(x)$ is implemented with a deep CNN, hence the Deep Triplet Networks naming. Typically, the samples of the triplet (x, x^+, x^-) are referred to as *anchor*, *positive* and *negative*; the *anchor* and *positive* samples belong to the same class, while the *negative* sample belongs to a different class. A diagram of a Deep Triplet Network is depicted in Fig. 1.

2.3   Triplet Loss with Online Hard-Mining

The loss used to train Deep Triplet Networks, referred to as triplet loss, is defined as follows:

$$L(x, x^+, x^-) = max(d(x, x^+) - d(x, x^-) + m, 0) + \lambda(||x||_2 + ||x^+||_2 + ||x^-||_2) \tag{2}$$

where m is a margin that controls how much farther apart do we want the *negative* sample to be with respect to the *anchor* and *positive* sample, and λ is an hyperparameter that controls the amount of L_2 norm penalization of the embedding vectors.

We implement an online hard-mining triplet loss, which has been shown to be more efficient and help convergence [5]. Instead of computing the embeddings on the whole training set in an offline fashion and then mine the hard triplets, which satisfy $d(x, x^-) < d(x, x^+)$, we compute the embeddings on a mini-batch of B images and then create a valid triplet with the hardest positive and the hardest negative for each anchor within that mini-batch [3]. We choose a batch size of $B = 64$ as it provides a good balance between memory demand and a number of samples large enough to mine valid triplets among a variety of classes.

2.4   Pipeline for Image Classification with Deep Triplet Networks

We propose a pipeline for medical image volume classification based on Deep Triplet Networks. The pipeline, shown in Fig. 2, starts with a preprocessing and slice sampling step that normalizes the orientation and image intensities of the volume and samples slices along the acquisition plane, emphasizing the sampling density around the FOV center. Each slice is then passed through a CNN that consists of a ResNet-50 [1] initialized with pre-trained weights from ImageNet and trained with the triplet loss previously described. Then, the embedding vectors extracted per slice are projected to a lower-dimensional space using Principal Component Analysis (PCA), in order to remove the noisy components of the embedded representation [6]. The PCA-projected embeddings are then clustered with a Gaussian Mixture Model (GMM) via expectation maximisation (EM). Unlike other clustering algorithms, such as k-means, a GMM is capable of capturing non-spherical cluster structures and provides estimates of the likelihood of a sample belonging to the model due to its probabilistic nature. We set the number of components of the GMM equal to the number of classes, and create a cluster to label mapping function by assigning to each cluster the most common class. From a GMM we can extract the posterior probability of each slice, that is, the probability that a sample came from each of the components of the mixture. We leverage that property to implement a hard decision function in

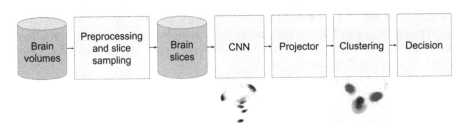

Fig. 2. Diagram of the end-to-end pipeline for image classification with Deep Triplet Networks

which each slice is assigned the class with maximum probability, and the volume is classified by majority voting.

3   Experiments

3.1   Hyperparameter Search

We use grid-search to obtain the optimal parameters of the model. The hyperparameters and options selected to optimize the network architecture are:

- Optimizer: ADAM, SGD with Nesterov momentum.
- Learning Rate: $1e^{-3}$, $1e^{-4}$, $1e^{-5}$.
- Learning Rate Decay: use a exponential decay with a decay rate of 0.9 every 1000 steps or not use decay.

The best performance was obtained when using SGD with Nesterov momentum as optimizer, a learning rate of $1e^{-3}$ and learning rate decay. We set in all experiments L_2 and L_1 regularization of weights to $1e^{-5}$ and $1e^{-6}$ respectively, the margin m of the triplet loss to 2, the L_2 penalization of the embeddings λ to 0.05, and the dimension of the embedding space to 64. We also perform random left-right and up-down flips as data augmentation. This configuration is used to evaluate the performance of the proposed model in all the subsequent experiments.

Furthermore, for each set of experiments, we evaluate the PCA projector using different number of projection components in order to select the best configuration. After evaluating the results, we select PCA with 9 components. The GMM is configured so that each component has its own general covariance matrix.

3.2   Few-Shot Learning

We compare the performance of our proposed Triplet Network (TN) classifier against a standard CNN classifier when training with all the available data (exp1) and training with restrictions on the number of slices of the few-shot classes (exp2). In the latter, we restrict the number of slices of the few-shot classes to only 150 slices, which corresponds to 10 volumes from which 5 slices have been sampled for each of the 3 orthogonal axes. The CNN classifier is based on the same architecture and pre-trained weights than the TN classifier, plus a fully-connected layer to directly predict the class from the imaging data.

In Table 1 we present the class-wise average of the precision, recall and F1-score, and the balanced accuracy for both experiments. The standard CNN classifier performs considerably well when trained with all the available data, but is unable to capture the relevant imaging traits of the few-shot classes when the training data is scarce. However, the TN classifier is able to produce an embedding space (Fig. 3) that separates the modalities into distinct clusters, allowing a better classification despite the under-representation of some classes.

Table 1. Classification metrics of the Triplet Network classifier (TN) and the standard CNN classifier (CNN). B: base classes; F: few-shot classes.

Model	Precision(B)	Recall(B)	F1-score(B)	Precision(F)	Recall(F)	F1-score(F)	Accuracy
CNN classifier - exp 1	0.98	0.99	0.9875	0.966	0.924	0.944	0.953
TN classifier - exp 1	1	0.938	0.965	0.89	0.996	0.93	**0.971**
CNN classifier - exp 2	0.782	0.995	0.887	1	0.332	0.396	0.626
TN classifier - exp 2	0.92	0.967	0.942	0.816	0.702	0.746	**0.819**

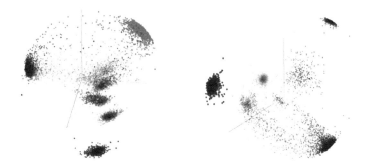

Fig. 3. Representation of the embedding space using the first three principal components of the evaluation embedding's projection on experiment 1 (left) and experiment 2 (right). Orange: T2, brown: T1, blue: CT, red: FDG-PET, purple: T2-FLAIR, yellow: T1-post, green: PD, pink: MRA, cyan: PASL. (Color figure online)

3.3   Robustness Against Noise

We measure the robustness of both classifiers when the dataset is corrupted with additive gaussian noise and salt and pepper noise. We consider the scenario where the model has been trained with data that has been randomly corrupted by noise and tested with corrupted samples (exp3), and the scenario where the model has been trained with curated data but is also tested with corrupted samples (exp4). Further, we also analyze the performance when limiting the number of instances of the few-shot classes in both exp3 and exp4, as described in the previous section.

In Table 2 we show the class-wise average of the precision, recall and F1-score, and the balanced accuracy for the experiments where the data is corrupted with additive gaussian noise and salt and pepper noise. When the noise applied is additive gaussian, in both experiments and both scenarios (with and without limiting few-shot classes), the TN classifier outperforms the CNN classifier, thus providing a more robust model. As expected, when the model has observed samples corrupted with noise during the training process the performance is better than when the training data is all curated. In the experiment using salt and pepper noise, when we use randomly corrupted samples during training the

CNN classifier performs better than the TN classifier, but the results of the network decrease considerably when the few-shot classes are limited, while our proposed model is able to maintain a good performance. Both networks achieve bad results when are trained with curated data and tested with samples with salt and pepper noise. It is interesting to observe that the performance of the CNN classifier is similar with both types of noise, while the TN classifier has decreased substantially its performance when the noise used is salt and pepper.

Table 2. Classification metrics of the few-shot classifier (Triplet) and the standard CNN classifier (Baseline) when trained with data corrupted noise (exp3) and trained with curated data but tested with corrupted volumes (exp4). B: base classes; F: few-shot classes.

Model	Precision(B)	Recall(B)	F1-score(B)	Precision(F)	Recall(F)	F1-score(F)	Accuracy
Noise	Gaussian						
CNN classifier - exp 3	0.99	0.987	0.987	0.956	0.93	0.938	0.955
TN classifier - exp 3	0.992	0.947	0.97	0.888	0.942	0.902	**0.97**
CNN classifier limit - exp 3	0.815	0.997	0.887	1	0.328	0.4	0.625
TN classifier limit - exp 3	0.942	0.965	0.952	0.658	0.62	0.622	**0.773**
CNN classifier - exp 4	0.85	0.742	0.735	0.964	0.478	0.638	0.596
TN classifier - exp 4	0.992	0.687	0.787	0.754	0.774	0.682	**0.737**
CNN classifier limit - exp 4	0.725	10.817	0.732	0.742	0.194	0.29	0.47
TN classifier limit - exp 4	0.927	0.67	0.765	0.634	0.678	0.588	**0.673**
Model	Precision(B)	Recall(B)	F1-score(B)	Precision(F)	Recall(F)	F1-score(F)	Accuracy
Noise	Salt and pepper						
CNN classifier - exp 3	0.982	0.985	0.982	0.946	0.916	0.93	**0.947**
TN classifier - exp 3	0.96	0.9375	0.945	0.658	0.738	0.668	0.827
CNN classifier limit - exp 3	0.765	0.99	0.87	0.914	0.31	0.384	0.625
TN classifier limit - exp 3	0.932	0.952	0.94	0.782	0.75	0.756	**0.839**
CNN classifier - exp 4	0.832	0.612	0.647	0.822	0.522	0.576	**0.561**
TN classifier - exp 4	0.912	0.49	0.6325	0.798	0.562	0.538	0.53
CNN classifier limit - exp 4	0.785	0.505	0.602	0.616	0.26	0.25	**0.47**
TN classifier limit - exp 4	0.722	0.49	0.545	0.64	0.396	0.448	0.44

3.4 Investigation of Uncertainty Measures

We investigate the use of the estimated log-likelihood of a sample on the GMM model as a measure of uncertainty. To do so, we obtain a minimum log-likelihood threshold by taking the 1st percentile over the training data, which corresponds to a value of -12.44, and compare such threshold with the estimated log-likelihood of samples: (a) that come from one of the classes on our dataset; (b) that come from classes not represented in our dataset (e.g. volumes with binary masks or derived images).

In Fig. 4 we can see examples of the proposed experimental setting. We observe that a sample from a class represented in the dataset (in our case, a T1 volume from the test split) presents a log-likelihood value above the proposed threshold. However, samples from classes not represented in the dataset (concretely, a segmentation map, a filtered image and a probability map) have a log-likelihood value lower than the proposed threshold.

This basic observation serves as an initial validation of the possibility of having uncertainty estimates using the combination of a Deep Triplet Network and a GMM model, thus having the capability of discerning out-of-sample modalities.

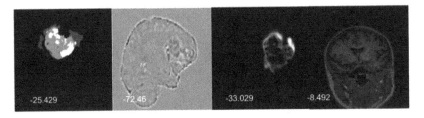

Fig. 4. Three samples of classes not represented in our dataset and a T1 slice, with their corresponding log-likelihood.

4   Conclusions

We have provided evidence that Deep Triplet Networks are a viable solution for modality classification in a few-shot setting. The proposed model, when trained with 30 times less instances of the rarer classes, surpasses substantially the performance of a CNN classifier trained under the same conditions. We have also concluded that the creation of an embedding space following a triplet network strategy increases the robustness against noise when compared to a standard CNN classifier. This is due to the fact that the results are not remarkably altered when the data is corrupted, regardless of whether the model has been trained with all the available samples or limiting the number of instances. Finally, we have explored the use of log-likelihood estimates of our model as a measure of uncertainty by evaluating such measure on samples not belonging to our dataset. We have found that this measure can effectively serve as an initial basis for uncertainty estimation, hence it can make our model more robust to unseen examples. This observation is preliminary and further investigation and development is required. Future work will focus on this topic, as well as extending the proposed model to alternative problems, such as disease staging.

References

1. He, K., Zhang, X., Ren, S., Sun, J.: Deep residual learning for image recognition. CoRR abs/1512.03385 (2015). http://arxiv.org/abs/1512.03385
2. He, K., Zhang, X., Ren, S., Sun, J.: Delving deep into rectifiers: surpassing human-level performance on imagenet classification. In: Proceedings of the IEEE International Conference on Computer Vision, pp. 1026–1034 (2015)
3. Hermans, A., Beyer, L., Leibe, B.: In defense of the triplet loss for person re-identification. ArXiv arXiv:1703.07737 (2017)
4. Hoffer, E., Ailon, N.: Deep metric learning using triplet network. In: ICLR (2014)
5. Schroff, F., Kalenichenko, D., Philbin, J.: Facenet: a unified embedding for face recognition and clustering. In: 2015 IEEE Conference on Computer Vision and Pattern Recognition (CVPR), pp. 815–823 (2015)
6. Wang, W., Carreira-Perpinan, M.A.: The role of dimensionality reduction in classification. In: Twenty-Eighth AAAI Conference on Artificial Intelligence (2014)

A Convolutional Neural Network Method for Boundary Optimization Enables Few-Shot Learning for Biomedical Image Segmentation

Erica M. Rutter[1,2(✉)], John H. Lagergren[1], and Kevin B. Flores[1]

[1] Center for Research in Scientific Computation, Department of Mathematics, North Carolina State University, Raleigh, USA
{jhlagerg,kbflores}@ncsu.edu
[2] Department of Applied Mathematics, University of California, Merced, Merced, USA
erutter2@ucmerced.edu

Abstract. Obtaining large amounts of annotated biomedical data to train convolutional neural networks (CNNs) for image segmentation is expensive. We propose a method that requires only a few segmentation examples to accurately train a semi-automated segmentation algorithm. Our algorithm, a convolutional neural network method for boundary optimization (CoMBO), can be used to rapidly outline object boundaries using orders of magnitude less annotation than full segmentation masks, i.e., only a few pixels per image. We found that CoMBO is significantly more accurate than state-of-the-art machine learning methods such as Mask R-CNN. We also show how we can use CoMBO predictions, when CoMBO is trained on just 3 images, to rapidly create large amounts of accurate training data for Mask R-CNN. Our few-shot method is demonstrated on ISBI cell tracking challenge datasets.

Keywords: Biomedical image segmentation · Few shot learning · Convolutional neural network

1 Introduction

Convolutional neural networks (CNNs) have recently been used to automate the segmentation of biomedical images [3], enabling an increase in the speed and accuracy of diagnosis, histology, and cell image analysis. However, creating segmentation training data for CNNs is a time intensive process requiring expert human annotation by clinicians or scientists. Thus, there is a need for methods to reduce the annotation burden by (1) drastically decreasing the amount of data

Electronic supplementary material The online version of this chapter (https://doi.org/10.1007/978-3-030-33391-1_22) contains supplementary material, which is available to authorized users.

© Springer Nature Switzerland AG 2019
Q. Wang et al. (Eds.): DART 2019/MIL3ID 2019, LNCS 11795, pp. 190–198, 2019.
https://doi.org/10.1007/978-3-030-33391-1_22

required to accurately train CNNs for segmentation, or (2) semi-automating the segmentation process while requiring minimal expert annotation. Recently, a novel method was proposed for using CNNs to improve segmentation accuracy by optimizing the task of tracing the boundary of objects in biomedical images [9]. This work found that using CNNs for optimizing boundary tracing accuracy better ensured contiguity of segmented regions and resulted in hyper-accurate cell segmentations. A unique aspect of the boundary optimization method is that the number of training examples obtained from a training image and its mask is equal to the number of pixels on the boundary of any object in the image. This is because the input to the CNN for boundary optimization is a small patch of the training image centered around any pixel on the boundary of an object, and the output is the prediction of the relative pixel displacements of the next m pixels in the trace (see Fig. 1, right panel). Thereby, a single segmentation training example can potentially yield hundreds or thousands (depending on the image size) of training examples for the task of boundary optimization. In this work, we investigated whether this property of boundary optimization could be leveraged to create accurate CNN-based segmentation methods for tasks (1) and (2) above with using only a few training images.

Contributions:

- We show that our **Co**nvolutional neural network **m**ethod for **bo**undary optimization (CoMBO) can be used to accurately segment biomedical images using just 3 training examples. To make predictions, this method requires an extremely minimal amount of human annotation, i.e., a single pixel per object.
- Provide a comparison of CoMBO with Mask R-CNN [3] and U-net [8].
- We show that CoMBO predictions can be used to rapidly create accurate training data for Mask R-CNN. The Mask R-CNN model trained on CoMBO predictions is just as accurate as a Mask R-CNN model trained on human annotations.

Related Work (Few-Shot Learning): Our work is related to the task of training a method for image segmentation with only a few training examples, i.e., few-shot learning. Unlike the task of one or few-shot image classification, the concept of one or few-shot image segmentation is relatively new [2,5,6,10]. Importantly, many previous methods for few-shot segmentation have been developed with a large margin of error and for multiple classes, since the focus has not been on biomedical imaging. Shaban et al. [10] created the first one-shot semantic segmentation network. Many few-shot segmentation techniques rely on using pre-trained networks [2,6], which may not be as applicable to medical imaging datasets. Other few-shot techniques consider multi-class segmentation, thus leveraging the existence of multiple images (one per class). Michaelis et al. [5] created a one-shot segmentation algorithm in clutter, but their method is best suited towards an instance where there is only one target in the image to segment, while there may be many targets to segment in a biomedical image.

2   Methods

In contrast to previous few-shot segmentation learning approaches, our method does not use transfer learning or pre-training. By formulating the learning task as a boundary optimization task, we naturally create many image-label pairs upon which to train a CNN for our algorithm. Our method modifies a previously developed CNN-based algorithm for object tracing described in [9].

The input to the CNN is a 64×64 patch of an image with a previously 'traced' boundary overlaid (Fig. 1, left panel). The CNN itself consists of three repeating blocks, each of which has 3 3×3 convolutional layers followed by a max-pooling layer. The final layer is an 8×8 convolutional layer. The number of filters for each repeating block is 32, 64, and 128, while the final layer has 60 filters. The output of the CNN is the next predicted 30 pixel horizontal and vertical displacements of the boundary relative to the center of the image (Fig. 1, middle). These horizontal and vertical displacements are then overlaid on the image as the cell boundary (Fig. 1, right panel cyan). A key modification we make to the algorithm in [9] is that we use the predicted displacements to move the trace multiple steps instead of one step at a time. This has resulted in higher accuracies, since the algorithm can 'skip' over problematic areas, while also speeding up forward passes by an order of magnitude. We do this by using a Bresenham line to connect the predicted pixel locations, thus ensuring a smooth outline of a cell. The number of steps to trace at each iteration is treated as a hyper-parameter selected using the validation data.

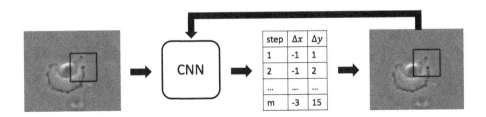

Fig. 1. Schematic of the tracing algorithm. Weak annotation shown as a red dot. The CNN takes as input the black patch, returns the next m predicted pixel locations, which are overlaid on the image in cyan. (Color figure online)

To trace an object in an image, we first choose an initial trace location (Fig. 1, left panel, red dot). In previous work [9] this initialization point was determined via output from other convolutional neural networks (U-Net). Due to the inaccuracies of such estimations in the few-shot setting, we instead utilize weak annotations provided by the user, namely a single pixel on the boundary of each object. Although annotating full segmentations for each object is laborious, clicking on an initial starting location for each object in an image is relatively quick and simple: for a dataset with approximately 25–30 objects per image, we were able to provide starting locations for approximately 12 images in 8 min. Once the initialization is begun, we pass the 64 × 64 image patch around the starting location through the CNN.

The forward pass on an image consists of (i) choosing an initial location (weak annotation by the user), (ii) iteratively using the CNN to trace the outline of the object, and (iii) stopping the iteration when the trace is greater than a certain length and the final pixel predictions are within a small distance to the initial pixel location.

One natural question arising from this algorithm is what happens for non-ideal tracing patterns? There are two such possible cases: either the CNN predicts a trace in the direction it just came from, or the trace deviates far from the true object boundary. We generate training data to always train counter-clockwise to ensure that traces do not go back in the direction they came from. We use a large patch size and, more importantly, predict the next thirty pixel displacements. By predicting multiple steps ahead, we can 'skip' areas in which the tracing algorithm might go awry. By including an adequate level of image context via a large patch size, the true boundary location is usually included in the image patch being passed to the CNN and the prediction can direct the trace back toward the boundary. We have not experienced a trace going off-course, but we include Supplementary Figure S1 which shows that the CNN predicts a trajectory that recovers from an initial pixel location off the boundary.

3   Experiments

Data: We evaluated our methodology on two grayscale light microscopy image data sets from the ISBI cell tracking benchmarks [4,11]: (1) GFP-GOWT1 mouse stem cells (Fluo-N2DH-GOWT1), and (2) Glioblastoma-astrocytoma U373 cells (PhC-C2DH-U373). From each data set, we used k images for training, 1 image for validation, and tested on the remaining images. Images from these datasets were prepared by zero-padding with 32 pixels (to ensure 64 × 64 patches for the CNN could be generated at the edge of the image). We found that this simplifies the algorithm in [9], which used symmetric padding, by helping to keep the trace away from the padded region when it reaches the edge of an image. Only images that had corresponding masks were used for training, validation, and testing (8 images for the GFP-GOWT1 dataset and 34 images for the U373 dataset). We performed 5-fold cross-validation for all experiments. In order to reduce stochasticity associated with initial pixel locations for the traces, the results from CoMBO are reported as the mean of 10 random initial locations for each object boundary. We perform the following series of augmentations at random to produce 48 augmented images per training image: up-down flips, left-right flips, rotations between $-45°$ and $75°$, shears between $-10°$ and $30°$, Gaussian blurring, and additive Gaussian noise.

Evaluation Metrics: Several metrics are used to assess the accuracy of our segmentations, since recent work showed that altering evaluation metrics can vastly change how algorithms are ranked [7]. To evaluate the accuracy of both the semantic segmentation and predicted cell morphology we calculated the Jaccard score, Dice Similarity Coefficient, Hausdorff distance, and mean surface distance (MSD).

Baseline: We compare the performance of our approach to Mask R-CNN, a well known method for instance segmentation [3]. Although Mask R-CNN is not formulated specifically for few-shot learning, we use it as a baseline comparison because there are not many other published few-shot segmentation algorithms. Moreover, Mask R-CNN is one of the best-performing benchmark segmentation algorithms. To make Mask R-CNN more adept at the few-shot segmentation task, we start training Mask R-CNN from weights that were pre-trained on imagenet [1]. We fine-tuned Mask R-CNN for each dataset and k-shot experiment for 400 epochs.

4   Results

We consider few-shot learning on 1, 3, and 5 training images. For each of these sets, an additional image is used for validation. We compare results with a pre-trained Mask R-CNN fine-tuned on the same number of images. Figure 2 displays the median ($\pm$ standard deviation) of the Jaccard scores and mean surface distances (MSD) for the GFP-GOWT1 dataset and the U373 dataset.

For the GFP-GOWT1 dataset, we found that CoMBO performs significantly better for all k-shot experiments in both Jaccard score and MSD. Furthermore, we observe lower standard deviations in the CoMBO model, implying that CoMBO was much less sensitive to the choice of training data. CoMBO was especially better at predicting accurate cell morphology in the few-shot setting, as reflected in the MSD and Hausdorff metrics. The evaluation metrics (Jaccard, Dice, MSD, and Hausdorff Distance) are reported for the GFP-GOWT1 dataset in Supplementary Table S1.

For the U373 data, we found that CoMBO was significantly better than Mask R-CNN using just 3 images for training (Fig. 2, right). Moreover, the CoMBO algorithm appears to reach convergence in Jaccard scores (and MSD) with only 5 images, i.e., training on more images did not appear to improve segmentation accuracy.

Since CoMBO is a semi-automated method, we investigated whether it could be used to rapidly generate data that was accurate enough to train Mask R-CNN. If CoMBO predictions are accurate enough for this purpose, then it would show that it could be used to effectively take the human out of the loop, eliminating the need for any human annotation. To test this, we used the 3-shot trained CoMBO that had the median Jaccard score for the U373 dataset to predict masks for the remaining images (approximately 30 images). We note that this would require minimal human annotation for each image, i.e., one pixel on the boundary of each object to initialize the predicted trace. We then generated masks from the CoMBO traces and used these data to train Mask R-CNN. We found that Mask R-CNN trained on data from CoMBO traces was able to achieve similar accuracy

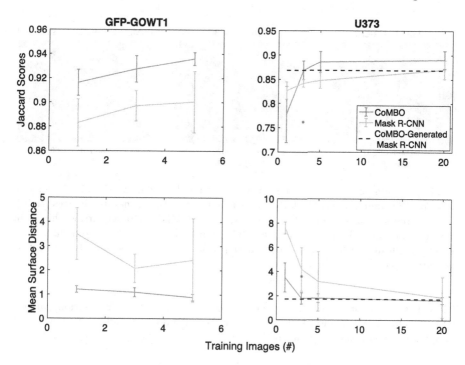

Fig. 2. Median Jaccard scores (top) and mean surface distances (bottom) for the GFP-GOWT1 dataset (left) and the U373 dataset (right). Blue=CoMBO, Red = Mask R-CNN, and the dashed black line represents Mask R-CNN retrained on images traced by CoMBO. Error bars denote standard deviation, outliers (*) were removed from standard deviation calculations. (Color figure online)

as using ground-truth masks (Fig. 2, right). These results suggest that CoMBO can be used to quickly and accurately annotate large datasets for fully automated machine learning methods. Figure 3 displays an example segmentation from the U373 testing set for 3-shot Mask R-CNN (left), 3-shot CoMBO (middle), and the Mask R-CNN trained on CoMBO-generated trainined data (right). This example shows how using the predicted masks from the 3-shot CoMBO to train Mask R-CNN is able to fix the false positives and improve both the Jaccard score and MSD.

Few-shot segmentation results for the U373 dataset are shown in Table 1 for all four accuracy metrics we considered. At all k-shot levels, CoMBO performed significantly better in the Hausdorff distance and MSD metrics. Mask R-CNN had a higher Jaccard and Dice scores for 1-shot segmentation. However, CoMBO had significantly higher Jaccard and Dice scores when trained on 3 and 5 images, and on the full dataset. Similar results for the GFP-GOWT1 dataset are reported in Supplementary Table S1.

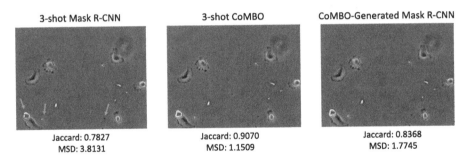

3-shot Mask R-CNN   **3-shot CoMBO**   **CoMBO-Generated Mask R-CNN**

Jaccard: 0.7827   Jaccard: 0.9070   Jaccard: 0.8368
MSD: 3.8131   MSD: 1.1509   MSD: 1.7745

Fig. 3. An example image from the U373 test set for the 3-shot Mask R-CNN (left), 3-shot CoMBO (middle) and Mask R-CNN trained on CoMBO-generated images (right). =Ground Truth, Blue=Mask R-CNN, Red=CoMBO. Orange arrows highlight areas in which CoMBO is more accurate. The 3-shot Mask R-CNN had difficulty accurately segmenting cells, both by having false positive cells and inaccurately segmenting the leftmost cell. (Color figure online)

Table 1. Performance of algorithms on the testing set averaged over five train/val/test data splits for CoMBO and Mask R-CNN for the U373 dataset. Bold denotes the best score within each k-shot experiment.

k-shot	Method	Jaccard score mean (std)	Dice coefficient mean (std)	Mean surface distance mean (std)	Hausdorff distance mean (std)
1-shot	Mask R-CNN	**0.8192** (0.01796)	**0.8986** (.01780)	7.3651 (0.4886)	137.3790 (11.9108)
	CoMBO	0.7866 (.05795)	0.8754 (.03905)	**3.4096** (1.1970)	**36.0004** (12.0755)
3-shot	Mask R-CNN	0.8434 (0.007609)	0.9135 (0.01078)	5.2904 (1.7850)	97.1921 (48.9499)
	CoMBO	**0.8679** (0.01906)	**0.9276** (0.01172)	**1.9130** (0.4637)	**25.0281** (5.7986)
5-shot	Mask R-CNN	0.8451 (0.01645)	0.9140 (0.003871)	4.7925 (2.4530)	81.9223 (60.8722)
	CoMBO	**0.8745** (0.02126)	**0.9313** (0.01369)	**1.9041** (0.3538)	**24.0791** (5.7986)
Full	Mask R-CNN	0.86278 (0.01924)	0.9246 (0.01430)	2.6368 (1.6806)	30.1077 (18.8510)
	CoMBO	**0.8914** (0.01831)	**0.9416** (0.01057)	**1.5586** (0.2866)	**18.5223** (2.0231)
	Retrained Mask R-CNN	0.8685	0.9294	1.7458	14.0817

5   Discussion

We found that our CoMBO algorithm for image segmentation is able to achieve accurate segmentations with 3 or fewer training images. We speculate that CoMBO is able to achieve high accuracy with a few training images because it transforms a small training data set, i.e., a few image/segmentation pairs, into thousands of training examples for a boundary optimization CNN task. It does so at the cost of requiring minimal user input, i.e., clicking a single pixel on the boundary of each object in an image. However, we also found that the predicted segmentations from CoMBO were accurate enough to create training data for Mask R-CNN [3], a fully automated segmentation method. The accuracy of Mask R-CNN trained on CoMBO data matched the use of ground-truth data.

Future work will include extending CoMBO to multi-class segmentation and also augmenting this method to handle instance segmentation, perhaps by using Mask R-CNN predictions as an additional channel for each patch input to the CNN. Using other few-shot algorithms to determine a starting location along the cell boundary would also enable a fully-automated few-shot segmentation learning approach.

References

1. Abdulla, W.: Mask R-CNN for object detection and instance segmentation on keras and tensorflow (2017). https://github.com/matterport/Mask_RCNN
2. Caelles, S., Maninis, K.K., Pont-Tuset, J., Leal-Taixé, L., Cremers, D., Van Gool, L.: One-shot video object segmentation. In: CVPR 2017. IEEE (2017)
3. He, K., Gkioxari, G., Dollár, P., Girshick, R.: Mask R-CNN. In: Proceedings of the IEEE International Conference on Computer Vision, pp. 2961–2969 (2017)
4. Maška, M., et al.: A benchmark for comparison of cell tracking algorithms. Bioinformatics 30(11), 1609–1617 (2014)
5. Michaelis, C., Bethge, M., Ecker, A.: One-shot segmentation in clutter. In: International Conference on Machine Learning, pp. 3546–3555 (2018)
6. Milan, A., et al.: Semantic segmentation from limited training data. In: 2018 IEEE International Conference on Robotics and Automation (ICRA), pp. 1908–1915. IEEE (2018)
7. Reinke, A.: How to exploit weaknesses in biomedical challenge design and organization. In: Frangi, A.F., Schnabel, J.A., Davatzikos, C., Alberola-López, C., Fichtinger, G. (eds.) MICCAI 2018. LNCS, vol. 11073, pp. 388–395. Springer, Cham (2018). https://doi.org/10.1007/978-3-030-00937-3_45
8. Ronneberger, O., Fischer, P., Brox, T.: U-Net: convolutional networks for biomedical image segmentation. In: Navab, N., Hornegger, J., Wells, W.M., Frangi, A.F. (eds.) MICCAI 2015. LNCS, vol. 9351, pp. 234–241. Springer, Cham (2015). https://doi.org/10.1007/978-3-319-24574-4_28

9. Rutter, E.M., Lagergren, J.H., Flores, K.B.: Automated object tracing for biomedical image segmentation using a deep convolutional neural network. In: Frangi, A.F., Schnabel, J.A., Davatzikos, C., Alberola-López, C., Fichtinger, G. (eds.) MICCAI 2018. LNCS, vol. 11073, pp. 686–694. Springer, Cham (2018). https://doi.org/10.1007/978-3-030-00937-3_78

10. Shaban, A., Bansal, S., Liu, Z., Essa, I., Boots, B.: One-shot learning for semantic segmentation. arXiv preprint arXiv:1709.03410 (2017)

11. Ulman, V., et al.: An objective comparison of cell-tracking algorithms. Nat. Methods **14**, 1141 (2017). https://doi.org/10.1038/nmeth.4473

Transfer Learning from Partial Annotations for Whole Brain Segmentation

Chengliang Dai[1]([✉]), Yuanhan Mo[1], Elsa Angelini[2], Yike Guo[1], and Wenjia Bai[1,3]

[1] Data Science Institute, Imperial College London, London, UK
c.dai@imperial.ac.uk
[2] ITMAT Data Science Group, Imperial College London, London, UK
[3] Department of Brain Sciences, Imperial College London, London, UK

Abstract. Brain MR image segmentation is a key task in neuroimaging studies. It is commonly conducted using standard computational tools, such as FSL, SPM, multi-atlas segmentation etc, which are often registration-based and suffer from expensive computation cost. Recently, there is an increased interest using deep neural networks for brain image segmentation, which have demonstrated advantages in both speed and performance. However, neural networks-based approaches normally require a large amount of manual annotations for optimising the massive amount of network parameters. For 3D networks used in volumetric image segmentation, this has become a particular challenge, as a 3D network consists of many more parameters compared to its 2D counterpart. Manual annotation of 3D brain images is extremely time-consuming and requires extensive involvement of trained experts. To address the challenge with limited manual annotations, here we propose a novel multi-task learning framework for brain image segmentation, which utilises a large amount of automatically generated partial annotations together with a small set of manually created full annotations for network training. Our method yields a high performance comparable to state-of-the-art methods for whole brain segmentation.

1 Introduction

Magnetic resonance imaging (MRI) plays an important role in human brain studies due to its good performance on presenting anatomy, pathology and function of the brain. Accurate segmentation of brain MRI scans is a prerequisite for measuring volume, thickness and shape of brain structure, which allows researchers to track and study the development, ageing and diseases of the brain [1]. Brain image segmentation is a time-consuming process when conducted manually, which typically takes several hours for a single subject. Therefore computational tools including FSL [2], SPM [3], MALP-EM [4] etc have been developed to automatically segment brain MRI scans and to enable large-scale population-based

© Springer Nature Switzerland AG 2019
Q. Wang et al. (Eds.): DART 2019/MIL3ID 2019, LNCS 11795, pp. 199–206, 2019.
https://doi.org/10.1007/978-3-030-33391-1_23

imaging studies. Most of these computational tools segment the scans by performing linear and nonlinear registration between a manually annotated brain atlas and a target scan and then propagating the atlas. Despite the efficiency they bring, these tools still suffer problems such as expensive computational cost and potential failures in image registration. Furthermore, strict pre-processing steps including brain stripping and bias correction are required to improve the reliability of these computational tools.

Neural networks have been explored and widely used for brain segmentation in recent years. Comparing to conventional brain image segmentation pipelines that are registration-based, network-based methods use pairs of images and manual annotations to train a discriminative model for inferring the segmentation of a new scan. Such difference brings a few advantages: (i) pre-processing can be potentially simplified [5]; (ii) processing time is significantly reduced without sacrificing the segmentation accuracy. Segmenting brain with network-based models also has drawbacks as these models require massive amount of annotated data for model training. The limited amount of annotations for brain images has become one of the biggest challenges for applying neural networks to brain image segmentation.

Previous works have been exploring ways for training image segmentation networks with limited annotations. A common approach is to fine-tune a pre-trained network from large image datasets like ImageNet [6]. In [7], an encoder-decoder model is pre-trained with auxiliary labels generated by FreeSurfer and then fine-tuned with an error corrective boosting loss. In [8], a multi-task image segmentation model is investigated to learn features that can be shared between MRI scans of different parts of human body. Generative adversarial networks (GANs) are adopted in [9] for data augmentation, which indicates a better performance than conventional augmentation methods.

Here we propose a novel brain image segmentation network, which leverages a massive set of automatically generated partial annotations (sub-cortical segmentations from FSL) for network pre-training and then perform transfer learning onto a small set of full annotations (manual whole brain segmentations). Compared to [7], our method is conducted in 3D but with less convolutional

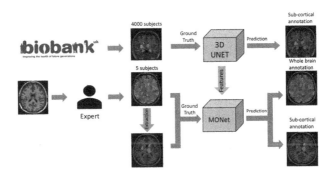

Fig. 1. Two-stage training scheme: Stage 1: pre-training; Stage 2: joint training.

layers. We demonstrate how features learnt from partial annotations in the source domain can be adapted to the target domain. With very limited annotations, our method achieves a performance comparable to state-of-the-art methods for brain image segmentation.

2 Method

Our work adopts a two-stage training scheme as illustrated in Fig. 1. Stage 1 pre-trains the segmentation network using a large set of automatically generated partial annotations. Stage 2 fine-tunes the network by jointly training on partial annotations and a small set of full annotations.

2.1 Pre-training with Partial Annotations

In this work, partial annotation refers to segmentation that only covers part of the brain structures. In our case, it refers to segmentation of 15 sub-cortical structures automatically generated by FSL. Full annotation refers to segmentation of whole brain structures manually annotated by human experts, which is a superset of partial annotation and consists of 138 structures. Since partial annotations are automatically generated, it is easy to acquire many of them. On the other hand, acquiring full annotations is more difficult as it requires extensive manual labour.

A 3D U-Net is employed for pre-training on partial annotations, using categorical cross-entropy as the loss function,

$$\mathcal{L} = -\sum_{v} g_l^w(v) \log p_l^w(v) \tag{1}$$

where $p_l^w(v)$ is the the predictive probability of partial segmentation belonging to class l at voxel v and $g^w(v)$ is the probability of it belonging to its actual class.

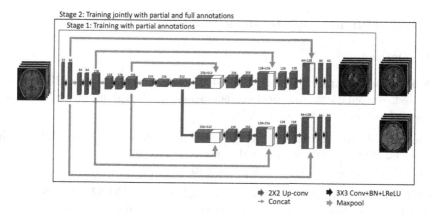

Fig. 2. Network architectures used in stage one and two training.

2.2   Joint Training with Full Annotations

We employ a multi-task learning framework for the second stage. The encoder is consistent with the architecture used in the first stage. Two decoders are used, so that the two tasks (partial segmentation and full segmentation) can be jointly trained. We refer our method as the multi-output network (MO-Net). The encoder and both decoders are loaded with the pre-trained parameters. Multi-output design encourages the encoder to learn shared features for partial segmentation and full segmentation. The partial segmentation used for joint training is extracted from the full segmentation, which are manual segmentations of the whole brain. Since manual segmentations have always been considered as 'gold standard' and should be more reliable than segmentations from automatic tools, the trained MO-Net should also be able to provide more accurate partial segmentation than the one trained in the first stage. The multi-output design given in Fig. 2 is similar to the one described in [5], which allows the network to learn jointly from two segmentation maps in order to achieve more accurate prediction and to have the potential to provide segmentation output for various annotation protocols. However, the difference is that we use a modified U-Net instead of ResNet and FCN adopted in [5], and our network is loaded with the parameters learnt from the pre-training stage.

A weighted loss that combines the overall loss of two decoders of MO-Net for joint training is formulated as,

$$\mathcal{L}_{MO-Net} = -\sum_v \lambda_s g^s(v) \log p_m^s(v) - \sum_v \lambda_w g^w(v) \log p_l^w(v) \qquad (2)$$

where $p_m^s(v)$ is the predictive probability of full segmentation belonging to class m at voxel v and $g^s(v)$ is the probability of it belonging to its actual class. λ_s and λ_w are the weights for overall loss function. To balance between the learning tasks for partial segmentation and full segmentation, we assign 0.5 to both losses in the overall loss function.

3   Experiments and Results

3.1   Datasets

UK Biobank Dataset (UKBB). 4,000 MRI brain scans from the UK Biobank are used. Automatic sub-cortical segmentations of 15 regions by FSL are used as partial annotations for pre-training.

Hammers Adult Atlases (HAA). The HAA dataset [10,11] contains brain atlases for 20 subjects with manual annotations for 67 regions. The dataset is split into 5/2/13 for training, validation and test.

MICCAI 2012 Multi-atlas Labelling Challenge (MALC). The MALC dataset [12] contains MRI scans from 30 subjects (15 subjects for training) with manual annotations for the whole brain for 138 regions and 132 regions are used for performance evaluation. The dataset also includes 5 follow-up scans, but they are excluded in our work. The dataset is split into 15/2/13 for training, validation and testing.

The manual annotations from the HAA and MALC datasets are regarded as ground truth in evaluation.

3.2   Preprocessing and Training

The typical brain image resolution is 256^3, with isotropic spatial resolution of $1\,mm^3$. All images were rigidly registered to MNI space and normalized to zero mean and unit standard deviation. For training the network, 3D patches of size 128^3 were randomly drawn from the brain images. Batch size was set to 1 due to the limitation of GPU memory. Random elastic deformation was applied to the 3D patches for data augmentation. Cropping and augmentation were performed on-the-fly. Adam optimiser with a starting learning rate of 0.001 was used for both stages of network training. Leaky rectified linear unit (LeakyReLU) with a negative slope of 0.01 is applied as the activation function. For the proposed method, pre-training was ran for 3 epochs and joint training was ran for 200 epochs. We also trained a standard U-Net as a baseline method for comparison.

3.3   Results

We evaluated the performance of MO-Net in terms of Dice score. For comparison, two versions of U-Nets were trained, one trained from scratch (U-Net (FS)) and the other fine-tuned (U-Net (FT)) on MALC and HAA respectively. For evaluating whole brain segmentation performance on MALC, we also compared our result to SLANT8 and SLANT27 [13], which is based on fine-tuning 8 and 27 3D U-Nets pre-trained with 5111 subjects for different locations of brain.

As shown in Tables 1 and 2, our method outperformed the U-Net trained from scratch by 26% on MALC dataset and 19% on HAA dataset. MO-Net also shows slight improvements over fine-tuned U-Net, SLANT8 and SLANT27 on both MALC and HAA datasets. We further compared to QuickNAT [7] on the same 25 brain structures as in their paper on the MALC dataset. The result is given in Table 3. MO-Net outperformed the fine-tuned U-Net, SLANT8 and SLANT27 by a small margin, although the performance is inferior to QuickNAT.

Table 1. Whole brain segmentation accuracy on MALC.

Method	Dice (mean ± std)
U-Net (FS)	0.623 ± 0.095
U-Net (FT)	0.782 ± 0.043
SLANT8 [13]	0.768 ± 0.011
SLANT27 [13]	0.776 ± 0.012
MO-Net	$\mathbf{0.785 \pm 0.070}$

Table 2. Whole brain segmentation accuracy on HAA.

Method	Dice (mean ± std)
U-Net (FS)	0.706 ± 0.032
U-Net (FT)	0.821 ± 0.019
MO-Net	$\mathbf{0.843 \pm 0.037}$

Table 3. Segmentation accuracy for 25 structures on MALC.

Method	Dice (mean ± std)
U-Net (FS)	0.775 ± 0.035
U-Net (FT)	0.809 ± 0.021
SLANT9 [13]	0.817 ± 0.036
SLANT27 [13]	0.823 ± 0.037
QuickNAT [7]	0.901 ± 0.045
MO-Net	0.838 ± 0.049

Table 4. Segmentation accuracy for 15 sub-cortical structures on MALC.

Method	Dice (mean ± std)
U-Net (FS)	0.649 ± 0.145
U-Net (FT)	0.835 ± 0.062
FSL	0.637(9 failed) ± 0.216
MO-Net	0.826 ± 0.029

Table 5. Segmentation accuracy for 15 sub-cortical structures on HAA.

Method	Dice (mean ± std)
U-Net (FS)	0.612 ± 0.103
U-Net (FT)	0.874 ± 0.053
FSL	0.763 ± 0.043
MO-Net	**0.879 ± 0.091**

For sub-cortical segmentation, we compared our result to FSL FIRST and U-Net. The proposed method MO-Net shows similar Dice score performance to fine-tuned U-Net and it is better than FSL and U-Net trained from scratch. The result is shown in Tables 1 and 4.

A box-plot of Dice scores comparing MO-Net with U-Net trained from scratch and fine-tuned on HAA for 8 brain structures is given in Fig. 3 showing the improvement of adopting our method. A qualitative result of whole brain and sub-cortical segmentation from MO-Net is given in Fig. 4, which shows better segmentation accuracy for certain structures comparing with U-Net and FSL (Table 5).

The result has demonstrated that a CNN-based model pre-trained with partial segmentation can achieve better accuracy for whole brain segmentation. The performance of MO-Net in terms of Dice scores is comparable to 3D U-Net based approaches in [13] on MALC with less strict training data, although inferior to [7] probably due to the deeper network they adopted. We believe the performance of our approach has the potential to be improved with a more advanced CNN design in the future. In general, multi-task learning helps the model to improve the generalization and in our case, to learn features shared by partial segmentation and full segmentation, which can possibly make our encoder more robust. Such claim would need more experiments to prove in the future.

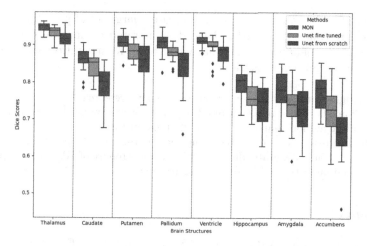

Fig. 3. Box-plot of Dice scores of MO-Net, U-Net fine-tuned and U-Net trained from scratch on HAA for 8 brain structures on the left hemisphere.

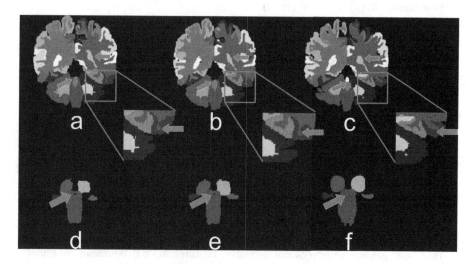

Fig. 4. Visual inspection of whole brain segmentation and sub-cortical segmentation on MALC: Ground truth of full (a) and partial (d) brain segmentation from the expert, full (b) and partial (e) brain segmentation from MO-Net, full (c) segmentation from fine-tuned U-Net, and sub-cortical (f) segmentation from FSL. Red arrows indict regions where MO-Net looks consistent with manual annotations and outperforms other methods. (Color figure online)

4   Conclusion

In this paper, we propose a method that combines transfer learning and multi-task learning to address the small data learning problem. Our method takes advantage of existing automatic tool to create a large set of partial annotations for model pre-training which has been demonstrated to improve segmentation accuracy. The preliminary result on whole brain segmentation shows a good potential of the proposed method.

Acknowledgements. This research is independent research funded by the NIHR Imperial Biomedical Research Centre (BRC). The views expressed in this publication are those of the author(s) and not necessarily those of the NHS, NIHR or Department of Health. The research is conducted using the UK Biobank Resource under Application Number 18545. We gratefully acknowledge the support of NVIDIA Corporation with the donation of the GPU used for this research.

References

1. Douaud, G., Groves, A.R., Tamnes, C.K., Westlye, L.T., Duff, E.P., et al.: A common brain network links development, aging, and vulnerability to disease. Proc. Natl. Acad. Sci. **111**(49), 17648–17653 (2014)
2. Jenkinson, M., Beckmann, C.F., Behrens, T.E., Woolrich, M.W., Smith, S.M.: FSL. NeuroImage **62**(2), 782–790 (2012)
3. Ashburner, J., Friston, K.J.: Voxel-based morphometry - the methods. NeuroImage **11**(6), 805–821 (2000)
4. Ledig, C., et al.: Robust whole-brain segmentation: application to traumatic brain injury. Med. Image Anal. **21**(1), 40–58 (2015)
5. Rajchl, M., Pawlowski, N., Rueckert, D., Matthews, P.M., Glocker, B.: NeuroNet: fast and robust reproduction of multiple brain image segmentation pipelines. In: International Conference on Medical Imaging with Deep Learning (MIDL) (2018)
6. Tajbakhsh, N., et al.: Convolutional neural networks for medical image analysis: full training or fine tuning? IEEE Trans. Med. Imaging **35**(5), 1299–1312 (2016)
7. Roy, A.G., Conjeti, S., Navab, N., Wachinger, C., Alzheimer's Disease Neuroimaging Initiative: QuickNAT: a fully convolutional network for quick and accurate segmentation of neuroanatomy. NeuroImage **186**, 713–727 (2019)
8. Moeskops, P., et al.: Deep learning for multi-task medical image segmentation in multiple modalities. In: International Conference on Medical Image Computing and Computer Assisted Intervention, pp. 478–486 (2016)
9. Shin, H.C., et al.: Medical image synthesis for data augmentation and anonymization using generative adversarial networks. In: International Workshop on Simulation and Synthesis in Medical Imaging, pp. 1–11 (2018)
10. Hammers, A., et al.: Three-dimensional maximum probability atlas of the human brain, with particular reference to the temporal lobe. Hum. Brain Mapp. **19**(4), 224–247 (2003)
11. Gousias, I.S., et al.: Automatic segmentation of brain MRIs of 2-year-olds into 83 regions of interest. NeuroImage **40**(2), 672–684 (2008)
12. Landman, B., Warfield, S.: MICCAI 2012 workshop on multi-atlas labeling. In: Medical Image Computing and Computer Assisted Intervention Conference (2012)
13. Huo, Y., et al.: 3D whole brain segmentation using spatially localized atlas network tiles. NeuroImage **194**, 105–119 (2019)

Learning to Segment Skin Lesions
from Noisy Annotations

Zahra Mirikharaji[✉], Yiqi Yan, and Ghassan Hamarneh

School of Computing Science, Simon Fraser University, Burnaby, Canada
{zmirikha,yiqiy,hamarneh}@sfu.ca

Abstract. Deep convolutional neural networks have driven substantial advancements in the automatic understanding of images. Requiring a large collection of images and their associated annotations is one of the main bottlenecks limiting the adoption of deep networks. In the task of medical image segmentation, requiring pixel-level semantic annotations performed by human experts exacerbate this difficulty. This paper proposes a new framework to train a fully convolutional segmentation network from a large set of cheap unreliable annotations and a small set of expert-level clean annotations. We propose a spatially adaptive reweighting approach to treat clean and noisy pixel-level annotations commensurately in the loss function. We deploy a meta-learning approach to assign higher importance to pixels whose loss gradient direction is closer to those of clean data. Our experiments on training the network using segmentation ground truth corrupted with different levels of annotation noise show how spatial reweighting improves the robustness of deep networks to noisy annotations.

1 Introduction

Skin cancer is one of the most common type of cancers, and early diagnosis is critical for effective treatment [10]. In recent years, computer aided diagnosis based on dermoscopy images has been widely researched to complement human assessment. Skin lesion segmentation is the task of separating lesion pixels from background. Segmentation is a nontrivial task due to the significant variance in shape, color, texture, etc. Nevertheless, segmentation remains a common precursor step for automatic diagnosis as it ensures subsequent analysis (i.e. classification) concentrates on the skin lesion itself and discards irrelevant regions.

Since the emergence of fully convolutional networks (FCN) for semantic image segmentation [5], FCN-based methods have been increasingly popular in medical image segmentation. Particularly, U-Net [9] leveraged the encoder-decoder architecture and applied skip-connections to merge low-level and high-level convolutional features, so that more refined details can be preserved. FCN and U-Net have become the most common baseline models, on which many different proposed variants for skin lesion segmentation were based. Venkatesh et al. [14] and Ibtehaz et al. [3] modified U-Net, designing more complex residual

© Springer Nature Switzerland AG 2019
Q. Wang et al. (Eds.): DART 2019/MIL3ID 2019, LNCS 11795, pp. 207–215, 2019.
https://doi.org/10.1007/978-3-030-33391-1_24

connections within each block of the encoders and the decoders. Yuan et al. [17] and Mirikharaji et al. [6] introduced, in order, a Jaccard distance based and star-shape loss functions to refine the segmentation results of the baseline models employing cross-entropy (CE) loss. Oktay et al. [7] proposed an attention gate to filter the features propagated through the skip connections of U-Net.

Despite the success of the aforementioned FCN-based methods, they all assume that reliable ground truth annotations are abundant, which is not always the case in practice, not only because collecting pixel-level annotation is time-consuming, but also since human-annotations are inherently noisy. Further, annotations suffer from inter/intra-observer variation even among experts as the boundary of the lesion is often ambiguous. On the other hand, as the high capacity of deep neural networks (DNN) enable them to memorize a random labeling of training data [18], DNNs are potentially exposed to overfitting to noisy labels. Therefore, treating the annotations as completely accurate and reliable may lead to biased models with weak generalization ability. This motivates the need for constructing models that are more robust to label noise.

Previous works on learning a deep classification model from noisy labels can be categorized into two groups. Firstly, various methods were proposed to model the label noise, together with learning a discriminative neural network. For example, probabilistic graphical models were used to discover the relation between data, clean labels and noisy labels, with the clean labels treated as latent variables related to the observed noisy label [12,16]. Sukhbaatar et al. [11] and Goldberger et al. [2] incorporated an additional layer in the network dedicated to learning the noise distribution. Veit et al. [13] proposed a multi-task network to learn a mapping from noisy to clean annotations as well as learning a classifier fine-tuned on the clean set and the full dataset with reduced noise.

Instead of learning the noise model, the second group of methods concentrates on reweighting the loss function. Jiang et al. [4] utilized a long short-term memory (LSTM) to predict sample weights given a sequence of their cost values. Wang et al. [15] designed an iterative learning approach composed of a noisy label detection module and a discriminative feature learning module, combined with a reweighting module on the softmax loss to emphasize the learning from clean labels and reduce the influence of noisy labels. Recently, a more elaborate reweighting method based on a meta-learning algorithm was proposed to assign weights to classification samples based on their gradient direction [8]. A small set of clean data is leveraged in this reweighting strategy to evaluate the noisy samples gradient direction and assign more weights to sample whose gradient is closer to that of the clean dataset.

In this work, we aim to extend the idea of example reweighting [8] explored previously for the classification problem to the task of pixel-level segmentation. We propose the first deep robust network to target the segmentation task by considering the spatial variations in the quality of pixel-level annotations. We learn spatially adaptive weight maps associated with training images and adjust the contribution of each pixel in the optimization of deep network. The importance weights are assigned to pixels based on the pixel-wise loss gradient directions.

A meta-learning approach is integrated at every training iteration to approximate the optimal weight maps of the current batch based on the CE loss on a small set of skin lesion images annotated by experts. Learning the deep skin lesion segmentation network and spatially adaptive weight maps are performed in an end-to-end manner. Our experiments show how efficient leveraging of a small clean dataset makes a deep segmentation network robust to annotation noise.

2   Methodology

Our goal is to leverage a combination of a small set of expensive expert-level annotations as well as a large set of unreliable noisy annotations, acquired from, e.g., novice dermatologists or crowdsourcing platforms, into the learning of a fully convolutional segmentation network.

FCN's Average Loss. In the setting of supervised learning, with the assumption of the availability of high-quality clean annotations for a large dataset of N images and their corresponding pixel-wise segmentation maps, $\mathcal{D} : \{(X(i), Y(i)); i = 1, 2, \ldots, N\}$, parameters θ of a fully convolutional segmentation network are learned by minimizing the negative log-likelihood of the generated segmentation probability maps in the cost function $\mathcal{L}$:

$$\mathcal{L}(X, Y; \theta) = -\frac{1}{N} \Sigma_{i=1}^{N} \frac{1}{P} \Sigma_{p \in \Omega_i} y_p \log Pr(y_p | x_p; \theta) \tag{1}$$

where P is the number of pixels in an image, Ω_i is the pixel space of image i, x_p and y_p refer, in order, to the image pixel p and its ground truth label, and Pr is the predicted probability. As the same level of trust in the pixel-level annotations of this clean training data annotations is assumed, the final value of the loss function is averaged equally over all pixels of the training images.

FCN's Weighted Loss. As opposed to the fully supervised setting, when the presence of noise in most training data annotations is inevitable while only a limited amount of data can be verified by human experts, our training data comprises of two sets: $\mathcal{D}^c : \{(X^c(i), Y^c(i)); i = 1, 2, \ldots, K\}$ with verified clean labels and $\mathcal{D}^n : \{(X^n(i), Y^n(i)); i = 1, 2, \ldots, M \gg K\}$ with unverified noisy labels. We also assume that $\mathcal{D}^c \subset \mathcal{D}^n$. Correspondingly, we have two losses, $\mathcal{L}^c$ and $\mathcal{L}^n$. Whereas $\mathcal{L}^c$ has equal weighting, $\mathcal{L}^n$ penalizes a log-likelihood of the predicted pixel probabilities but *weighted* based on the amount of noise:

$$\mathcal{L}^c(X^c(i), Y^c(i); \theta) = -\frac{1}{P} \Sigma_{p \in \Omega_i} y_p^c \log Pr(y_p^c | x_p^c; \theta), \tag{2}$$

$$\mathcal{L}^n(X^n(i), Y^n(i); \theta, W(i)) = -\Sigma_{p \in \Omega_i} y_p^n w_{ip} \log Pr(y_p^n | x_p^n; \theta) \tag{3}$$

where w_{ip} is the weight associated with pixel p of image i. All the weights of the P pixels of image i are collected in a spatially adaptive weight map

$W(i) = \{w_{i1}, \ldots, w_{ip}, \ldots, w_{iP}\}$, and weight maps associated with all M noisy training images X^n are collected in $W = \{W(1), \ldots, W(M)\}$.

Model Optimization. The deep noise-robust network parameters θ are now found by optimizing the weighted objective function $\mathcal{L}^n$ (as opposed to equal weighting in (1)) on the noisy annotated data $\mathcal{D}^n$, as follows:

$$\theta^* = \arg\min_{\theta} \Sigma_{i=1}^{M} \mathcal{L}^n(X^n(i), Y^n(i); \theta, W(i)). \tag{4}$$

Optimal Spatially Adaptive Weights. The optimal value of unknown parameters W is achieved by minimizing the expectation of negative log-likelihoods in the meta-objective function $\mathcal{L}^c$ over the clean training data $\mathcal{D}^c$:

$$W^* = \arg\min_{W, W \geqslant 0} \frac{1}{K} \Sigma_{i=1}^{K} \mathcal{L}^c(X^c(i), Y^c(i); \theta^*(W)). \tag{5}$$

Efficient Meta-training. Solving (5) to optimize the spatially adaptive weight maps W for each update step of the network parameter θ in (4) is inefficient. Instead, an online meta-learning approach is utilized to approximate W for every gradient descent step involved in optimizing θ (4). At every update step t of θ (4), we pass a mini-batch b_n of noisy data forward through the network and then compute one gradient descent step toward the minimization of $\mathcal{L}^n$:

$$\hat{\theta} = \theta_t - \alpha \nabla_\theta \Sigma_{i=1}^{|b_n|} \mathcal{L}^n(X^n(i), Y^n(i); \theta_t, W_0(i)) \tag{6}$$

where α is the gradient descent learning rate and W_0 in the initial spatial weight maps set to zero. Next, a mini-batch b_c of clean data is fed forwarded through the network with parameters $\hat{\theta}$ and the gradient of $\mathcal{L}^c$ with respect to the current batch weight maps $W^B = \{W(1), \ldots, W(|b_n|)\}$ is computed. We then take a single step toward the minimization of $\mathcal{L}^c$, as per (5), and pass the output to a rectifier function as follows:

$$U^B = W_0^B \Big|_{W_0^B = 0} - \eta \nabla_{W^B} \frac{1}{|b_c|} \Sigma_{i=1}^{|b_c|} \mathcal{L}^c(X^c(i), Y^c(i); \hat{\theta}(W)), \tag{7}$$

$$W^B = g(\max(\mathbf{0}, U^B)). \tag{8}$$

where η is a gradient descent learning rate, max is an element-wise max and g is the normalization function. Following the average loss over a mini-batch samples in training a deep network, g normalizes the learned weight maps such that $\Sigma_{i=1}^{|b_n|} \Sigma_{p \in \Omega_i} w_{ip} = 1$.

Equations (7) and (8) clarify how the learned weight maps prevents penalizing the pixels whose gradient direction is not similar to the direction of gradient on the clean data. A negative element u_{ip} in U (associated with pixel p of image i) implies a positive gradient $\nabla_{w_{ip}} \mathcal{L}^c$ in (7), meaning that increasing the assigned weight to pixel p, w_{ip}, increases the $\mathcal{L}^c$ loss value on clean data.

So by rectifying the values of u_{ip} in (8), we assign zero weights w_{ip} to pixel p and prevent penalizing it in the loss function. In addition, the rectify function makes the $\mathcal{L}^n$ loss non-negative (cf. (3)) and results in more stable optimization.

Once the learning of spatially adaptive weight maps is performed, a final backward pass is needed to minimize the reweighted objective function and update the network parameters from θ_t to θ_{t+1}:

$$\theta_{t+1} = \theta_t - \alpha \nabla_{\theta_t} \Sigma_{i=1}^{|b_n|} \mathcal{L}^n(X^n(i); \theta_t, W^B). \tag{9}$$

3   Experiments and Discussion

Data Description. We validated our spatially adaptive reweighting approach on data provided by the International Skin Imaging Collaboration (ISIC) in 2017 [1]. The data consists of 2000 training, 150 validation and 600 test images with their corresponding segmentation masks. The same split of validation and test data are deployed for setting the hyper-parameters and reporting the final results. We re-sized all images to 96×96 pixels and normalized each RGB channel with the per channel mean and standard deviation of training data.

To create noisy ground truth annotations, we consider a lesion boundary as a closed polygon and simplify it by reducing its number of vertices: Less important vertices are discarded first, where the importance of each vertex is proportional to the acuteness of the angle formed by the two adjacent polygon line segments and their length. 7-vertex, 3-vertex and 4-axis-aligned-vertex polygons are generated to represent different levels of annotation noise for our experiments. To simulate an unsupervised setting, as an extreme level of noise, we automatically generated segmentation maps that cover the whole image (excluding a thin band around the image perimeter). Figure 1 shows a sample lesion image and its associated ground truth as well as generated noisy annotations.

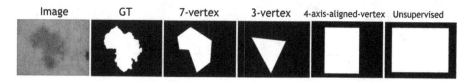

Fig. 1. A skin image and its clean and various noisy segmentation maps.

Implementation. We utilize PyTorch framework to implement our segmentation reweighting network. We adopt the architecture of fully convolutional network U-Net [9] initialized by a random Gaussian distribution. We use the stochastic gradient descent algorithm for learning the network parameters from scratch as well as the spatial weight maps over the mini-batch of sizes $|b_n| = 2$ and $|b_c| = 10$. We set the initial learning rate for both α and η to 10^{-4} and divide by 10 when the validation performance stops improving. We set the momentum and weight decay to 0.99 and 5×10^{-5}, respectively. Training the deep reweighting network took three days on our 12 GB GPU memory.

Spatially Adaptive Reweighting vs. Image Reweighting and Fine-Tuning. We compare our work with previous work on noisy labels which assign a weight per training images [8]. In addition, one popular way of training a deep network when a small set of clean data as well as a large set of noisy data are available is to pre-train the network on the noisy dataset and then fine-tune it using the clean dataset. By learning the spatially adaptive weight maps proposed in this work, we expect to leverage clean annotations more effectively for segmentation task and achieve an improved performance. We start with $|\mathcal{D}^n| = 2000$ images annotated by 3-vertex polygons and gradually replace some of the noisy annotation with expert-level clean annotations, i.e., increase $|\mathcal{D}^c|$. We report the Dice score on the test set in Fig. 2. The first (leftmost) point on the fine-tuning curve indicates the result of U-Net when all annotation are noisy and the last point corresponds to a fully-supervised U-Net. When all annotation are either clean or noisy, training the reweighting networks are not applicable. We observe a consistent improvement in the test Dice score when the proposed reweighting algorithm is deployed. In particular, a bigger boost in improvement when the size of the clean annotation is smaller signifies our method's ability to effectively utilize even a handful of clean samples.

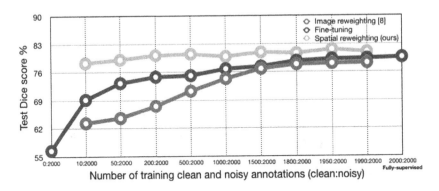

Fig. 2. Test Dice score comparison for fine-tuning, per image reweighting [8] and, spatially adaptive reweighting (ours) models.

Size of the Clean Dataset. Figure 2 shows the effect of the clean data size, $|\mathcal{D}^c|$, on the spatial reweighting network performance. Our results show leveraging just 10 clean annotations in the proposed model improves the test Dice score by 21.79% in comparison to training U-Net on all noisy annotations. Also, utilizing 50 clean annotations in the spatial reweighting algorithm achieves a test Dice score ($\sim$80%) almost equal to that of the fully supervised approach. With only $\sim$100 clean image annotations, the spatial reweighting method outperforms the fully-supervised with 2000 clean annotations. Incrementing $|\mathcal{D}^c|$ from 50 to 1990, the reweighting approach improves the test Dice score by about 2%, questioning whether a 2% increase in accuracy is worth the $\sim$40-fold increase in annotation effort. Outperforming the supervised setting using spatial reweighting algorithm suggests that the adaptive loss reweighting strategy works like a regularizer and improves the generalization ability of the deep network.

Robustness to Noise. In our next experiment, we examine how the level of noise in the training data affect the performance of the spatial reweighting network in comparison to fine-tuning. We utilized four sets of (i) 7-vertex; (ii) 3-vertex; (iii) 4-axis-aligned-vertex simplified polygons as segmentation maps; and (iv) unsupervised coarse segmentation masks where each set corresponds to a level of annotation noise (Fig. 1). Setting $|\mathcal{D}^c| = 100$ and $|\mathcal{D}^n| = 1600$,

Table 1. Dice score using fine-tuning and reweighting methods for various noise levels.

	Noise type	Fine-tuning	Proposed reweighting
A	No noise (fully-supervised)	78.63%	Not applicable
B	7-vertex	76.12%	80.72%
C	4-axis-aligned-vertex	75.04%	80.29%
D	3-vertex	73.02%	79.45%
E	Maximal (unsupervised)	70.45%	73.55%

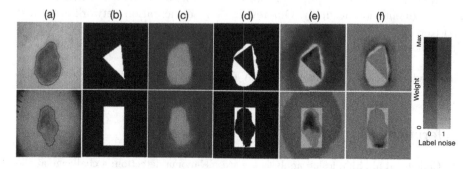

Fig. 3. (a) Sample skin images and expert lesion delineations (thin black contour), (b) noisy ground truth, (c) network output, (d) the erroneously labelled pixels (i.e. noisy pixels) and learned weight maps in iterations (e) 1K and (f) 100K overlaid over the noisy pixel masks using the following coloring scheme: Noisy pixels are rendered via the blue channel: mislabelled pixels are blue, and weights via the green channel: the *lower* the weight the greener the rendering. The cyan color is produced when mixing green and blue, i.e. when low weights (green) are assigned to mislabelled pixels (blue). Note how the cyan very closely matches (d), i.e. mislabelled pixels are ca. null-weighted. (Color figure online)

the segmentation Dice score of test images for reweighting and fine-tuning approaches are reported in Table 1. We observe that deploying the proposed reweighting algorithm for 3-vertex annotations outperforms learning from accurate delineation without reweighting. Also, increasing the level of noise, from 7-vertex to 3-vertex polygon masks in noisy data, results in just ∼1% Dice score drop when deploying reweighting compared to ∼3% drop in fine-tuning.

Qualitative Results. To examine the spatially adaptive weights more closely, for some sample images, we overlay the learned weight maps, in training iterations 1K and 100K, over the incorrectly annotated pixels mask (Fig. 3). To avoid overfitting to annotation noise, we expect the meta-learning step to assign zero weights to noisy pixels (the white pixels in Fig. 3(d)). Looking into Fig. 3(e, f) confirms that the model consistently learns to assign zero (or very close to zero) weights to noisy annotated pixels (cyan pixels), which ultimatly results in the prediction of the segmentation maps in Fig. 3(c) that, qualitatively, closely resemble the unseen expert delineated contours shown in Fig. 3(a).

4   Conclusion

By learning a spatially-adaptive map to perform pixel-wise weighting of a segmentation loss, we were able to effectively leverage a limited amount of cleanly annotated data in training a deep segmentation network that is robust to annotation noise. We demonstrated, on a skin lesion image dataset, that our method can greatly reduce the requirement for careful labelling of images without sacrificing segmentation accuracy. Our reweighting segmentation network is trained end-to-end, can be combined with any segmentation network architecture, and does not require any additional hyper-parameter tuning.

Acknowledgments. We thank NVIDIA Corporation for the donation of Titan X GPUs used in this research and Compute Canada for computational resources.

References

1. Codella, et al.: Skin lesion analysis toward melanoma detection: a challenge at the 2017 ISBI. arXiv:1710.05006 (2017)
2. Goldberger, J., Ben-Reuven, E.: Training deep neural-networks using a noise adaptation layer. In: ICLR (2017)
3. Ibtehaz, N., Rahman, M. S.: Multiresunet: rethinking the U-Net architecture for multimodal biomedical image segmentation. arXiv preprint arXiv:1902.04049 (2019)
4. Jiang, et al.: Mentornet: regularizing very deep neural networks on corrupted labels. arXiv preprint arXiv:1712.05055 (2017)
5. Long, et al.: Fully convolutional networks for semantic segmentation. In: IEEE CVPR, pp. 3431–3440 (2015)

6. Mirikharaji, Z., Hamarneh, G.: Star shape prior in fully convolutional networks for skin lesion segmentation. In: Frangi, A.F., Schnabel, J.A., Davatzikos, C., Alberola-López, C., Fichtinger, G. (eds.) MICCAI 2018. LNCS, vol. 11073, pp. 737–745. Springer, Cham (2018). https://doi.org/10.1007/978-3-030-00937-3_84

7. Oktay, et al.: Attention U-Net: learning where to look for the pancreas. In: MIDL (2018)

8. Ren, et al.: Learning to reweight examples for robust deep learning. In: ICML (2018)

9. Ronneberger, et al.: U-Net: convolutional networks for biomedical image segmentation. In: Navab, N., Hornegger, J., Wells, W.M., Frangi, A.F. (eds.) MICCAI 2015. LNCS, vol. 9351, pp. 234–241. Springer, Cham (2015). https://doi.org/10.1007/978-3-319-24574-4_28

10. Siegel, et al.: Cancer statistics. CA. Cancer J. Clin. **67**(1), 7–30 (2017)

11. Sukhbaatar, et al.: Learning from noisy labels with deep neural networks. arXiv preprint arXiv:1406.2080 (2014)

12. Vahdat, A.: Toward robustness against label noise in training deep discriminative neural networks. In: NIPS, pp. 5596–5605 (2017)

13. Veit, et al.: Learning from noisy large-scale datasets with minimal supervision. In: IEEE CVPR, pp. 839–847 (2017)

14. Venkatesh, et al.: A deep residual architecture for skin lesion segmentation. In: OR 2.0 Context-Aware Operating Theaters, Computer Assisted Robotic Endoscopy, Clinical Image-Based Procedures, and Skin Image Analysis, pp. 277–284 (2018)

15. Wang, et al.: Iterative learning with open-set noisy labels. In: IEEE CVPR, pp. 8688–8696 (2018)

16. Xiao, et al.: Learning from massive noisy labeled data for image classification. In: IEEE CVPR, pp. 2691–2699 (2015)

17. Yuan, et al.: Automatic skin lesion segmentation using deep fully convolutional networks with jaccard distance. IEEE TMI **36**(9), 1876–1886 (2017)

18. Zhang, et al.: Understanding deep learning requires rethinking generalization. In: ICLR (2017)

A Weakly Supervised Method for Instance Segmentation of Biological Cells

Fidel A. Guerrero-Peña[1,2], Pedro D. Marrero Fernandez[2], Tsang Ing Ren[2], and Alexandre Cunha[1(✉)]

[1] Center for Advanced Methods in Biological Image Analysis – CAMBIA, California Institute of Technology, Pasadena, CA, USA
cunha@caltech.edu
[2] Center for Informatics, Federal University of Pernambuco, Recife, PE, Brazil

Abstract. We present a weakly supervised deep learning method to perform instance segmentation of cells present in microscopy images. Annotation of biomedical images in the lab can be scarce, incomplete, and inaccurate. This is of concern when supervised learning is used for image analysis as the discriminative power of a learning model might be compromised in these situations. To overcome the curse of poor labeling, our method focuses on three aspects to improve learning: (i) we propose a loss function operating in three classes to facilitate separating adjacent cells and to drive the optimizer to properly classify underrepresented regions; (ii) a contour-aware weight map model is introduced to strengthen contour detection while improving the network generalization capacity; and (iii) we augment data by carefully modulating local intensities on edges shared by adjoining regions and to account for possibly weak signals on these edges. Generated probability maps are segmented using different methods, with the watershed based one generally offering the best solutions, specially in those regions where the prevalence of a single class is not clear. The combination of these contributions allows segmenting individual cells on challenging images. We demonstrate our methods in sparse and crowded cell images, showing improvements in the learning process for a fixed network architecture.

Keywords: Instance segmentation · Weakly supervised · Cell segmentation · Microscopy cells · Loss modeling

1 Introduction

In developmental cell biology studies, one generally needs to quantify temporal signals, *e.g.* protein concentration, on a per cell basis. This requires segmenting individual cells in many images, accounting to hundreds or thousands of cells per

We thank the financial support from the Beckman Institute at Caltech to the Center for Advanced Methods in Biological Image Analysis – CAMBIA (FAG, AC) and from the Brazilian funding agencies FACEPE, CAPES and CNPq (FAG, PF, TIR).

© Springer Nature Switzerland AG 2019
Q. Wang et al. (Eds.): DART 2019/MIL3ID 2019, LNCS 11795, pp. 216–224, 2019.
https://doi.org/10.1007/978-3-030-33391-1_25

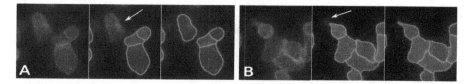

Fig. 1. Incomplete (A) and inaccurate (B) annotations of training images might be harmful for supervised learning as the presence of similar regions with erratic annotations might puzzle the optimization process. Our formulation is able to segment well under uncertainty as shown in the examples in the right panels of A and B above.

experiment. Such data availability suggests carrying on large annotation efforts, following the common wisdom that massive annotations are beneficial for fully supervised training to avoid overfitting and improve generalization. However, full annotation is expensive, time consuming, and it is often inaccurate and incomplete when it is done at the lab, even by specialists (see Fig. 1).

To mitigate these difficulties and make the most of limited training data, we work on three fronts to improve learning. In addition to the usual data augmentation strategies (rotation, cropping, etc.), we propose a new augmentation scheme which modulates intensities on the borders of adjacent cells as these are key regions when separating crowded cells. This scheme augments the contrast patterns between edges and cell interiors. We also explicitly endow the loss function to account for critically underrepresented and reduced size regions so they can have a fair contribution to the functional during optimization. By adopting large weights on short edges separating adjacent cells we increase the chances of detecting them as they now contribute more significantly to the loss. In our experience, without this construction, these regions are poorly classified by the optimizer – weights used in the original U-Net formulation [9] are not sufficient to promote separation of adjoining regions. Further, adopting a three classes approach [4] has significantly improved the separation of adjacent cells which are otherwise consistently merged when considering a binary foreground and background classification strategy. We have noticed that complex shapes, *e.g.* with small necks, slim invaginations and protrusions, are more difficult to segment when compared to round, mostly convex shapes [10]. Small cells, tiny edges, and slim parts, equally important for the segmentation result, can be easily dismissed by the optimizer if their contribution is not explicitly accounted for and on par with other more dominant regions.

Previous Work. In [6] the authors propose a weakly semantic segmentation method for biomedical images. They include prior knowledge in the form of constraints into the loss function for regularizing the size of segmented objects. The work in [11] proposes a way to keep annotations at a minimum while still capturing the essence of the signal present in the images. The goal is to avoid excessively annotating redundant parts, present due to many repetitions of almost identical cells in the same image. In [8] the authors also craft a tuned loss function applied to improve segmentation on weakly annotated gastric cancer images.

The instance segmentation method for natural images Mask R-CNN [5] uses two stacked networks, with detection followed by segmentation. We use it for comparisons on our cell images. Others have used three stacked networks for semantic segmentation and regression of a watershed energy map allowing separating nearby objects [1].

2   Segmentation Method

Notation. Let $S = \{(x_j, g_j)\}_{j=1}^N$ be a training instance segmentation set where $x_j \colon \Omega \to \mathbb{R}^+$ is a single channel gray image defined on the regular grid $\Omega \in \mathbb{R}^2$, and $g_j \colon \Omega \to \{0, \ldots, m_j\}$ its instance segmentation ground truth map which assigns to a pixel $p \in \Omega$ a unique label $g_j(p)$ among all $m_j + 1$ distinct instance labels, one for each object, including background, labeled 0. For a generic (x, g), $V_i = \{p \mid g(p) = i\}$ contains all pixels belonging to instance object i, hence forming the connected component of object i. Due to label uniqueness, $V_i \cap V_j = \emptyset, i \neq j$, *i.e.* a pixel cannot belong to more than one instance thus satisfying the panoptic segmentation criterion [7]. Let $h \colon \Omega \to \{0, \ldots, C\}$ be a semantic segmentation map, obtained using g, which reports the semantic class of a pixel among the $C + 1$ possible semantic classes, and $y \colon \Omega \to \mathbb{R}^{C+1}$ its one hot encoding mapping. That is, for vector $y(p) \in \mathbb{R}^{C+1}$ and its l-th component $y_l(p)$, we have $y_l(p) = 1$ iff $h(p) = l$, otherwise $y_l(p) = 0$. We call $n_l = \sum_{p \in \Omega} y_l(p)$ the number of pixels of class l, and $\eta_k(p), k \geqslant 1$, the $(2k+1) \times (2k+1)$ neighborhood of a pixel $p \in \Omega$. In our experiments we adopted $k = 2$.

From Instance to Semantic Ground Truth. We formulate the instance segmentation problem as a semantic segmentation problem where we obtain object segmentation and separation of cells at once. To transform an instance ground truth to a semantic ground truth, we adopted the three semantic classes scheme of [4]: image background, cell interior, and touching region between cells. This is suitable as the intensity distribution of our images in those regions is multi-modal. We define our semantic ground truth h as

$$h(p) = \begin{cases} 0 & \text{if } g(p) = 0 & - \text{ background} \\ 2 & \text{if } \sum_{p' \in \eta_k(p)} [g(p') \neq g(p)] \cdot [g(p') \neq 0] > 1 & - \text{ touching} \\ 1 & \text{otherwise} & - \text{ cell} \end{cases} \quad (1)$$

where $[\cdot]$ refers to Iverson bracket notation [2]: $[b] = 1$ if the boolean condition b is true, otherwise $[b] = 0$. Equation 1 assigns class 0 to all background pixels, it assigns class 2 to all pixels whose neighborhood η_k contains at least one pixel of another connected component, and it assigns class 1 to cell pixels not belonging to touching regions.

Touching Region Augmentation. Touching regions have the lowest pixel count among all semantic classes, having few examples to train the network. They are in general brighter than their surroundings, but not always, with varying values along its length. To train with a larger gamut of touching patterns, including

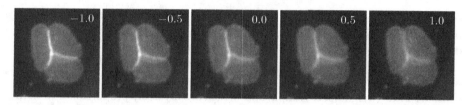

Fig. 2. Contrast modulation around touching regions. Separating adjacent cells is one of the major challenges in crowded images. To leverage learning, we feed the network with a variety of contrasts around touching regions. We do so by modulating their intesities while keeping adjacencies the same. In this example, an original image ($a = 0$) has its contrast increased (decreased) around shared edges when we set $a < 0$ ($a > 0$). - see our formulation in Sect. 2.

weak edges, we augment existing ones by modulating their pixel values according to the expression $x_a(p) = (1 - a) \cdot x(p) + a \cdot \tilde{x}(p)$, only applied when $h(p) = 2$, where $\tilde{x}$ is the 7×7 median filtered image of x. When $a < 0$ ($a > 0$) we increase (decrease) contrast. During training, we have random values of $a \sim U(-1,1)$. An example of this modulation is shown in Fig. 2.

Loss Function. U-Net [9] is an encoder–decoder network for biomedical image segmentation with proven results in small datasets, and with cross entropy being the most commonly adopted loss function. The weighted cross entropy [9] is a generalization where a pre–computed weight map assigns to each pixel its importance for the learning process,

$$\mathcal{L}(y, z) = - \sum_{l=0}^{C} \sum_{p \in \Omega} \omega_{\beta,\nu,\sigma}(p) \cdot y_l(p) \cdot \log z_l(p) \tag{2}$$

where $\omega_{\beta,\nu,\sigma}(p)$ is the parameterized weight at pixel p, and $z_l(p)$ the computed probability of p belonging to class l for ground truth $y_l(p)$.

Let $R(u) = u^+$ be the rectified linear function, ReLu, and $\varphi_\beta(u) = R(1 - u/\beta), u \in \mathbb{R}$, a rectified inverse function saturated in $\beta \in \mathbb{R}^+$. We propose the Triplex Weight Map, W^3, model

$$\omega_{\beta,\nu,\sigma}(p) = \begin{cases} \nu/n_0 + \nu \cdot \varphi_\beta\left(\phi_h(p)\right)/n_1 & \text{if } h(p) = 0 \\ \nu/n_1 + \nu \cdot \varphi_\beta\left(\phi_K(p)\right) & \text{if } h(p) = 1, p \in \Gamma \\ \nu/n_1 + \omega_{\beta,\nu,\sigma}(\zeta_\Gamma(p)) \cdot \exp(-\phi_\Gamma^2(p)/\sigma^2) & \text{if } h(p) = 1, p \notin \Gamma \\ \nu/n_2 & \text{if } h(p) = 2 \end{cases} \tag{3}$$

where Γ represents cell contour; n_l is the number of pixels of class l; ϕ_h is the distance transform over h that assigns to every pixel its Euclidean distance to the closest non-background pixel; ϕ_K and ϕ_Γ are, respectively, the distance transforms with respect to the skeleton of cells and cell contours; and $\zeta_\Gamma : \Omega \to \Omega$ returns the pixel in contour Γ closest to a given pixel p, thus $\zeta_\Gamma(p) \in \Gamma$. The W^3 model sets $\omega_{\beta,\nu,\sigma}(p) = \nu/n_0$ for all background pixels distant at least β to a cell contour. This way, true cells that are eventually not annotated and located beyond β from annotated cells have very low importance during training – by design, weights on non annotated regions are close to zero.

The recursive expression for foreground pixels (third line in Eq. 3) creates weights using a rolling Gaussian with variance σ^2 centered on each pixel of the contour. These weights have amplitudes which are inversely proportional to their distances to cell skeleton, resulting in large values for slim and neck regions. The parameter ν is used for setting the amplitude of the Gaussians. The weight at a foreground pixel is the value of the Gaussian at the contour point closest to this pixel. The touching region is assigned a constant weight for class balance, larger than all other weights.

From Semantic to Instance Segmentation. After training the network for semantic segmentation, we perform the transformation from semantic to panoptic, instance segmentation. First, a decision rule $\hat{h}$ over the output probability map z is applied to hard classify each pixel. The usual approach is to classify with *maximum a posteriori* (MAP) where the semantic segmentation is obtained with $\hat{h}(p) = \arg\max_l z_l(p)$. However, since pixels in the touching and interior cell regions share similar intensity distributions, the classifier might be uncertain in the transition zone between these regions, where it might fail to assign the right class for some, sometimes crucial, pixels in these areas. A few misclassified pixels can compromise the separation of adjacent cells (see Fig. 3). Therefore, we cannot solely rely on MAP as our hard classifier. An alternative is to use a thresholding (TH) strategy as a decision rule, where parameters γ_1 and γ_2 control, respectively, the class assignment of pixels: $\hat{h}(p) = 2$ if $z_2(p) \geq \gamma_2$, and $\hat{h}(p) = 1$ if $z_1(p) \geq \gamma_1$ and $z_2(p) < \gamma_2$, and 0 otherwise. Finally, the estimated instance segmentation $\hat{g}$ labels each cell region $\hat{V}_i$ and it distributes touching pixels to their closest components,

$$\hat{g}(p) = \begin{cases} 0 & \text{if } \hat{h}(p) = 0 \\ i & \text{if } \hat{h}(p) = 1 \text{ and } p \in \hat{V}_i \\ \hat{g}(\zeta_\Gamma(p)) & \text{if } \hat{h}(p) = 2 \end{cases} \tag{4}$$

Another alternative for post-processing is to segment using the Watershed Transform (WT) with markers. It is applied on the topographic map formed by the subtraction of touching and cell probability maps, $z_2 - z_1$. Markers are comprised of pixels in the background and cell regions whose probabilities are larger than given thresholds τ_0 and τ_1, $\{p | z_0(p) \geq \tau_0 \text{ or } z_1(p) \geq \tau_1\}$. High values for these should be safe, *e.g.* $\tau_0 = \tau_1 = 0.8$.

3   Experiments and Results

Training of our triplex weight map method, W^3, is done using U-Net [9] initialized with normally distributed weights according to the Xavier method [3]. We compare it to the following methods: Lovász-Softmax loss function ignoring

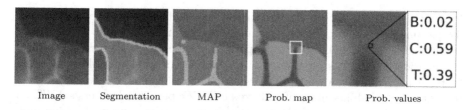

Image   Segmentation   MAP   Prob. map   Prob. values

Fig. 3. Poor classification. *Maximum a posteriori*, MAP, does not separate adjacent cells due to poor probabilities in the junctions shown above. The misclassification of just a few pixels renders a wrong cell topology. Probability maps are shown as RGB images with Background (red), Cell (green) and Touching (blue) classes. (Color figure online)

the background class, LSMAX [2]; weighted cross entropy using class balance weight map, BWM; U-Net with near object weights [9] adapted to three classes, UNET; and the per-class average combination of the probability maps from BWM, UNET, and W^3, followed by a softmax, named COMB. We also compared our results with those obtained by Mask R-CNN, MRCNN [5]. The use of COMB is motivated by ensemble classifiers where one tries to combine the predictions of multiple classifiers to achieve a prediction which is potentially better than each individual one. We plan to explore other choices beyond averaging.

We trained all networks over a cell segmentation dataset containing 28 images of size 1024×1024 with weak supervision in the form of incomplete and inaccurate annotations. We use the optimizer Adam with initial learning rate $lr = 10^{-4}$. The number of epochs and minibatch size were, respectively, 1000 and 1. We augmented data during training by random mirroring, rotating, warping, gamma correction, and touching contrast modulation, as in Fig. 2.

We follow [7] to assess results. For detection, we use the Precision (P05) and the Recognition Quality (RQ) of instances with Jaccard index above 0.5. For segmentation, we use Segmentation Quality (SQ) computed as the average Jaccard of matched segments. For an overall evaluation of both detection and segmentation, we use the Panoptic Quality (PQ) metric, $PQ = RQ \cdot SQ$.

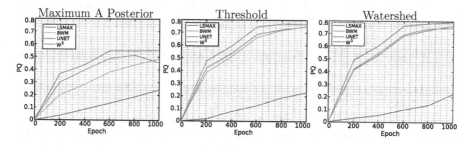

Fig. 4. Panoptic Quality (PQ) training values for all methods we compare to W^3, except COMB, using *Maximum a Posteriori* (MAP), Thresholded Maps (TH) and Watershed Transform (WT) post-processing. W^3 converges faster to a better solution.

Panoptic Segmentation Performance. We performed an exploration over the parameter space for the two parameters used in the TH and WT postprocessing methods. Table 1 shows a comparison of different post-processing strategies considering the best combination of parameters for Thresholds (TH) and Watershed (WT). For Mask R-CNN we used the same single threshold TH on the instance probability maps of all boxed cells. We performed watershed WT on each boxed cell region with seeds extracted from the most prominent background and foreground regions in the probability maps. Although Lovász-Softmax seems to be a promising loss function, we believe that the small training dataset and minibatch size negatively influenced its performance. For most values of thresholds used in the TH post-processing, the average combination (COMB) improved the overall result due to the reduction of False Positives (see P05 column). Also, in most cases, our W^3 approach obtained better SQ values than other methods suggesting a better contour adequacy. Because touching and cell intensity distributions overlap, a softer classification was obtained for these regions. MAP did not achieve the same performance of other approaches (Fig. 3). The behavior in Table 1 remained the same during training as shown in Fig. 4.

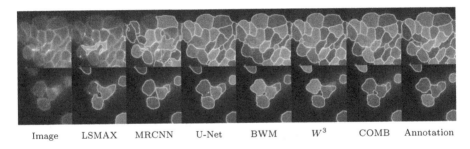

Image   LSMAX   MRCNN   U-Net   BWM W^3 COMB   Annotation

Fig. 5. Segmentation results for packed cell clusters obtained using methods described in Sect. 3. Colors serve to show cell separation. Note the superiority of our W^3.

Examples of segmenting crowded cells with various methods are shown in Fig. 5. In our experiments, MRCNN was able to correctly segment isolated and nearly adjacent cells (second row), but it sometimes failed in challenging high-density clusters. BWM and U-Net tend to misclassify background pixels in neighboring cells (second row) with estimated contours generally beyond cell boundaries. W^3 had a better detection and segmentation performance with improvement of contour adequacy over COMB.

We believe our combined efforts of data augmentation, loss formulation with per pixel geometric weights, and multiclass classification enabled our trained neural networks to correctly segment cells even from domains it has never seen. For example, we have never trained with images of meristem and sepal cells but we still obtain good quality cell segmentation for these as shown in Fig. 6. These solutions might be further improved by training with a few samples from these domains.

Table 1. Metric values for different post processing schemes and segmentation methods. Numbers are average values obtained for the best combination of threshold parameters for both TH and WT post processing methods. Tests were done on 7 images, totaling 138 cells, with 14 clusters containing from 2 to approximately 32 cells. Metric values obtained with TH and WT are higher than those obtained with MAP showing that our post procesing schemes improve results. Overall, our W^3 and COMB outperform other segmentation methods for almost all metrics, except P05, when thresholding and watershed classification schemes are adopted.

Methods	MAP				TH				WT			
	P05	RQ	SQ	PQ	P05	RQ	SQ	PQ	P05	RQ	SQ	PQ
MRCNN	**0.9188**	**0.8617**	0.8002	**0.6892**	**0.9343**	0.8767	0.8012	0.7019	**0.9343**	0.8767	0.8019	0.7026
LSMAX	0.3871	0.3236	0.7455	0.2408	0.4348	0.3119	0.7171	0.2286	0.4000	0.3149	0.7073	0.2237
BWM	0.6756	0.5580	0.8674	0.4858	0.8583	0.8504	0.8769	0.7476	0.8193	0.8405	0.8831	0.7437
U-Net	0.6801	0.5381	0.8418	0.4556	0.8413	0.8508	0.8791	0.7492	0.8708	0.8600	0.8850	0.7621
W^3 (Ours)	0.7384	0.6305	**0.8721**	0.5513	0.8477	0.8439	**0.8994**	0.7604	0.9028	**0.8775**	**0.8995**	0.7896
COMB (Ours)	0.7587	0.6129	0.8698	0.5351	0.8952	**0.8851**	0.8908	**0.7889**	0.8925	0.8759	0.8944	0.7837

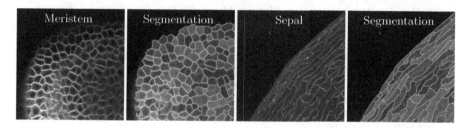

Fig. 6. Zero-shot panoptic segmentation of meristem and sepal images with our W^3 method exclusively trained with cell images from different domains.

4   Conclusions

We proposed a weakly supervised extension to the weighted cross entropy loss function that enabled us to effectively segment crowded cells. We used a semantic approach to solve a panoptic segmentation task with a small training dataset of highly cluttered cells which have incomplete and inaccurate annotations. A new contrast modulation was proposed as data augmentation for touching regions allowing us to perform an adequate panoptic segmentation. We were able to segment images from domains other than the one used for training the network. The experiments showed a better detection and contour adequacy of our method and a faster convergence when compared to similar approaches.

References

1. Bai, M., Urtasun, R.: Deep watershed transform for instance segmentation. In: Proceedings of IEEE CVPR, pp. 5221–5229 (2017)
2. Berman, M., Rannen Triki, A., Blaschko, M.B.: The Lovász-Softmax loss: a tractable surrogate for the optimization of the intersection-over-union measure in neural networks. In: Proceedings of IEEE CVPR, pp. 4413–4421 (2018)

3. Glorot, X., Bengio, Y.: Understanding the difficulty of training deep feedforward neural networks. In: Proceedings of 13th AISTATS, pp. 249–256 (2010)
4. Guerrero-Pena, F.A., Fernandez, P.D.M., Ren, T.I., Yui, M., Rothenberg, E., Cunha, A.: Multiclass weighted loss for instance segmentation of cluttered cells. In: 2018 25th IEEE ICIP, pp. 2451–2455. IEEE (2018)
5. He, K., Gkioxari, G., Dollár, P., Girshick, R.: Mask R-CNN. In: Proceedings of IEEE ICCV, pp. 2961–2969 (2017)
6. Kervadec, H., et al.: Constrained-CNN losses for weakly supervised segmentation. Med. Image Anal. **54**, 88–99 (2019)
7. Kirillov, A., He, K., Girshick, R., Rother, C., Dollár, P.: Panoptic Segmentation. arXiv preprint arXiv:1801.00868 (2018)
8. Liang, Q., et al.: Weakly-supervised biomedical image segmentation by reiterative learning. IEEE J. Biomed. Health Inf. **23**(3), 1205–1214 (2018)
9. Ronneberger, O., Fischer, P., Brox, T.: U-net: convolutional networks for biomedical image segmentation. In: Navab, N., Hornegger, J., Wells, W.M., Frangi, A.F. (eds.) MICCAI 2015. LNCS, vol. 9351, pp. 234–241. Springer, Cham (2015). https://doi.org/10.1007/978-3-319-24574-4_28
10. Schmidt, U., Weigert, M., Broaddus, C., Myers, G.: Cell detection with star-convex polygons. In: Frangi, A.F., Schnabel, J.A., Davatzikos, C., Alberola-López, C., Fichtinger, G. (eds.) MICCAI 2018. LNCS, vol. 11071, pp. 265–273. Springer, Cham (2018). https://doi.org/10.1007/978-3-030-00934-2_30
11. Yang, L., Zhang, Y., Chen, J., Zhang, S., Chen, D.Z.: Suggestive annotation: a deep active learning framework for biomedical image segmentation. In: Descoteaux, M., Maier-Hein, L., Franz, A., Jannin, P., Collins, D.L., Duchesne, S. (eds.) MICCAI 2017. LNCS, vol. 10435, pp. 399–407. Springer, Cham (2017). https://doi.org/10.1007/978-3-319-66179-7_46

Towards Practical Unsupervised Anomaly Detection on Retinal Images

Khalil Ouardini[1,2], Huijuan Yang[2], Balagopal Unnikrishnan[2],
Manon Romain[2,3], Camille Garcin[1,2], Houssam Zenati[1,2], J. Peter Campbell[4],
Michael F. Chiang[4], Jayashree Kalpathy-Cramer[5], Vijay Chandrasekhar[2],
Pavitra Krishnaswamy[2], and Chuan-Sheng Foo[2(✉)]

[1] CentraleSupelec, Gif-sur-Yvette, France
khalil.ouardini@student.ecp.fr
[2] Institute for Infocomm Research, A*STAR, Singapore, Singapore
{pavitrak,foo_chuan_sheng}@i2r.a-star.edu.sg
[3] École Polytechnique, Palaiseau, France
[4] Oregon Health & Science University, Portland, USA
[5] Massachusetts General Hospital, Harvard Medical School, Boston, USA

Abstract. Supervised deep learning approaches provide state-of-the-art performance on medical image classification tasks for disease screening. However, these methods require large labeled datasets that involve resource-intensive expert annotation. Further, disease screening applications have low prevalence of abnormal samples; this class imbalance makes the task more akin to anomaly detection. While the machine learning community has proposed unsupervised deep learning methods for anomaly detection, they have yet to be characterized on medical images where normal vs. anomaly distinctions may be more subtle and variable. In this work, we characterize existing unsupervised anomaly detection methods on retinal fundus images, and find that they require significant fine tuning and offer unsatisfactory performance. We thus propose an efficient and effective transfer-learning based approach for unsupervised anomaly detection. Our method employs a deep convolutional neural network trained on ImageNet as a feature extractor, and subsequently feeds the learned feature representations into an existing unsupervised anomaly detection method. We show that our approach significantly outperforms baselines on two natural image datasets and two retinal fundus image datasets, all with minimal fine-tuning. We further show the ability to leverage very small numbers of labelled anomalies to improve performance. Our work establishes a strong unsupervised baseline for image-based anomaly detection, alongside a flexible and scalable approach for screening applications.

Keywords: Unsupervised deep learning · Transfer learning · Anomaly detection · Retinal images

K. Ouardini and H. Yang—Equal contribution.
P. Krishnaswamy and C.-S. Foo—Equal contribution.
Supplementary Material: http://s000.tinyupload.com/?file_id=50006502228459557624.

Q. Wang et al. (Eds.): DART 2019/MIL3ID 2019, LNCS 11795, pp. 225–234, 2019.
https://doi.org/10.1007/978-3-030-33391-1_26

1   Introduction

Deep learning approaches offer state-of-the-art performance for a variety of medical image classification tasks. However, a major challenge in practical translation of these methods is that model training and/or fine-tuning requires thousands of images labelled by domain experts or clinical specialists. Such labelling is laborious, expensive, inefficient, and difficult to scale across diverse settings and applications. Moreover, expert raters can have discordant opinions [5,9], resulting in noisy or biased labels. Accordingly, there has been increasing interest in semi-supervised approaches for medical image classification [10,13], but less work on unsupervised learning.

For disease screening, normal samples usually have higher prevalence than abnormal samples. Thus, the classification task is akin to a rare anomaly detection task. We focus on unsupervised methods to detect anomalies for medical image-based screening. The machine learning community has developed many methods for unsupervised anomaly detection on natural image datasets like CIFAR-10 and SVHN [3,16,19,20]. However, the tasks of detecting anomalies on natural vs. medical images are distinct. Medical images exhibit greater variability due to the heterogeneity in abnormality presentation across patients or cohorts, and differences in acquisition devices or parameters. Further, anomalies in medical images tend to have finer resolution or more localized features. Yet, there has been limited focus on unsupervised anomaly detection methods for medical image datasets.

In this work, we characterize a range of unsupervised anomaly detection methods on natural image benchmarks (CIFAR-10, SVHN) and medical image datasets. For the latter, we employ fundus images obtained to screen for Diabetic Retinopathy (DR) and Retinopathy of Prematurity (ROP). We compare and contrast performance to find that existing methods have relatively unsatisfactory performance on medical image datasets. We further find that the unsupervised methods often require significant fine tuning and intensive computational resources, and therefore have limited practical applicability.

To overcome these challenges, we introduce a simple yet effective transfer learning method for unsupervised anomaly detection on medical images. Our method leverages the expressive representations learned by deep learning based classifiers trained on large image collections (like ImageNet). We extract features learned with these models and feed them into Isolation Forests [11], which offer efficient and robust anomaly detection for high-dimensional data with minimal tuning requirements. We perform extensive experiments and show that this approach outperforms baselines on both data types, with more significant gains on medical image datasets. We further show how to use a small collection of labeled anomalous samples, akin to a "validation set" to improve performance by selecting the best feature representation. As such, our work provides a strong baseline for unsupervised image-based anomaly detection, and a flexible and scalable approach for screening applications.

2   Methods

2.1   Task Definition

We consider two experimental settings. First, we assume the training data comprises only of normal images and focus on identifying images that fall out-of-distribution. We term this as Novelty Detection. Second, we relax this assumption, and consider the fully unsupervised scenario where the training set contains normal images alongside a small number of anomalies. We term this as Anomaly Detection. We now describe our method and the baselines.

2.2   Transfer Learning for Anomaly Detection

Figure 1 illustrates our method, which leverages the feature representations learned by networks trained on large, diverse image collections. The basic approach consists of (1) computing feature representations with a pre-trained network, and (2) training an anomaly detection algorithm on top of the computed representations. Implementing this general approach requires choosing (1) the pre-trained network, (2) how representations are derived (e.g., choice of layer), (3) an anomaly detection algorithm, and (4) tuning hyperparameters of the anomaly detection algorithm. We detail these choices below.

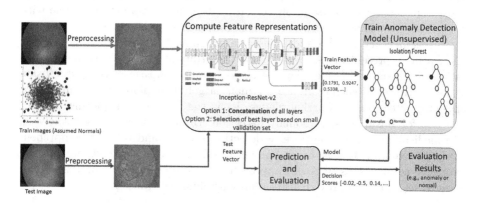

Fig. 1. Overview of proposed transfer learning-based anomaly detection method. Training images are assumed to come from a distribution of primarily normal images. We compute feature representations using a pre-trained deep learning model, and use the resulting feature vectors to train an unsupervised anomaly detection model. During testing, we transform images into feature space and use the trained model for anomaly detection.

Choice of Network: In our experiments, we used the Inception-ResNet-v2 network [18] trained on the ImageNet ILSVRC-2012-CLS dataset [15], as it is one of the best performing networks for such tasks; our results were similar when using the Inception-v3 network (Supplementary Table 17).

Deriving Representations: We evaluated two strategies for deriving the representations.

1. *Computing a representation from all layers:* Previous work suggests that features from convolutional layers earlier in the network can contain very discriminative features [12]. To harness the power of these features, we derive representations including these earlier convolutional layers as well. For computational tractability, the outputs of these layers are first spatially averaged and then concatenated to the output of the other fully connected layers to produce a representation from the whole network.
2. *Picking the best representation using a validation set:* If annotated anomalies are available, they could be used to pick the best performing representation (from a single network layer/module) by evaluating model performance on a constructed validation set including these anomalies.

Anomaly Detection Algorithm: We chose the Isolation Forest method as it is fast, handles high-dimensional data well, does not require much tuning, and works well whether the training set consists only of normal data, or is mixed with some anomalies.

Hyperparmeters for Anomaly Detection Algorithm: We used the scikit-learn implementation of Isolation Forests with default parameters, in line with our goal of proposing a method requiring minimal fine-tuning.

Supplementary Sects. 8 and 9 describe the impact of the choices of network and feature representations. We note that the utility of transfer-learned representations has been demonstrated across a wide range of *supervised* computer vision tasks [2]. However, such approaches remain largely unexplored for unsupervised anomaly detection. To our knowledge, [1] is the only work exploring transfer learning for unsupervised anomaly detection. However, they focused solely on non-medical images in the novelty detection setting, and did not comprehensively benchmark against other competing methods. In contrast, we provide extensive comparisons to recent approaches on retinal fundus images and offer ways to select and improve feature representations for transfer.

2.3 Baselines

We evaluate a range of methods including shallow models (one-class SVM [17], Isolation Forest (IF) [11]), deep anomaly detection methods based on autoencoders (DAGMM [3], DSEBM [20]) and generative adversarial networks (AnoGAN [16]), as well as recently emerging unsupervised methods based on geometric transformations (DeepGEO, [6]) and SVDD based representations (DeepSVDD, [14]). For medical datasets, we include a supervised baseline: we finetune an Inception Resnet V2 [18] network that is initialized with ImageNet weights for "normal" vs. "abnormal" classification. Supplementary Sect. 1 details the baselines and associated hyperparameters.

3   Experiments

Here, we detail datasets with definition of the anomalies in each case, and provides evaluation results across the datasets and methods for the two settings.

3.1   Datasets

Figure 2 shows an overview of data types and illustrates example normal vs. anomalous images in the different datasets. Supplementary Fig. 1 provides more examples highlighting the variations. Supplementary Table 10 breaks down the statistics.

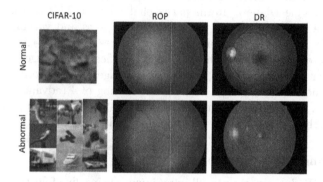

Fig. 2. Overview of datasets. The upper panel shows normal images while the lower panel shows abnormal images. These examples show the differences between natural and medical images, and highlight the nuanced nature of medical image anomaly detection.

Natural Image Datasets (SVHN, CIFAR-10): We used the official training and testing sets for SVHN and CIFAR-10. K denotes the number of classes in the dataset. Following previous works [6,14,19], we design K different experiments where samples from each label are alternately considered as "normal" and are used for training. We use 25% of the training set as a validation set and evaluate each model on the official test set containing anomalies at a ratio of $(K-1)/K$ (i.e, 90% for CIFAR-10 and SVHN). The only preprocessing was rescaling the images to $[0, 1]$.

Retinopathy of Prematurity (ROP): ROP is an eye disease affecting premature babies, and is graded as "pre-plus" and "plus" based on the extent of retinal arterial tortuosity and venous dilation at the posterior pole [4]. As ROP is a leading cause of childhood blindness, there is a need for automated systems to regularly screen for "plus" disease, a key determinant for treatment. We obtained posterior pole retinal RGB photographs as part of the ongoing 'Imaging & Informatics in ROP' (i-ROP) cohort study. Each image was annotated as "normal", "pre-plus" or "plus" by at least three independent experts, and a consensus reference standard label was assigned [4]. We squared cropped to cut the neutral background and resized images to 256 pixels, before subtracting the local average color to reduce differences in lighting. Pixel values were rescaled to [0,1]. Our experiments consider two scenarios: (1) "normal" vs. "plus" anomalies (total 4707 images, denoted as ROP by default), and (2) "normal" vs. "pre-plus" and "plus" anomalies (total 5511 images, denoted as ROP (All Grades)).

Diabetic Retinopathy (DR): DR is diagnosed based on the presence of microaneurysms, hemorrhages, hard exudates, microvascular abnormalities and neovascularization in retinal fundus photographs [7]. Due to the high prevalence of diabetes, there is a need to screen patients regularly. We obtained color retinal fundus photographs annotated with severity ratings from licensed clinicians as part of the Kaggle Diabetic Retinopathy challenge [8]. This is a large dataset from multiple sites with diverse patient demographics and varying acquisition conditions. It includes several poor quality images with over-exposed, out-of-focus and artefactual images, hence poses significant challenges for anomaly detection. For our experiments, we denoted images with severity rating of 0 (healthy) as normal and images with severity rating of 4 (advanced symptoms) as anomalous. We randomly sampled subsets of 3912 training and 7829 testing images from the official dataset, and preprocessed in the same way as for ROP.

3.2   Training and Evaluation

Except the DR dataset, we ran all experiments using five-fold cross-validation and quantify performance using the cross-validated area under the ROC curve (averaged across 5 seeds) and the corresponding standard deviation. AUROC is the common metric of choice for both anomaly detection papers [6,14,19] and medical applications [4,7]. We present the area under the precision-recall curve and the recall in Supplementary Tables 12–14.

3.3   Novelty Detection Setting

Results in the novelty detection setting are presented in Table 1. Our model outperforms all the baselines on CIFAR-10. We present results on a more challenging CIFAR-100 dataset in Supplementary Table 11. On SVHN, all methods perform only slightly better than random guessing, with a small advantage to DeepSVDD. The slightly lower performance for our method is likely due to a domain shift between the source (ImageNet) and target (SVHN) datasets. This is consistent with the fact that transfer learning performance can drop with dissimilarity between source and target datasets [2]).

On both the medical imaging datasets, our method outperforms every unsupervised baseline by a wide margin of around 20%. In all cases, however, the supervised classifier has better performance than the best unsupervised method. We repeated the ROP experiments on the more challenging setting that includes all grades of anomalies ("pre-plus" and "plus"). The results, in Supplementary Table 15, show similar trends.

Table 1. Area under the ROC curve in % with standard deviation in novelty detection setting. Results are averaged over the number of classes for natural images (see Sect. 3.1) and over 5 runs for medical images.

Natural images

	IF	DAGMM	AnoGAN	DSEBM	DeepSVDD	DeepGEO	Ours
CIFAR-10	59.4 ± 11	57.5 ± 10	57.6 ± 12	58.8 ± 11	64.8	86.0	**88.2 ± 6.6**
SVHN	51.4 ± 0.9	51.8 ± 1.2	53.3 ± 3.1	57.1 ± 2.8	**57.3 ± 3.3**	–	55.4 ± 4.1

Medical images

	IF	AnoGAN	DSEBM	DeepSVDD	DAGMM	Ours	Supervised
ROP	55.1 ± 5.0	49.5 ± 4.4	49.6 ± 3.9	57.5 ± 2.4	58.1 ± 6.2	**77.0 ± 3.8**	**97.3 ± 2.0**
DR	44.0 ± 0.5	44.2 ± 1.1	43.1 ± 0.2	46.4 ± 1.3	52.0 ± 0.1	**74.5 ± 1.7**	**94.5 ± 2.7**

3.4 Utilizing Small Numbers of Labeled Anomalies to Improve Performance

While it is difficult to curate large labeled datasets with sizeable numbers of anomalous samples for supervised learning, it is often feasible to obtain small numbers of labeled anomalies. We therefore explored whether it is possible to use such small "validation" sets to improve the choice of feature representation and anomaly detection performance. These experiments are done in the Novelty Detection setting. For the CIFAR-10 and ROP datasets, we compiled a small collection of N annotated anomalous samples, with N set as 3% of the total dataset size. We then evaluated representations from each of the blocks in the pre-trained network on this validation set, and chose the representation with best validation AUC. We employ these chosen representations to obtain evaluation results on the test set (Table 2). This strategy is especially useful for the medical image datasets (unlike for CIFAR-10 where gains are limited). In particular, we observed 6% AUC gain on the ROP dataset with just 4 annotated anomalies. Supplementary Sect. 10 provides further detailed results from individual blocks for varying sizes of the validation sets and for the complex ROP (AllGrades) task. Overall, these results suggest that our method could offer significant gains for medical domain end-users who are able to invest in limited resources to label a few examples.

Table 2. Averaged area under the ROC curve (over 5 runs) in % with standard deviation for different representations.

Representation	Concatenation	Best (picked) representation
CIFAR-10	**88.2 ± 6.6**	**88.2 ± 6.6**
ROP	77.0 ± 3.8	**82.6 ± 6.5**

3.5   Anomaly Detection Setting

We now consider how robust our method is to inclusion of varying proportions of anomalies in the training data. These evaluations correspond to the fully unsupervised Anomaly Detection setting. Table 3 illustrates the robustness of our method to varying numbers of anomalies mixed in to the training set for the CIFAR-10 and ROP datasets. We see that on CIFAR-10, test AUC decreases gradually as the proportion of anomalous samples in the training set increases. As CIFAR-10 has a high 90% proportion of anomalies, it provides an opportunity to understand how the performance of our method changes with varying anomaly proportions. For ROP, we expanded the training set to include up to 3% anomalies, to mimic the prevalence of disease in screening applications. Our results show that the performance is robust to inclusion of anomalous samples. We include evaluation against other baselines in Supplementary Table 16, and show that our method exhibits robust performance gains over competing methods even in the fully unsupervised setting.

Table 3. Area under the ROC curve (over 5 runs) for different anomaly ratios ρ in training set

ρ	1%	2%	3%	5%	10%	15%	20%	25%
CIFAR10	–	–	–	**86.8**	85.3	84.2	82.8	81.1
ROP	75.4	**76.9**	75.5	–	–	–	–	

4   Discussion and Conclusion

In this work, we characterized a range of unsupervised anomaly detection methods from the machine learning literature on medical images, and proposed a simple, efficient and effective transfer learning method to overcome prevailing limitations in this area. Our proposed method significantly outperforms competing methods on two computer vision benchmarks and two medical imaging datasets. Importantly, our method is flexible, and can effectively leverage very small numbers of labelled anomalies to improve performance. While our work offers a step towards closing the performance gap between unsupervised and supervised anomaly detection methods, we recognize the need for further performance improvements before they become suitable for clinical use. We anticipate that the first applications could lie in processes for more efficient labeling before diagnostic decision support applications can take shape.[1]

Acknowledgement. This project was supported by funding from the Deep Learning 2.0 program at the Institute for Infocomm Research (I2R), A*STAR, Singapore; and

---

[1] Link to code: https://github.com/khalilouardini/towards-practical-unsupervised-AD.

partially supported by SERC Strategic Funding (A1718g0045) research grants from the US National Institutes of Health (NIH grants R01EY19474, P30EY010572, and K12EY027720) and the US National Science Foundation (NSF grants SCH-1622679 and SCH-1622542); unrestricted departmental funding from the Oregon Health Sciences University, and a Career Development Award from Research to Prevent Blindness (New York, NY). We acknowledge helpful discussions with James M. Brown and Ken Chang (MGH) on datasets and experiment planning.

References

1. Andrews, J.T.A., Tanay, T., Morton, E.J., Griffin, L.D.: Transfer representation-learning for anomaly detection. In: ICML Anomaly Detection Workshop (2016)
2. Azizpour, H., Razavian, A.S., Sullivan, J., Maki, A., Carlsson, S.: Factors of transferability for a generic convnet representation. IEEE Trans. Pattern Anal. Mach. Intell. **38**(9), 1790–1802 (2016)
3. Bo, Z., et al.: Deep autoencoding Gaussian mixture model for unsupervised anomaly detection. In: International Conference on Learning Representations (2018)
4. Brown, J.M., et al.: Automated diagnosis of plus disease in retinopathy of prematurity using deep convolutional neural networks. JAMA Ophthalmol. **136**(7), 803–810 (2018)
5. Campbell, J.P., Kalpathy-Cramer, J., Dulanto-Reinoso, C.M., Montero-Mendoza, C., et al.: Plus disease in retinopathy of prematurity: a continuous spectrum of vascular abnormality as a basis of diagnostic variability. Ophthalmology **123**(11), 2338–2344 (2016)
6. Golan, I., El-Yaniv, R.: Deep anomaly detection using geometric transformations. In: Advances in Neural Information Processing Systems 31, pp. 9758–9769 (2018)
7. Gulshan, V., Peng, L., Mega, J.L., Webster, D.R., et al.: Development and validation of a deep learning algorithm for detection of diabetic retinopathy in retinal fundus photographs. JAMA **316**(22), 2402–2410 (2016)
8. Kaggle: Diabetic Retinopathy Detection (2015)
9. Krause, J., et al.: Grader variability and the importance of reference standards for evaluating machine learning models for diabetic retinopathy. Ophthalmology **125**(8), 1264–1272 (2018)
10. Lecouat, B., Chang, K., Kalpathy-Cramer, J., Krishnaswamy, P., et al.: Semi-supervised deep learning for abnormality classification in retinal images. CoRR abs/1812.07832 (2018)
11. Liu, F.T., Ting, K.M., Zhou, Z.H.: Isolation forest. In: Proceedings of the 2008 Eighth IEEE International Conference on Data Mining, pp. 413–422 (2008)
12. Liu, L., Shen, C., van den Hengel, A.: The treasure beneath convolutional layers: cross-convolutional-layer pooling for image classification. In: 2015 IEEE Conference on Computer Vision and Pattern Recognition (CVPR), pp. 4749–4757, June 2015
13. Madani, A., Ong, J.R., Tibrewal, A., Mofrad, M.R.K.: Deep echocardiography: data-efficient supervised and semi-supervised deep learning towards automated diagnosis of cardiac disease. npj Digit. Med. **1**(1), 59 (2018)
14. Ruff, L., Vandermeulen, R., Müller, E., Kloft, M., et al.: Deep one-class classification. In: Proceedings of the 35th International Conference on Machine Learning. Proceedings of Machine Learning Research, vol. 80, pp. 4393–4402 (2018)
15. Russakovsky, O., et al.: Imagenet large scale visual recognition challenge. CoRR abs/1409.0575 (2014)

16. Schlegl, T., Seeböck, P., Waldstein, S.M., Schmidt-Erfurth, U., Langs, G.: Unsupervised anomaly detection with generative adversarial networks to guide marker discovery. In: Niethammer, M., et al. (eds.) IPMI 2017. LNCS, vol. 10265, pp. 146–157. Springer, Cham (2017). https://doi.org/10.1007/978-3-319-59050-9_12
17. Schölkopf, B., Williamson, R., Smola, A., Shawe-Taylor, J., Platt, J.: Support vector method for novelty detection. In: Proceedings of the 12th International Conference on Neural Information Processing Systems, pp. 582–588 (1999)
18. Szegedy, C., Ioffe, S., Vanhoucke, V., Alemi, A.: Inception-v4, inception-resnet and the impact of residual connections on learning. CoRR abs/1602.07261 (2016)
19. Zenati, H., Romain, M., Foo, C., Lecouat, B., Chandrasekhar, V.: Adversarially learned anomaly detection. In: 2018 IEEE International Conference on Data Mining (ICDM), pp. 727–736 (2018)
20. Zhai, S., Cheng, Y., Lu, W., Zhang, Z.: Deep structured energy based models for anomaly detection. In: International Conference on Machine Learning, pp. 1100–1109 (2016)

Fine Tuning U-Net for Ultrasound Image Segmentation: Which Layers?

Mina Amiri[1]([✉]) [ID], Rupert Brooks[1,2] [ID], and Hassan Rivaz[1] [ID]

[1] Concordia University, Montreal, Canada
amirim@encs.concordia.ca
[2] Nuance Communications, Montreal, Canada

Abstract. Fine-tuning a network which has been trained on a large dataset is an alternative to full training in order to overcome the problem of scarce and expensive data in medical applications. While the shallow layers of the network are usually kept unchanged, deeper layers are modified according to the new dataset. This approach may not work for ultrasound images due to their drastically different appearance. In this study, we investigated the effect of fine-tuning different layers of a U-Net which was trained on segmentation of natural images in breast ultrasound image segmentation. Tuning the contracting part and fixing the expanding part resulted in substantially better results compared to fixing the contracting part and tuning the expanding part. Furthermore, we showed that starting to fine-tune the U-Net from the shallow layers and gradually including more layers will lead to a better performance compared to fine-tuning the network from the deep layers moving back to shallow layers. We did not observe the same results on segmentation of X-ray images, which have different salient features compared to ultrasound, it may therefore be more appropriate to fine-tune the shallow layers rather than deep layers. Shallow layers learn lower level features (including speckle pattern, and probably the noise and artifact properties) which are critical in automatic segmentation in this modality.

Keywords: Ultrasound imaging · Segmentation · Transfer learning · U-Net

1 Introduction

Training a deep convolutional neural network (CNN) from scratch is challenging, especially in medical applications, where annotated data is scarce and expensive. An alternative to full training is transfer learning, where a network which has been trained on a large dataset is fine-tuned for another application. When the new dataset is small, the recommended approach in fine-tuning is to keep the first layers of the network unchanged, and to fine-tune the last layers [14]. It is shown that first layers of a CNN represent more low-level features, while more semantic and high-level features are recognized by deeper layers [4]. Therefore,

Q. Wang et al. (Eds.): DART 2019/MIL3ID 2019, LNCS 11795, pp. 235–242, 2019.
https://doi.org/10.1007/978-3-030-33391-1_27

fine-tuning the deepest layers originates from the assumption that basic features of the datasets (associated with shallow layers) are similar, and more specific features of the datasets (associated with deeper layers) should be tuned in order to get acceptable results in a different application. This assumption may not hold true in some medical applications. For instance, in ultrasound imaging the presence of wave-tissue interactions such as scattering lead to creation of speckles, which may not be present in natural images or images from other medical modalities.

Ultrasound imaging is a standard modality for many diagnostic and monitoring purposes, and there has been significant research into developing automatic methods for segmentation of ultrasound images [5,11]. U-Net [7] for instance has been shown to be a fast and precise solution for medical image segmentation, and has successfully been adapted to segment ultrasound images too [1,8,10,12]. In this study, we investigate the effect of fine-tuning different layers of a U-Net network for the application of ultrasound image segmentation. We hypothesize that ultrasound-specific patterns are learned in shallow layers which disentangle the information in speckle pattern. Therefore, fine-tuning these layers is critical in fine-tuning the weights learned from another domain.

2   Methodology

This section provides an overview of the datasets used in this study, details of pre training and fine-tuning the U-Net, and the performance metrics used to validate our results.

2.1   Datasets

In order to pre-train the network, we used the XPIE dataset which contains 10000 segmented natural images [9]. The images in this dataset are not gray scale. In order to have a more similar pre-training dataset to ultrasound dataset, we converted these images into black and white prior to feeding to the network. We used 40 epochs to train the network, and 10% of the data was considered as the validation set. Figure 1 shows a few examples of this dataset. The pre-trained network was then used for the task of segmentation of ultrasound B-mode images. The ultrasound imaging dataset contains 163 images of the breast with either benign lesions or malignant tumors [13]. In order to investigate whether the results are specific to the ultrasound imaging, we repeated the analysis for a chest X-ray dataset with the total of 240 images [2], wherein we used the pre-trained network to segment both lungs.

Data Augmentation. As the size of ultrasound and X-ray datasets was small, we implemented data augmentation techniques to improve the network performance, invariance and robustness. For these datasets, the network should be robust to shift, rotation, flipping, shearing and zooming. We generated smooth

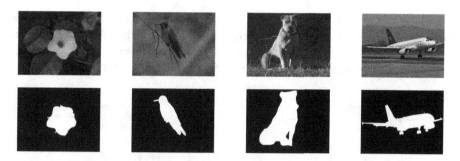

Fig. 1. Some examples from the XPIE dataset and the associated masks. These images have very different appearances when compared to X-ray or ultrasound images.

deformations of images using random and small degrees of all these transformations. In total, we had 600 images including the original images to train the network. In the case of natural images, we did not augment the data.

2.2   Analysis

We used the same U-Net architecture introduced in the original paper [7] except that we used up-sampling in the expanding path. The network consists of blocks of two convolutional layers with ReLU activation, followed by either a maxpooling or an upsampling operation. There are 64 filters in both layers in the first block. Following each maxpooling operation, the number of filters doubles, while after each upsampling operation, the number of filters is halved. A 1×1 convolutional layer with sigmoid activation is used as the last layer to map the feature vector to the interval of 0 and 1. For evaluation purposes, pixels with the value above 0.5 were considered as 1, and pixels with the value below 0.5 were considered as 0. We did not use batch normalization, but we used the dropout technique after the contracting path.

We first trained a U-Net using the XPIE dataset. The parameters of this pre-trained network was then utilized as an initial point to retrain the network for ultrasound or X-ray image segmentation. All images were resized to 256×256 pixels and were normalized to [0,1]. To examine whether fine-tuning shallow or deep layers differ significantly, we divided the U-Net into two parts: contracting (up to the 10th convolutional layer) and expanding (from 10th convolutional layer to the end). While freezing one part, we fine-tuned the other part using the ultrasound B-mode images as the training data. We then switched the frozen and trainable parts.

Next, we repeated the same approach but in a finer manner. We grouped all layers between two consecutive maxpooling or up-sampling layers in to one block (Fig. 2). Each block therefore consisted of two convolutional layers. We started by fine-tuning the first block (first two layers) while freezing all other layers. We then included other blocks in the fine-tuning procedure one-by-one, until the whole network was trained (from shallow to deep layers). We repeated the same procedure in the opposite direction; we started fine-tuning the deepest block while freezing the remaining of the network, and then included more blocks in fine-tuning until the whole network was trained (from deep to shallow layers). The same analysis was done for the chest X-ray dataset to segment the lungs.

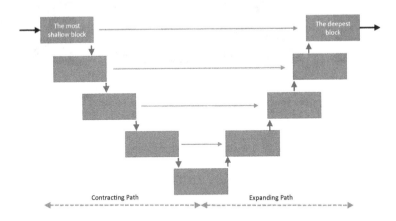

Fig. 2. Schematic of U-Net. Each box represents one block of layers. Red, green and blue arrows respectively represent maxpooling, upsampling and copy-crop-concatenating. (Color figure online)

2.3   Performance Metrics

We used 5-fold cross validation to evaluate the performance of the network. All the data was randomly divided into five folds, with four folds used for training and the 5th fold used for validation. The procedure was repeated five times so that all five folds served as the validation set. To evaluate the performance of the network in segmenting the images, we used Dice score, pixel error and rand score. Dice score equals twice the number of elements correctly predicted as the mask (2 * TP) divided by the sum of the number of elements in the ground-truth mask (TP + FN) and the predicted mask (TP + FP). Pixel error is the percentage of voxels falsely predicted by the network, and rand score is a measure of similarity between two clusterings by considering pairs that are assigned in the same or different clusters in the predicted and ground-truth image [6]. In this study, we used the rand score adjusted for chance clustering.

3   Results

Training the contracting part and freezing the expanding part led to better results compared to freezing the contracting part and fine-tuning the expanding part (Dice score: 0.80 ± 0.03 vs. 0.72 ± 0.04, pixel error: $1.4\% \pm 0.5$ vs.

1.9% ± 0.6, rand score: 0.78 ± 0.03 vs. 0.71 ± 0.05). It is interesting to note that the number of parameters in the contacting path is almost half the number of parameters in the expanding path, but still we get better results by training fewer number of parameters. Figure 3 represents some examples of the results on the test set. Contrary to ultrasound images, chest X-ray images resulted in an almost equal evaluation scores when segmenting lungs, by applying the same fine-tuning procedure (Dice score: 0.98 for both scenarios, pixel error: 1.1% vs. 1.3%, rand score: 0.95 for both scenarios).

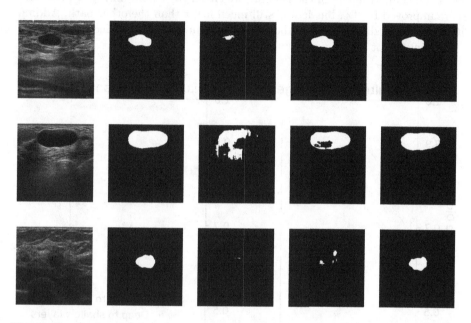

Fig. 3. Comparison of the two scenarios on a few examples. From left to right: the original image, the ground truth mask, the predicted mask by the pre-trained network, the predicted mask when the expanding part is fine-tuned, the predicted mask when the contracting part is fine-tuned. First row: both scenarios work well. Second row: fine-tuning the contracting path outperforms the other scenario. Third row: fine-tuning the contracting path performs much better than the other scenario.

When we investigated fine-tuning in a more rigorous manner (including blocks of layers one-by-one), better performance was achieved moving from shallow to deep layers compared to moving from deep to shallow layers. Figure 4 shows the average Dice score for the two directions of fine-tuning. Note that the middle part of Fig. 4 corresponds to the results reported in the previous paragraph; blue graph: fine-tuning the contracting path and freezing the expanding path, red graph: fine-tuning the expanding path and freezing the contracting path.

As the number of parameters in the expanding part of the network is much higher than the contracting part, it would be expected that the expanding part of the network trains more slowly than the contracting part, and it would therefore affect the results. We used a fixed number of epochs (20 epochs) for fine-tuning the network in all studied scenarios. Although the network was stable after 20 epochs, we added 20 more epochs (40 epochs in total now) to examine the impact of number of epochs on the segmentation performance. The changes in Dice score were below 1% for all cases except for the case when the deepest block of layers was trained and the rest of the network was fixed (first point in Fig. 4); the Dice score improved by 3%, but it was still much lower than the other path. Adding 10 more epochs did not change the results anymore. Thus, the effect of the speed of training is not a major one.

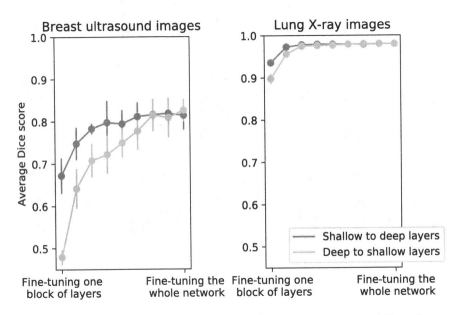

Fig. 4. Average Dice score for two different scenarios for ultrasound and X-ray images. Error bars depict the standard deviation of the mean among the five folds. (Color figure online)

In order to see what features are seen by different layers of the network, we employed Keras-Vis [3] to visualize the input image which maximize the activation in each neuron. Several low-level patterns were recognized for shallow layers (mostly edges), while high-level maps are more detailed and complex shapes. Figure 5 shows some examples in different neurons of shallow and deep layers.

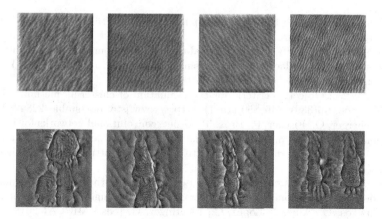

Fig. 5. Some examples of images which maximize the activation in a network trained on ultrasound images, top: in the fourth layer, bottom: in the deepest convolutional layer.

4   Discussion and Conclusions

We showed that in breast ultrasound image segmentation using U-Net, fine-tuning shallow layers of a pre-trained network outperforms fine-tuning deep layers, when a small number of images are available. It could be due to the presence of specific low-level patterns such as speckles in this modality, which are associated with shallow layers of the network.

It is important to note that U-Net is not a simple feedforward architecture. The notion of deep and shallow is ambiguous in a U-Net, because there are short and long paths from the input to the output. In this study, we considered the depth of a layer to be the longest possible path to reach it. Some differences in the behavior could potentially be related to the difference in architecture of a U-Net. However, given that the behaviour on non-ultrasound data is similar to previously reported results, we believe the primary cause of the differences are due to the character of the image.

Acknowledgment. This work was supported by in part by Natural Science and Engineering Research Council of Canada (NSERC) Discovery Grant RGPIN-2015-04136.

References

1. Alsinan, A.Z., Patel, V.M., Hacihaliloglu, I.: Automatic segmentation of bone surfaces from ultrasound using a filter-layer-guided CNN. Int. J. Comput. Assist. Radiol. Surg. (2019). https://doi.org/10.1007/s11548-019-01934-0
2. van Ginneken, B., Stegmann, M., Loog, M.: Segmentation of anatomical structures in chest radiographs using supervised methods: a comparative study on a public database. Med. Image Anal. **10**(1), 19–40 (2006)
3. Kotikalapudi, R., contributors: keras-vis (2017). https://github.com/raghakot/keras-vis

4. LeCun, Y., Bengio, Y., Hinton, G.: Deep learning. Nature **521**, 436 (2015). https://doi.org/10.1038/nature14539

5. Looney, P., et al.: Fully automated, real-time 3D ultrasound segmentation to estimate first trimester placental volume using deep learning. JCI Insight **3**(11) (2018). https://insight.jci.org/articles/view/120178

6. Rand, W.M.: Objective criteria for the evaluation of clustering methods. J. Am. Stat. Assoc. **66**(336), 846–850 (1971). http://www.jstor.org/stable/2284239

7. Ronneberger, O., Fischer, P., Brox, T.: U-net: convolutional networks for biomedical image segmentation. In: International Conference on Medical Image Computing and Computer Assisted Intervention (MICCAI) (2015). http://arxiv.org/abs/1505.04597

8. Wang, N., et al.: Densely deep supervised networks with threshold loss for cancer detection in automated breast ultrasound. In: Frangi, A.F., Schnabel, J.A., Davatzikos, C., Alberola-López, C., Fichtinger, G. (eds.) MICCAI 2018. LNCS, vol. 11073, pp. 641–648. Springer, Cham (2018). https://doi.org/10.1007/978-3-030-00937-3_73

9. Xia, C., Li, J., Chen, X., Zheng, A., Zhang, Y.: What is and what is not a salient object? Learning salient object detector by ensembling linear exemplar regressors. In: 2017 IEEE Conference on Computer Vision and Pattern Recognition (CVPR), pp. 4399–4407, July 2017. https://doi.org/10.1109/CVPR.2017.468

10. Yang, J., Faraji, M., Basu, A.: Robust segmentation of arterial walls in intravascular ultrasound images using dual path U-Net. Ultrasonics **96**, 24–33 (2019). http://www.sciencedirect.com/science/article/pii/S0041624X18308059

11. Yang, X., et al.: Towards automatic semantic segmentation in volumetric ultrasound. In: Descoteaux, M., Maier-Hein, L., Franz, A., Jannin, P., Collins, D.L., Duchesne, S. (eds.) MICCAI 2017. LNCS, vol. 10433, pp. 711–719. Springer, Cham (2017). https://doi.org/10.1007/978-3-319-66182-7_81

12. Yap, M.H., et al.: Breast ultrasound lesions recognition: end-to-end deep learning approaches. J. Med. Imaging **6**, 011007 (2018)

13. Yap, M.H., et al.: Automated breast ultrasound lesions detection using convolutional neural networks. IEEE J. Biomed. Health Inf. **22**, 1218–1226 (2018)

14. Yosinski, J., Clune, J., Bengio, Y., Lipson, H.: How transferable are features in deep neural networks? In: Proceedings of the 27th International Conference on Neural Information Processing Systems, NIPS 2014, vol. 2 (2014). http://arxiv.org/abs/1411.1792

Multi-task Learning for Neonatal Brain Segmentation Using 3D Dense-Unet with Dense Attention Guided by Geodesic Distance

Toan Duc Bui[1], Li Wang[1($\boxtimes$)], Jian Chen[2], Weili Lin[1], Gang Li[1($\boxtimes$)], and Dinggang Shen[1,3($\boxtimes$)]

[1] Department of Radiology and Biomedical Research Imaging Center,
University of North Carolina at Chapel Hill, Chapel Hill, NC, USA
{li_wang,gang_li,dgshen}@med.unc.edu
[2] School of Information Science and Engineering, Fujian University of Technology,
Fuzhou 350118, China
[3] Department of Brain and Cognitive Engineering, Korea University,
Seoul 02841, Republic of Korea

Abstract. The deep convolutional neural network has achieved outstanding performance on neonatal brain MRI tissue segmentation. However, it may fail to produce reasonable results on unseen datasets that have different imaging appearance distributions with the training data. The main reason is that deep learning models tend to have a good fitting to the training dataset, but do not lead to a good generalization on the unseen datasets. To address this problem, we propose a multi-task learning method, which simultaneously learns both tissue segmentation and geodesic distance regression to regularize a shared encoder network. Furthermore, a dense attention gate is explored to force the network to learn rich contextual information. By using three neonatal brain datasets with different imaging protocols from different scanners, our experimental results demonstrate superior performance of our proposed method over the existing deep learning-based methods on the unseen datasets.

Keywords: Neonatal brain segmentation · Multi-task learning · Attention · Geodesic distance

1 Introduction

Brain tissue segmentation is a fundamental step in the baby brain MRI analysis. However, due to the low tissue contrast in the early infantile phase, accurate and automatic segmentation of the neonatal brain is still a challenge. Many efforts [2,10,14] have been proposed to improve segmentation accuracy. Over the past few years, deep convolutional neural network (DCNN) is considered as a potentially promising approach for infant brain segmentation. The DCNN aims to

Q. Wang et al. (Eds.): DART 2019/MIL3ID 2019, LNCS 11795, pp. 243–251, 2019.
https://doi.org/10.1007/978-3-030-33391-1_28

learn a supervised model from relevant features in the training images. A benchmark for infant brain segmentation based on DCNN can be found in [14], where the DCNN methods demonstrated great success, in comparison with non-deep learning based methods. However, these methods achieve a good segmentation accuracy only on the testing datasets that have the similar imaging appearance as the training dataset, but may fail to produce reasonable results, when the testing data have different imaging appearance (i.e., from different acquisition conditions). The main reason is that these deep learning models tend to have a good fitting to the training dataset, but they generally do not lead to good generalization on unseen data [5].

Multi-task learning [1] has been proposed to improve the generalization of the DCNN by forcing a single model to learn several related tasks at once. For instance, Myronenko [9] added a variational autoencoder branch for image reconstruction and jointly trained it with segmentation branch to regularize the shared encoder for brain tumor segmentation. Dangi et al. [4] proposed multi-task learning for cardiac MR image segmentation by jointly learning a segmentation network and a Euclidean distance map regression network. Wang et al. [13] employed the Euclidean distance to refine the segmentation result for infant brains. However, the Euclidean distance uses ground-truth label information to compute the distance to the tissue boundary, thus it does not leverage the rich image contextual information. Contrary to the Euclidean distance, the geodesic distance [3] allows encoding both spatial regularization and contrast-sensitivity. Wang et al. [12] demonstrated the effectiveness of the geodesic distance over the Euclidean distance for the interactive segmentation. However, it is not designed for multi-task learning.

In this paper, we propose multi-task learning for neonatal brain segmentation. Instead of learning a single segmentation task, the proposed network simultaneously trains both the tissue segmentation task and a geodesic distance regression task together to regularize the shared encoder network. Meanwhile, we observe that the regression features can be used to further refine the segmentation result. Hence, we further concatenate the segmentation features and the regression features together followed by three $3 \times 3 \times 3$ convolutions to produce a refined segmentation result. Furthermore, we propose a dense attention gate (DAG) to guide the network to focus on learning the contextual information. The DAG utilizes contextual information from high-level features to provide unambiguous information for the correct category as the guidance of low-level features.

2 Method

2.1 Dense Attention Gate (DAG)

Let $\mathbf{U}^l = [u_1^l, u_2^l, \cdots, u_{C_l}^l]$ be a feature map at the lth layer, where $u_i^l \in \mathbb{R}^{D \times H \times W}$ and C_l is the number of channel. A statistic vector $\mathbf{z}^l = [z_1^l, z_2^l, \cdots, z_{C_l}^l]$ is achieved by the global average pooling [8], and each element z_i^l of vector $\mathbf{z}^l$ is computed as $z_i^l = \frac{1}{D \times H \times W} \sum_{d=1}^{D} \sum_{h=1}^{H} \sum_{w=1}^{W} u_i^l(d, h, w)$. Since high-level features often have a larger number of channels, we apply $1 \times 1 \times 1$ convolution to reduce the number of channels to C_l. It provides a balance of important features among different levels. An attention vector $\mathbf{a}^l$ at the layer l^{th} is formulated via a sigmoid activation [6]:

$$\mathbf{a}^l = \sigma(\mathbf{F}(\mathbf{z}^l, \mathbf{W}_0^l)) \qquad (1)$$

where $\mathbf{W}_0^l = [\mathrm{w}_1, \mathrm{w}_2, ..., \mathrm{w}_{C_l}]$ is learnable weight for each element of the vector $\mathbf{z}^l$, and $\mathbf{F}(.)$ is a transformation function.

To integrate the contextual information from high-level features, we define our proposed dense attention gate (DAG) as follows:

$$\mathbf{a}_{DAG}^l = \sum_{i=l}^{n} \mathrm{w}_i \mathbf{a}^i \qquad (2)$$

where the dense attention vector $\mathbf{a}_{DAG}^{n-1}$ at the layer $(n-1)^{th}$ computes as follows: $\mathbf{a}_{DAG}^{n-1} = \mathrm{w}_n \mathbf{a}^n + \mathrm{w}_{n-1} \mathbf{a}^{n-1}$. In which, $\mathbf{a}^n = \sigma(\mathbf{F}(\mathbf{z}^n, \mathbf{W}_0^n))$ is the attention vector at the layer n^{th}. In the same way, the dense attention vector $\mathbf{a}_{DAG}^{n-2}$ at the layer $(n-2)^{th}$ calculates as follows: $\mathbf{a}_{DAG}^{n-2} = \mathrm{w}_n \mathbf{a}^n + \mathrm{w}_{n-1} \mathbf{a}^{n-1} + \mathrm{w}_{n-2} \mathbf{a}^{n-2} = \mathbf{a}_{DAG}^{n-1} + \mathrm{w}_{n-2} \mathbf{a}^{n-2}$. Thus, the Eq. 2 can be rewritten as follows:

$$\mathbf{a}_{DAG}^l = \mathbf{a}_{DAG}^{l-1} + \mathrm{w}_l \mathbf{a}^l \qquad (3)$$

The Eq. 3 indicates that the dense attention vector $\mathbf{a}_{DAG}^l$ at layer l^{th} can be computed via linear combination of the dense attention vector $\mathbf{a}_{DAG}^{l-1}$ at the higher level feature $l-1^{th}$ and the attention vector at the layer l^{th}. Hence, the dense attention vector $\mathbf{a}_{DAG}^l$ not only contains the information of the layer l^{th}, but also includes the contextual information of higher level features. We employ the weight $\mathbf{W}_1^l = [\mathrm{w}_l, \mathrm{w}_{l+1}, \cdots, \mathrm{w}_n]$ to learn the contribution of each high-level feature to the attention vector $\mathbf{a}_{DAG}^l$. Figure 1 shows our proposed dense attention gate, which aims to force the network to learn the contextual information of features. By using the contextual information from high-level features, our proposed DAG enables the network to emphasize useful information and ignore ambiguous information in the low-level features.

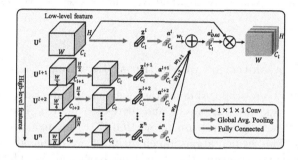

Fig. 1. Our proposed dense attention gate (DAG).

2.2 Geodesic Distance

Given an image $I : \Omega \to \mathbb{R}^{D \times H \times W}$ and a corresponding ground-truth label $Y : \Omega \to \mathbb{R}^{D \times H \times W}$. We use one-hot encoding scheme to convert the ground-truth label Y to M_i binary mask images where $M_i(d, h, w) = 1$ if $M_i(d, h, w)$ belongs to the class i^{th}; otherwise it takes 0 value, $i = 1, \cdots, C$, where C is the number of tissue classes. For the binary mask M_i, the geodesic distance [12] from a voxel x to the boundary of the mask M_i is defined:

$$GD(x, M_i, \nabla I) = \min_{x' \in M_i} d(x, x', \nabla I) \tag{4}$$

where $d(x, x', \nabla I) = \min_{\Gamma \in P(x, x')} \int_0^1 \sqrt{\Gamma'(s)^2 + \gamma^2 (\nabla I(s) \cdot u(s))^2} ds$, and $P(x, x')$ denotes a set of all possible paths between voxels x and x', and $\Gamma(s)$ is a path in the set, parameterized by $s \in [0, 1]$. The unit vector $u(s) = \frac{\Gamma'(s)}{\|\Gamma'(s)\|}$ presents the direction of the path. The factor γ controls the contribution of the image gradient $\nabla I(s)$ and the spatial distances, $\Gamma'(s)$. Note that the geodesic distance reduces to the Euclidean distance when setting $\gamma = 0$.

We define a signed geodesic distance map for the tissue i^{th}, $D_i(x)$, by taking negative value $-GD(.)$ if the voxel inside the tissue M_i, and positive value $GD(.)$ if the voxel outside the tissue. Figure 2 indicates an example of the signed geodesic distance for three classes. For a given voxel, the red color shows the voxels far away from the tissue boundary, while the blue color indicates the voxels close to the tissue boundary. By considering the geodesic distance, the network enables learning the spatial relationship for each voxel in each class.

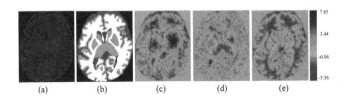

Fig. 2. An example of computing geodesic distance: (a) original T1-weighted image (I), (b) label image (Y), geodesic distance maps of (c) cerebrospinal fluid (CSF) class M_1, (d) gray matter (GM) class M_2, and (e) white matter (WM) class M_3. (Color figure online)

2.3 Network Architecture of Multi-task Learning

Figure 3 illustrates our proposed multi-task network architecture, which has two main branches: segmentation branch and regression branch. The segmentation branch is a 3D-Unet [2] with dense connection [7] to improve information flow between blocks. The segmentation branch includes two paths: an encoder and a decoder. The encoder path comprises four dense blocks, followed by max-pooling layers to enlarge the receptive field. To preserve the spatial resolution of feature

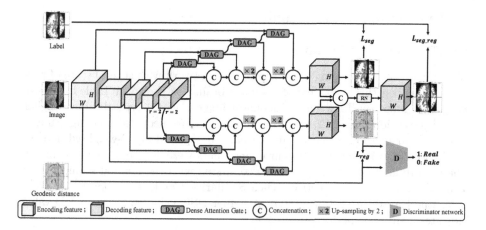

Fig. 3. Our proposed multi-task learning architecture for neonatal brain segmentation.

maps, we used dilated convolution with the rate of 2 for two last blocks. The proposed DAG is added on the skip connection to force the network to learn the contextual information. In the decoder path, 3D convolutions with stride of 2 are used to recover the input resolution. We apply a $1 \times 1 \times 1$ convolution to map the segmentation features to one of the four tissue classes, i.e., GM, WM, CSF and BG (background).

The regression branch shares the same encoder with the segmentation branch and has a similar decoding structure. Instead of pixel-wise classification, the distance regression learns pixel-wise regression. We use the mean square error loss to measure the difference between the estimated geodesic distance and the ground-truth distance. A discrimination network is added to encourage the regression network to produce similar output as the ground-truth distance. The features from two last layers of segmentation and regression branch are concatenated together, and then fed to a refinement network (RN) that consists of three convolutional layers $3 \times 3 \times 3$ to fuse the two features and provide a refinement segmentation result. By using the shared encoder, the proposed network enables learning a joint representation between segmentation and regression task. Hence, the regression task helps regularize the shared features and improves the generalization of the network, thus yielding a better segmentation on the unseen datasets. The proposed network not only provides the pixel-wise prediction, but also estimates the spatial distance of each pixel to the tissue boundary.

The proposed multi-task loss is thus defined as follows:

$$\mathcal{L} = \alpha_1 \mathcal{L}_{seg} + \alpha_2 \mathcal{L}_{reg} + \alpha_3 \mathcal{L}_D + \mathcal{L}_{seg\_reg} \tag{5}$$

where $\mathcal{L}_{seg}$ and $\mathcal{L}_{seg\_reg}$ are the cross-entropy losses, and $\mathcal{L}_{reg}$ and $\mathcal{L}_D$ denote the mean square error losses for distance regression and the discrimination network, respectively. The parameters α_i $(i = 1, \cdots, 3)$ control the balance among losses.

3 Experiments and Results

3.1 Datasets and Training

We compare the performance of our proposed network with several state-of-the-art baselines on three datasets of neonatal brains, as shown in Table 1. Herein, we mainly focus on T1-weighted neonatal images, which typically have higher spatial resolutions than T2-weighted images in most neonatal imaging studies. However, our method is generic and can also be applied in T2-weighted images. All T1-weighted images used in our experiments were acquired on 3T scanners. The performance of each method was compared with the manual segmentation using the following two metrics: Dice Similarity Coefficient (DSC) and 95th-percentile Hausdorff Distance (HD). A higher DSC value and a lower HD value indicates a superior performance.

Table 1. Datasets and imaging settings.

Datasets (# subject)	Scanners	Image resolutions	Imaging parameters (TR/TE)
Dataset A ($N = 25$)	GE	$0.9375 \times 0.9375 \times 1\,\mathrm{mm}^3$	$10.47/4.76\,\mathrm{ms}$
Dataset B ($N = 10$)	Siemens	$0.8 \times 0.8 \times 0.8\,\mathrm{mm}^3$	$2400/2.24\,\mathrm{ms}$
Dataset C ($N = 10$)	Siemens	$1 \times 1 \times 1\,\mathrm{mm}^3$	$1900/4.38\,\mathrm{ms}$

All networks were implemented and trained using Pytorch framework on the 12 GB Titan X GPU. We normalized the input image to zero mean and unit variance, and randomly cropped a sub-region with a size of $64 \times 64 \times 64$ before inputting them into the network. The Adam optimizer with a batch size of four were used to train the network. The initialization learning rate was set as 0.0002 and was decreased ten times every 4,000 epochs. The total number of iteration was 20,000 epochs. The balance weights were set as $\alpha_1 = 1$ and $\alpha_2 = \alpha_3 = 0.5$. We set $\gamma = 0.2$ for the geodesic distance map. We selected the dataset A as the training data and the two remaining datasets for the validation datasets.

3.2 Training and Testing Within the Same Dataset

We first evaluate the performance of those methods on the dataset A. We randomly select sixteen samples for training and four samples for validation and nine samples for testing. Table 2 shows the segmentation accuracy in term of DSC values for 3-fold cross validation and testing on the dataset A of different methods. We employ 3D-Unet [2] with dense connection [7] as a baseline model. The proposed architecture is built upon the baseline model and extended by including the regression branch. Meanwhile, the concurrent spatial and channel (ScSE) [11] is included to the baseline model for comparing with the proposed DAG block.

Table 2 reports the performance of the proposed method and the competing methods on validation and testing sets when training on the same dataset. Both proposed DAG and ScSE blocks provide better results in comparison with the baseline, demonstrating the advantage of the attention mechanism for neonatal brain segmentation. By adding the distance regression branch, the proposed network overcomes the existing methods in term of average DSC. From Table 2, we can conclude that these methods provide good generalization when the training and testing data are from the same scanning center.

Table 2. Performance comparison on 3-fold cross validation and testing using DSC.

	Method	CSF	GM	WM	Avg. DSC
Validation	3D-Unet [2] (Baseline)	97.59(0.39)	96.77(0.30)	98.43(0.28)	97.59
	Baseline + ScSE [11]	97.63(0.40)	96.83(0.29)	98.45(0.27)	97.64
	Baseline + DAG (Ours)	97.68(0.39)	96.97(0.28)	98.51(0.27)	97.72
	Baseline + DAG + DR (Ours)	97.80(0.41)	97.09(0.32)	98.55(0.28)	**97.81**
Testing	3D-Unet [2] (Baseline)	97.65(0.44)	96.85(0.33)	98.51(0.26)	97.67
	Baseline + ScSE [11]	97.71(0.44)	96.93(0.32)	98.54(0.26)	97.73
	Baseline + DAG (Ours)	97.75(0.49)	97.06(0.33)	98.59(0.26)	97.80
	Baseline + DAG + DR (Ours)	97.88(0.48)	97.18(0.35)	98.65(0.26)	**97.90**

ScSE: Spatial Channel Squeeze Exciation [11]; DAG: Dense Attention Gate, DR: Distance Regularization. Bold indicates a significant better performance with p-value < 0.05 using paired t-test

3.3 Training and Testing in Different Datasets

To demonstrate the effectiveness of the proposed multi-task learning, we further evaluate the proposed network on the unseen datasets: B and C. All testing images are resampled to the training resolution of $0.9375 \times 0.9375 \times 1$ mm^3.

Figure 4 illustrates the segmentation results obtained by different methods in all three datasets. The baseline method, 3D-Unet [2], provides a good result when testing and training data have the similar distribution, but has misclassification on the unseen datasets indicated by white rectangle as shown in Fig. 4 (b). This indicates that the existing methods have a poor generalization on the unseen datasets. In contrast, the proposed method provides better stability and generalization capability among different datasets as shown in Fig. 4(d).

Table 3 compares the mean and standard deviation of segmentation accuracy of those methods on the unseen datasets in term of DSC, and HD metrics. It is observed that the proposed multi-task learning provides a better generalization than the existing networks on unseen datasets, i.e., achieving more accurate segmentation. The proposed architecture not only improved DSC from 89.02% to 90.29%, but also reduced HD distance from 1.32 mm to 1.11 mm, compared with the existing methods. Since the all networks are trained on low resolution images (dataset A), thus they led to a low performance on the testing images with a high resolution (dataset B).

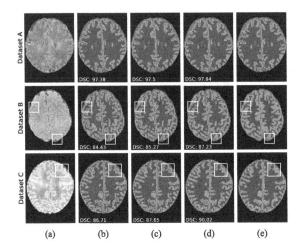

Fig. 4. An example of neonatal brain image: (a) axial slice of T1-weighted MRI from the dataset A (first row), the dataset B (second row) and the dataset C (third row), (b) results by 3D-Unet [2] (baseline), (c) results by baseline + SCSE [11], (d) results by our proposed method, and (e) the ground-truth results.

Table 3. Segmentation accuracy on different datasets.

	Method	DSC (%)	HD (mm)
Dataset B	3D-Unet [2] (Baseline)	84.55 (0.93)	2.28 (0.20)
	Baseline + ScSE [11]	84.98 (0.98)	2.07 (0.17)
	Baseline + DAG + DR (Ours)	**85.85 (1.19)**	**1.61 (0.12)**
Dataset C	3D-Unet [2] (Baseline)	89.02 (3.15)	1.32 (0.11)
	Baseline + ScSE [11]	89.15 (3.01)	1.29 (0.09)
	Baseline + DAG + DR (Ours)	**90.29 (2.43)**	**1.11 (0.06)**

4   Conclusion

We presented an effective of multi-task learning architecture that allows training segmentation and distance regression tasks simultaneously to address the generalization issue on unseen datasets in neonatal brain segmentation. We also proposed a dense attention gate to force learning the important features in the low level-features by using the information from high-level features. We show that the proposed multi-task learning network can provide a good generalization, yielding a better segmentation accuracy on unseen datasets.

Acknowledgment. This work was supported in part by NIH Grants MH107815, MH109773, MH116225, and MH117943.

References

1. Caruana, R.: Multitask learning. Mach. Learn. **28**(1), 41–75 (1997)
2. Çiçek, Ö., Abdulkadir, A., Lienkamp, S.S., Brox, T., Ronneberger, O.: 3D U-Net: learning dense volumetric segmentation from sparse annotation. In: Ourselin, S., Joskowicz, L., Sabuncu, M.R., Unal, G., Wells, W. (eds.) MICCAI 2016. LNCS, vol. 9901, pp. 424–432. Springer, Cham (2016). https://doi.org/10.1007/978-3-319-46723-8_49
3. Criminisi, A., Sharp, T., Blake, A.: GeoS: geodesic image segmentation. In: Forsyth, D., Torr, P., Zisserman, A. (eds.) ECCV 2008. LNCS, vol. 5302, pp. 99–112. Springer, Heidelberg (2008). https://doi.org/10.1007/978-3-540-88682-2_9
4. Dangi, S., Yaniv, Z., Linte, C.: A distance map regularized CNN for cardiac cine MR image segmentation. arXiv preprint arXiv:1901.01238 (2019)
5. Davatzikos, C.: Machine learning in neuroimaging: progress and challenges. NeuroImage **197**, 652 (2018)
6. Hu, J., Shen, L., Sun, G.: Squeeze-and-excitation networks. In: Proceedings of the IEEE CVPR, pp. 7132–7141 (2018)
7. Huang, G., Liu, Z., Van Der Maaten, L., Weinberger, K.Q.: Densely connected convolutional networks. In: Proceedings of the IEEE CVPR, pp. 4700–4708 (2017)
8. Lin, M., Chen, Q., Yan, S.: Network in network. arXiv preprint arXiv:1312.4400 (2013)
9. Myronenko, A.: 3D MRI brain tumor segmentation using autoencoder regularization. In: Crimi, A., Bakas, S., Kuijf, H., Keyvan, F., Reyes, M., van Walsum, T. (eds.) BrainLes 2018. LNCS, vol. 11384, pp. 311–320. Springer, Cham (2019). https://doi.org/10.1007/978-3-030-11726-9_28
10. Ronneberger, O., Fischer, P., Brox, T.: U-Net: convolutional networks for biomedical image segmentation. In: Navab, N., Hornegger, J., Wells, W.M., Frangi, A.F. (eds.) MICCAI 2015. LNCS, vol. 9351, pp. 234–241. Springer, Cham (2015). https://doi.org/10.1007/978-3-319-24574-4_28
11. Roy, A.G., Navab, N., Wachinger, C.: Concurrent spatial and channel squeeze & excitation in fully convolutional networks. arXiv preprint arXiv:1803.02579 (2018)
12. Wang, G., et al.: DeepIGeoS: a deep interactive geodesic framework for medical image segmentation. IEEE Trans. PAMI **41**(7), 1559–1572 (2018)
13. Wang, L., et al.: Volume-based analysis of 6-month-old infant brain MRI for autism biomarker identification and early diagnosis. In: Frangi, A.F., Schnabel, J.A., Davatzikos, C., Alberola-López, C., Fichtinger, G. (eds.) MICCAI 2018. LNCS, vol. 11072, pp. 411–419. Springer, Cham (2018). https://doi.org/10.1007/978-3-030-00931-1_47
14. Wang, L., et al.: Benchmark on automatic 6-month-old infant brain segmentation algorithms: the iSeg-2017 challenge. IEEE Trans. Med. Imaging **38**(9), 2219–2230 (2019)

Author Index

Printed in the United States
By Bookmasters